Praise for The Healing Kitchen

"*The Healing Kitchen* is the perfect cure for dinner dread. Its delicious and doable recipes are sure to please even picky family members and improve their health."

—KAREN CICERO, food and nutrition director, *Child* magazine

"There should be a copy of this book in every kitchen in America!"

—CATHERINE CASSIDY, editor-in-chief of *A Taste of Home* and former executive editor of *Prevention* magazine

"As a regular contributor to *diane, The Curves Magazine*, Ellen has changed lives with her powerful, moving stories. In her new book, *The Healing Kitchen*, she continues to change lives by offering many practical, simple methods for improving your health and your life. This well-researched book is jam-packed with common sense advice, utilizing everyday household items and ingredients most of us already have on our shelves."

—DIANE HEAVIN, cofounder, Curves International and publisher of *diane, The Curves Magazine*

"In this day and age of 'good' and 'bad' foods, phytochemicals, trans-fats, anti-oxidants and other such ambiguous nutrition concepts, we now have a fascinating book defining what and how to eat on a daily basis. *The Healing Kitchen* does a wonderful job of not only highlighting the foods that belong in a healthy kitchen, but also explaining why the foods are healing. A rich blend of science, research and practical information...to say nothing of positive recipes. Cookies with a purpose, anyone?"

—NANCY CLARK, MS, RD, Sports Nutrition Services, Boston, author of *Nancy Clark's Sports Nutrition Guidebook*

The
HEALING KITCHEN

*From tea tin to fruit basket,
breadbox to veggie bin—
how to unlock the curative powers
of foods that heal!*

ELLEN MICHAUD

WITH RECIPES BY

Anita Hirsch, MS, RD

BENBELLA BOOKS, INC.
Dallas, Texas

BenBella Books, Inc.
6440 N. Central Expressway, Suite 503
Dallas, TX 75206
www.benbellabooks.com
Send feedback to feedback@benbellabooks.com

Printed in the United States of America
10 9 8 7 6 5 4 3 2

Library of Congress Cataloging-in-Publication Data
Michaud, Ellen.
    The healing kitchen : from tea tin to fruit basket, breadbox to veggie bin--how to unlock the curative powers of foods that heal! / by Ellen Michaud, with recipes by Anita Hirsch.
        p. cm.
    Includes bibliographical references and index.
    ISBN 1-932100-53-9 (alk. paper)
    1. Functional foods. 2. Diet therapy—Popular works. 3. Nutrition. I. Hirsch, Anita, M.S. II. Title.

    QP144.F85M53 2005
    615.8'54--dc22

                                                                    2005004584

Proofread by Meghan Kuckelman and Stacia Seaman
Cover design by Laura Watkins
Cover photo by Laura Yeffeth
Text design and composition by John Reinhardt Book Design

Distributed by Independent Publishers Group
To order call (800) 888-4741
www.ipgbook.com

For special sales contact Robyn White at robyn@benbellabooks.com

The Healing Kitchen *is dedicated to all women who sense the sacred, healing place of food and nurture in our lives. In particular, it's dedicated to my mother, Florence Clay Watts; my stepmother, Edna Thulin Watts; my mother-in-law, Alyce Michaud; and my two aunts, Gladys Hughes and Ellen Johnson.*

These women have set a standard of individual strength, nurturance, and family commitment that will live for generations to come.

Contents

Acknowledgments

Every book is the product of many caring people—and *The Healing Kitchen* is no exception. In particular I'd like to thank the following, who shared their work, their time, and frequently bits and pieces of their lives:

Priscilla Benner, M.D., an incredibly caring physician from Pennsburg, Pennsylvania, who, in between saving the lives of thousands of Honduran children, took the time to bake cookies with me in her kitchen;

Nicolette Brady, M.S., a researcher in the University of Waikato Honey Research Unit, Australia, who shared her knowledge of manuka honey and its antimicrobial properties;

Bruce Chassey, Ph.D., head of nutrition and food science at the University of Illinois, who provided an inordinate amount of information on probiotics and their practical applications;

Connie Chipman, Penny Randal, and the entire Game Supper team, who fill the Bradford United Church of Christ Congregational hall full of good food, good people, and the Good Spirit every fall;

Steven K. Clinton, M.D., Ph.D., director of the Dana-Farber Cancer Institute and a professor at Harvard Medical School in Boston, who took time from a busy conference to explain the effects of lycopenes on prostate cancer;

Allan Conney, Ph.D., director of the Laboratory for Cancer Research at Rutgers University's College of Pharmacy in New Brunswick, New Jersey, for sharing his research on tea;

Louise Desaulniers, R.D., a nutritional consultant in Montreal, who taught me how to make healthy snacks;

T. Lyle and Betty Ferderber, organic farmers and millers near Pittsburgh, who showed me just why whole grain breads are healthier—and tastier!—than lesser bread products;

David Fitzpatrick, Ph.D., a researcher at the University of South Florida, who—even though he was in the midst of moving his lab—took the time to explain how plant chemicals affect arterial walls;

Gale Frank, Ph.D., R.D., a professor of nutrition at California State University at Long Beach, who in the midst of an overwhelming schedule of workshops, students, and courses, somehow made time to explain how snacking could contribute to healthy eating;

Najla Guthrie, Ph.D., and Elzbieta Kurowska, Ph.D., two researchers at the University of Western Ontario's Centre for Human Nutrition in Canada, who explained why orange juice is good for us;

Anita Hirsch, M.S., R.D., a consulting nutritionist who not only developed and tested—over and over and over again!—the recipes for this book, but who was always willing to explain why cookies bounced, veggies wilted, and bread fell as I experimented my way through *The Healing Kitchen*; who reviewed each chapter to make sure it was based on sound nutritional science and practice—and who volunteered her good sport of a husband, Sy, to eat every single variation of every single recipe;

Betsy Jacobs, chair of the New York chapter of the American Herb Society and former director of children's education at the Brooklyn Botanical Garden, who shared her knowledge of herbs, spices, and cooking;

Michael McBurney, Ph.D., a professor of nutrition at the University of Alberta, who explained how high-fiber diets affect the body's production of GLP-1;

John A. Milner, Ph.D., head of the nutrition department at Penn State University, who took time from a busy conference to explain the effects of garlic on a fatty diet;

John Pezzuto, Ph.D., director of collaborative research in the pharmaceutical sciences at the University of Illinois in Chicago, who explained the significance of resveratrol in grapes and peanuts;

Marla Reicks, Ph.D., R.D., an associate professor of nutrition at the University of Minnesota, who shared her research on ways to encourage women to eat more healthfully;

Keith Singletary, Ph.D., associate professor of food science at the University of Illinois, who explained his investigations into a wide variety of spices;

Stine Storsrud, Ph.D., a researcher at Sahlgrenska University Hospital in Sweden, who patiently explained the effects of an oat diet on those with celiac disease;

Walter Willet, Ph.D., head of nutrition at Harvard University, one of the first nutrition researchers to understand the role of "good" and "bad" fats in the diet—and who had the courage to stand firm when his conclusions ran counter to the prevailing academic winds;

Researchers and staff at the Functional Foods for Health Program at the University of Illinois, members of which took me by the hand over 15 years ago and showed me how the components in food could prevent disease.

In terms of actually getting the book done, I'd also like to thank my editor, Denise Foley, who had the heart to understand what I wanted to do and the guts to tell me when I was wrong; my publisher Glenn Yeffeth, who has the vision to try new things and make them a reality; Linda Rao, a former researcher at *Prevention* magazine, who gave me a hand with gathering the incredible amount of research that went into this book; and two wonderfully enthusiastic students, Tina Segan from Cedar Crest College and Steph Griffin from the University of Utah—both of whom helped Anita and me organize our offices and kitchens as the book got under way.

On a personal note, I'd also like to thank my friend Jane Knutila, who was always ready to hold my hand when the going got tough; my son Matthew, who aside from being the sunshine of my life provided me with unlimited tech support as computers crashed, programs disappeared, databases self-destructed, my memory evaporated, and the Internet slowed to a crawl; and my husband Wayne, who drove me thousands of miles from one interview to another and who was always willing to rate the latest culinary experiment on a scale of 1 to 10, figure out why my printer wouldn't print, and give me the loving support it takes to complete such a complex project.

Blessings to you all,

Ellen Michaud

Caveat

A key reason for writing this book is to help all of us understand that the foods we put in our mouths can have as powerful an effect on the body as drugs and other pharmaceuticals.

Sometimes those effects are good. Sometimes they're not. Because just as drugs and other pharmaceuticals have side effects, so can foods. In particular, they can trigger an allergic response that can be as life-threatening as a mugger on the street. And when certain foods are combined with prescription or over-the-counter drugs you may be taking for a particular condition, there can be unexpectedly dangerous consequences. Sometimes foods can potentiate drugs; other times they can weaken them.

For that reason, I want you to take this caveat very seriously: If you're prone to food allergies, or if you're taking any medication for any condition whatsoever, please check with your doctor before trying any of the foods described in this book. Further, please do not try to use the foods described here to treat medical problems on your own. If you suspect something's wrong, please consult your doctor.

This book is intended only as a reference, not a medical manual. The information in it is designed to help you make informed decisions—but it is not intended as a substitute for any treatment that may have been prescribed by your doctor.

Introduction

೫)(೫

In our childhood homes, the kitchen was always where we could find a cup of honeyed tea to soothe a scratchy throat, dry toast to settle a queasy stomach, or a bowl of chicken soup to clear a stuffy nose.

For most of us, those kitchens are long gone. Yet the healing kitchen of today more than retains its healthful, nurturing purpose—mostly because scientists working in laboratories around the world have led us to the understanding that the foods we serve in these kitchens can do more than counteract minor symptoms of illness and offer comfort. They can also prevent or fight powerful, life-threatening diseases as well: Alzheimer's, anxiety disorders, arthritis, cancer, adult-onset diabetes, digestive problems, diverticulitis, gallstones, gum disease, heart disease, high cholesterol, high blood pressure, kidney stones, liver disease, macular degeneration, osteoporosis, psoriasis, sinus infections, and stroke.

That's why meal planning is no longer a case of balancing the Four Basic Food Groups most of us learned in a high school home economics course. Instead, meal planning today means making sure that our spouses get the powerful nutrients from specific foods that buffer stress, help prevent heart disease, and block the maverick molecules that cause cancer.

It means making sure that our parents get the naturally occurring food chemicals—the new "nutriceuticals"—that reduce their chances of a heart attack and ease the pain of arthritis.

It means making sure that our children get the raw nutritional material they need to build the strong bones, healthy bodies, and sharp minds they need now and into adulthood.

And, for ourselves, meal planning means making sure that we get the nutrients we need to prevent breast cancer, clogged arteries, and the abnormal cell growth that leads to cervical cancer—as well as the energy we need to power our increasingly demanding lives.

The Healing Kitchen honors the kitchen as that central place of nurture and healing in the home and provides you with the tools you need to turn it into a place of preventive care. As you flip through the pages, you'll notice that we've divided the book into sections that match the way most of us divide up our kitchens. You'll find meat and poultry in the freezer, milk and shellfish in the refrigerator, fresh fruits and vegetables in the crisper. There're tea and honey on the countertop. The root vegetables are in the vegetable bin, spices are in the spice rack, and dried fruits are in the snack cupboard.

The bottom cupboard is loaded with beans, brown rice, nuts, seeds, oats, oils, and anything else we couldn't find room for somewhere else. And, of course, under the sink you'll find natural cleaning products to keep the surfaces of your kitchen as healthy as the food you prepare in it. There's even an herbal shampoo for your pets, since we all know that every dog and cat worth its organic flea collar is certain to be under your feet as soon as you open a cupboard door.

No one recipe is going to help you prevent or eliminate any one disease or condition all by itself. But consistently using recipes that have been specifically designed to include a wide variety of protective nutrients and naturally occurring phytochemicals will.

That's why we've designed this book to work in two ways: One, it lists every readily available food scientists have found to contain protective nutrients so you can find out what foods suit your needs. And two, it also contains bunches of spectacularly easy recipes that show you how to creatively use the foods you choose.

As you've probably already discovered, finding recipes that include all the protective nutrients scientists have recently uncovered isn't easy—especially if you must also meet the taste requirements of a thoroughly spoiled family as I do. In my case, the problem is this: My husband comes from a family of food brokers and restaurateurs. And those who worked at Chez Michaud, a historic landmark first in Paris, then in Philadelphia during the early part of the last century, passed to my husband certain standards for taste and texture that nearly got him returned to his mama during the early years of our marriage.

A lifetime of kids and dogs later, however, I fully realize that the only way to get him to eat healthful foods is to make them in creative dishes that meet his standards—or hand him creatively simple recipes that will allow him to prepare healthy food himself. That's why I asked consulting nutritionist Anita Hirsch, M.S., R.D.—the "grandmother" of healthy cooking who helped establish *Prevention* magazine's reputation for nourishing recipes—to develop recipes for *The Healing Kitchen.*

Anita's recipes are fabulous. Using my picky spouse and her own equally spoiled husband as guinea pigs, Anita has created what amounts to a new bible of healthy eating. Every one of her recipes contains not just one protective ingredient, but several. A recipe that illustrates how to cook artichokes, for example, includes not only that venerable vegetable with its ability to heal damaged livers, but also olive oil, garlic, onions, and scallops to prevent heart disease, and peppers and tomatoes to prevent cancer.

Think that's a lot? It is. And it all goes to show that every single recipe Anita created offers layers of subtle flavors and interesting textures that will please the most discerning palate. In short, there's not a recipe in this book that won't tickle your taste buds as it helps you stave off one disease or another.

To put Anita's recipes to work for your own picky eaters, simply leaf through the book and try whichever one catches your fancy. Or, if you're concerned about one particular disease or condition, locate it in The Recipe Finder that appears on p. 267, then prepare some of the recipes listed under it.

Want to look around?

Feel free. As they say in the southern parts of our hemisphere, *mi casa es su casa*—my home is yours.

Ellen Michaud
South Starksboro, Vermont

The Tea Tin

Every afternoon at 4 P.M., my grandmother—a tall woman with sturdy English bones and silver-dusted copper hair—would walk into her sunny kitchen and head for the stove.

There she'd pick up the kettle, fill it with fresh, cold water, and put it on a burner to boil.

Four o'clock was time for tea—for my mother, my grandmother and the generations of women before them. The habit was so ingrained that whether my father's work had landed us in Tokyo, San Francisco, Indianapolis, New York, or East Orange, New Jersey, my mother could set the kettle on to boil at precisely 4 P.M. and know that 100, 1,000, or 10,000 miles away, her mother would do precisely the same thing.

Decades later, I would remember those afternoons as my son Matthew and I sipped tea from the same thin, ivory cups. "Beige tea!" as he demanded from the age of two, was every afternoon at 4 P.M. in the kitchen.

But each generation reinterprets a family's rituals. And just as I had replaced my grandmother's sweet creamy tea and tarts with milky tea and fresh fruit, eventually Matthew reinterpreted our afternoon tea as well. Sugar got added to the tea, cheese and whole wheat crackers replaced the fruit, and the cheerful chatter of *Sesame Street* edged into our lives.

The one thread that remained constant from generation to generation was an ingrained appreciation for tea—for its sensual ability to carry a family's warmth, love, and strength down through the generations; for the sense of continuity it provided as each generation moved through wars, depressions, conflicts, and recessions; and for the reassuring sense of health and well-being it carried with every sip.

1

TEA TIN

BEST FOR HELPING YOU:

- Prevent cancer
- Prevent heart disease
- Lower blood pressure
- Relieve allergy symptoms
- Prevent cavities
- Lower cholesterol
- Prevent stroke
- Prevent heart attacks
- Stop anxiety
- Fight viral invaders
- Reduce the risk of Alzheimer's

Health in a Teacup

To my mother and grandmother, teatime was simply an afternoon break from the day's tasks that brought the family together. Neither woman knew that tea helped keep diabetes, high blood pressure, Alzheimer's, and a dozen forms of cancer off my family tree. It also helped stave off a familial propensity toward premature heart disease.

How? The answer lies in a warm, rainy, mountainous area centered between southeastern Asia: northeast India, southwestern China, northern Thailand, and eastern Myanmar.

Nearly 5,000 years ago, the aboriginal people living in the tangled tea jungles covering these hills began boiling the leaves of a wild camellia—*Camellia sinensis*—over smoky campfires and drinking the bitter result. They noticed that those who drank the tea stayed healthier than those who did not, so it wasn't long before the tea became used throughout the area as an all-purpose medicinal drink.

It would have been hard to choose a better tonic. Today scientists know that this primitive green tea contained epicatechin, epigallocatechin-3-galate, and epicatechin-3-gallate—three powerful antioxidants that, in the lab, have demonstrated their ability to intercept molecular mavericks that trigger the underlying disease processes for half a dozen different conditions, particularly cancer.

"We've found that green tea inhibits chemically induced and ultraviolet-induced colorectal, lung, and skin tumors in mice," confirms Allan Conney, Ph.D., director of the Laboratory for Cancer Research at Rutgers University's College of Pharmacy in New Brunswick, New Jersey. "Giving green tea to mice in their drinking water—in concentrations that people would normally drink—will inhibit tumor formation. And we've also found that we can actually stop tumor growth if we give the mice a 50 percent higher concentration of the tea."

That's a startling revelation, admits Dr. Conney, but scientists still have a lot more research to do before they can make specific recommendations.

"Right now," says the cautious researcher, "we know that green tea is good for mice and promising for humans. And we're trying to understand the mechanism by which it works."

The problem, he explains, is that scientists are still sorting out all the active constituents in tea, what each does on its own in the lab, and what each does when it occurs naturally with other constitu-

---

TEA BASICS

HOW TO BUY: For maximum effectiveness, green tea should be bought in small quantities and used as soon as possible. The same goes for herbal teas. Oolong and black teas, which can be stored for a year or so without losing their potency, can be purchased in larger quantities.

What kinds of teas should you buy? Loose, full-leaf teas that have been organically grown will contain more of the active plant ingredients than teas that have been pulverized into "tea dust"—the tea industry's nickname for the powdery stuff that fills a tea bag or a jar of instant tea.

HOW TO STORE: Tea should be stored in air tight containers that shield it from air, heat, humidity, light, and strong odors.

HOW TO USE: Bring eight ounces of water to a boil, then pour over loose tea leaves and cover. Steep green, oolong, or black teas anywhere from 5 to 10 minutes, depending on your flavor preference. Steep herbal teas from 5 to 15 minutes, or as directed on package labels. Cool slightly, then sip.

ents in tea. In one experiment, for example, mice given green tea with caffeine and exposed to cancer-causing ultraviolet light did not get tumors. Mice given green tea without caffeine did.

Whether this means that decaffeinated tea doesn't retain the healing properties of regular tea in its natural state is unknown. But it is a possibility—and one so significant that researchers in Dr. Conney's lab and at the National Institutes of Health are gearing up to begin human studies that will eventually tell us exactly how green tea does what it does.

Other scientists are following up on studies that indicate even more health benefits. Some, for example, have found that green tea may help control leukemia, while others have found that it may prevent cavities and act as a naturally occurring antihistamine to relieve allergy symptoms. The powerful antioxidants in green tea may also act as a magnet for the type of cholesterol—LDL cholesterol—that clogs your arteries and causes heart disease.

Not too long ago, for instance, a study of more than 2,000 Japanese workers between the ages of 49 and 55 revealed that those who regularly sipped 10 cups of green tea over the course of a day generally had a cholesterol level that was six points lower than the level of those who did not.

And as if that's not enough to put a teacup in your hand, a Chinese study recently published in the *Archives of Internal Medicine* reveals that daily consumption of oolong or green tea reduces the risk of high blood pressure between 46 and 65 percent.

Black Tea: Reduce Stroke by 69 Percent

Although those who lived in the tea jungles centuries ago were unaware of the specific health benefits of green tea, they knew enough to make tea a booming industry.

By the eighth century, tea was being roasted, formed into cakes, then crumbled into boiling kettles of water with onion, ginger, and orange added for flavor.

By the ninth century, dried leaves were being ground into a powder, then whisked into hot water to make a more pleasant-tasting beverage. Eventually, the tea—just a simple beverage made from a simple plant—began to take on complex social and spiritual dimensions: scholars traced its history, sociologists weighed its effects on the social fabric of an entire empire, philosophers created symbolic rituals to express its meaning, and potters kept their wheels humming in an effort to create one delicate china cup more exquisite than the next.

By the 17th or 18th century, tea producers had figured out how to alter the basic processing of tea leaves to create two new forms of the brew. "Oolong tea" was made when the leaves were dried, rolled, twisted, and steamed before packaging, and "black tea" was made when the leaves were dried, rolled, sifted, and then fermented for a longer period of time.

Until recently, black and oolong teas were thought to lack the healing qualities of their green cousins. But a group of Dutch researchers recently studied 552 men between the ages of 50 and 69 and found that those who drank five cups of black tea reduced their risk of stroke by 69 percent.

Other researchers found that both black and green teas contain apigenin, a naturally occurring chemical flavonoid that, in laboratory studies, reduces the number and incidence of tumors, decreases anxiety, fights viral invaders, and relaxes the heart's main artery, thus reducing chances of a heart attack. And although laboratory findings do not always prove true when they leave the lab and splash into your teacup, these findings did: a study at the Harvard School of Public Health found that men who had had a heart attack and who subsequently consumed large quantities of flavonoids from tea and other foods reduced their risk of a second attack by 47 percent.

Further, a second study, this one conducted by Dutch researchers, found that the more flavonoids ingested by a group of 805 men between the ages of 65 and 84, the less likely they were to die from a heart attack.

The major source of flavonoids in their diet was tea.

As with heart disease, the cancer-fighting effects of tea outside the lab were demonstrated when researchers at the University of Minnesota School of Public Health in Minneapolis studied 35,369 women between the ages of 55 and 69. Although tea drinking did not protect against all cancers, the researchers noticed that women who drank only two cups a day—two cups!—reduced their risk of mouth, esophageal, stomach, colon, and rectal cancer by a third. They were also 60 percent less likely to develop bladder cancer than those who drank other beverages.

An Infusion of Herbs

As news of its healthful benefits spread, tea lingered within China's borders only until emerging trade routes were able to carry its fragrant bouquet to the rest of the world.

By the 16th century, tea had conquered people in neighboring cultures more effectively than a legion of Mongolian warlords. Natives of India added condensed milk, sugar, cardamom, and other spices to make their own distinctive brew, while the Moroccans added mint and sugar. The Russians, trying to neutralize the smoky taste absorbed from campfires as the tea traveled long caravan routes through rugged terrain, clenched sugar cubes between their teeth as they drank it by the gallon.

By 1700, tea had circumnavigated the world. Japan had established its own tea gardens, England had opened its first teahouse, and even the "colonists" in America had begun to drink a green tea flavored with peaches and sugar.

Not all botanicals and herbs were added to tea for flavoring, however. Many were added because they had a reputation for curing one malady or another.

STUFF YOUR SOCKS WITH TEA

Instead of tossing spent tea leaves into the compost bin, keep an old canning jar within easy reach under the sink and toss the leaves inside.

When the jar is full, sprinkle the tea leaves on a cookie sheet. Put them in the sun and periodically shake the cookie sheet until the leaves are dry. Then stuff them in a pair of old socks, tie the socks shut, and stick them into your stinkiest shoes.

Twenty-four hours later, toss the socks into a trash can and take a sniff of your shoes. Ten to one you'll find that the shoes smell more like fresh herbs than moldy cheese.

In fact, many—chamomile, valerian, and echinacea, for example—had stood alone for nearly 5,000 years as curatives for everything from anxiety, nervous stomachs, and menstrual cramps to colds, liver disease, and infertility.

Called "simples," "tisanes," or "infusions" by the herbalists who created them, these herbal teas were made by steeping the dried leaves, roots, stems, and/or flowers of a particular plant in just-boiled water anywhere from 1 to 15 minutes. If the herb happened to taste bitter, as some of the more potent botanicals did, the herbalist masked the tea's natural flavor by adding one or two other herbs and a spoonful of honey.

Following are some of the most effective infusions. Just two cautions: any herb that's potent enough to heal is potent enough to harm. So if you're pregnant or suspect you might be allergic to any ingredient listed below, common sense says you should check with your doctor before you take so much as a sip.

CHAMOMILE TEA. One of the oldest and most popular herbal teas, chamomile is made from the dried flowers of *Matricaria recutita*. Herbalists have prescribed it, in one form or another, to reduce anxiety and soothe frazzled nerves for centuries. It's only recently, however, that laboratory studies have revealed that chamomile contains apigenin, a flavonoid that literally plugs itself into your nervous system.

The result is that a tea made from chamomile not only calms your nerves, it also reduces your response to stress.

What's more, a few small but intriguing lab studies indicate that chamomile may also enhance your ability to learn, lighten your mood, and relax coronary arteries, thus reducing your chances of a heart attack.

I generally drink chamomile tea every afternoon—just about the time the constant demands of my work generate so much stress that it's hard to concentrate. I drizzle in some honey to overcome late-afternoon fatigue, and this sweet, flowery infusion calms me down, picks me up, and gives me the energy I need for an extra hour or two of work.

To make an afternoon pick-me-up, bring six ounces of water to a boil, remove it from the stove or microwave, then steep one tablespoon of dried chamomile flowers in it for 10 minutes and drink. If you're using it as a before-bed drink to make you drowsy, some experts recommend that you increase the amount of dried chamomile to three tablespoons.

One caveat: If you're allergic to ragweed, daisies, or any other members of their botanical families, you may also be allergic to chamomile.

ECHINACEA TEA. One of nature's most potent immune system boosters, echinacea fights infections and reduces the symptoms of colds and flu by increas-

---

CHAMOMILE TEA

BEST FOR HELPING YOU:

Calm frazzled nerves

Reduce your response to stress

Lighten your mood

Reduce your chances of a heart attack

ECHINACEA TEA

BEST FOR HELPING YOU:

Fight infections

Reduce cold and flu symptoms

Heal minor burns

ing the number of white cells your body produces to fight viruses. Although some studies indicate that that has little effect in real life, other studies indicate that it can cut the length of a cold or the flu by 50 percent.

I usually start brewing echinacea tea at the first sign of a sore throat. In my family it always seems to keep us from getting any sicker—and the warm vapors relieve nasal congestion so certain young people will sleep through the night.

If you'd like to try it yourself, bring eight ounces of water to a boil, then slowly pour it over three tablespoons of loose tea. Let it steep for five minutes, then sip the tea slowly over the next hour. Two cups a day usually does the trick.

Scientists also report that echinacea can be used topically as a poultice of damp leaves wrapped in a porous cloth to speed the healing of minor burns. In that case, simply steep three ounces of echinacea in four cups of boiling water. Let the herbs cool until they're barely warm, then wrap them in a small piece of cotton cloth and apply to the burn. Leave on for 15 minutes, then remove. Unless your doctor tells you otherwise, leave the burn open to the air to speed healing.

THE TEA SHOP

Too many of us base our feelings about green or black tea on the cheap, highly processed teas we get from teabags sold in grocery stores or in restaurants. To experience the rich, full flavor of tea as the Chinese emperors did, buy a loose, quality tea from local gourmet shops, health food stores, or department stores. And because such teas are sometimes hard to find, here are several mail order houses that sell only the best:

CHARLESTON TEA PLANTATION. 6617 Maybank Highway, Wadmalaw Island, South Carolina 29487. 800-443-5987. The Plantation produces American Classic Tea, the only black tea produced in the United States. Grown without insecticides or fungicides, it is served in the White House.

I'TCHIK HERBAL TEA. P.O. Box 730, Crow Agency, Montana 59022. 406-638-2515. I'Tchik Herbal Tea is produced by Theresa Sends-Part-Home on the Crow Indian Reservation in Montana. Many of the herbs are organically grown. Their Council of Elders tea is the only tea I have found anywhere that contains wild cherry bark as its primary ingredient.

THE REPUBLIC OF TEA. 8 Digital Drive, Suite 100, Novato, California 94949. 800-298-4TEA. The Republic of Tea arguably offers the widest range of teas found in the United States—including 5 black teas, 8 black tea blends, 2 oolong teas, 7 green teas and 10 herbal teas—including Mate Latte, a blend of mate with cocoa and almonds. The wide range of green teas available allows you to gradually acquire a taste for green tea by moving from a mild sencha tea, such as Spring Cherry, to a more potent hojicha tea, such as Big Green Hojicha.

THE WINDHAM TEA CLUB. 12 Wilson Road, Windham, New Hampshire 03087. 800-565-7527. Join the Windham Tea Club and they'll send you a different tea every month—either green, oolong, or black. One month it might be a sencha tea from Japan; another month it might be a black tea from Northern Formosa.

EUCALYPTUS TEA. The leaf from which eucalyptus tea is made contains eucalyptol, a naturally occurring decongestant that also kills several types of bacteria and viruses. If you live in California, where eucalyptus trees flourish, you can make tea from a handful of fresh-picked leaves tossed into a pot of just-boiled water. The rest of us will have to make do with the dried version sold in our local health food or drugstore. Simply take one teaspoon of the loose, dried leaf, crush it between your fingers, and drop it into a cup of just-boiled water. Steep the brew for 10 minutes. Drink once or twice a day when you have an upper respiratory infection or head cold.

You can also crush a handful of the dried leaves under running water in the bathtub, then inhale the fragrant steam as you bathe. Not only will it help clear a stuffy head, it will also soothe irritated bronchial passages and, perhaps, make you dream of the eucalyptus-carpeted redwood forests along the California coast.

I tried this recently during a cold, and it was wonderful—until I had to clean all those eucalyptus leaves out of the tub. Next time I wanted to soak my cold in eucalyptus, I stole my son's Spider-man bath mitt, filled it full of tea leaves, tied it off with an elastic band I normally use to pull back my hair, and threw the whole thing into the tub. It worked perfectly. And the clean-up was easy: I let the mitt dry, then shook all the tea leaves out into the compost bucket.

GINGER TEA. For those who suffer from motion sickness or common, garden-variety nausea, ginger is a gift. A study at the American Phytotherapy Research Laboratory in Salt Lake City, Utah, revealed that those who take ginger before they travel will have less nausea and dizziness than even those who took dimenhydrinate—better known as Dramamine.

Other studies suggest that ginger may help prevent stomach ulcers, reduce headache or arthritic pain, inhibit the clumping of platelets that can lead to a heart attack, and even lower high blood cholesterol. Ginger is not recommended for morning sickness during pregnancy, however, since scientists suspect that it may also cause the uterine contractions that can cause a miscarriage.

Ginger contains a number of active constituents that might be involved in its therapeutic action. One in particular is gingerol, an oily substance that makes up between 5 and 10 percent of the ginger plant itself. Another is zingibain, a powerful enzyme that makes up as much as 2 percent of the root—or rhizome, as it is actually classified.

Ginger tea is available in most health food and drug stores in individual bags. But the most effective—and least expensive—way to brew a cup of ginger tea is to grate two teaspoons of fresh ginger root into a cup of just-boiled water. Since many of ginger's therapeutic constituents are contained in volatile oils that will evapo-

---

EUCALYPTUS TEA

BEST FOR HELPING YOU:

Loosen congestion

Kill bacteria and viruses

GINGER TEA

BEST FOR HELPING YOU:

Soothe nausea

Banish dizziness

Prevent stomach ulcers

Reduce headache pain

Reduce arthritic pain

Lower cholesterol

Prevent heart attacks

rate, immediately cover the tea. Then let the ginger steep for 10 minutes, strain the tea, and sip. Your taste buds will tell you just how much more potent the freshly grated root is than its bagged counterpart.

GINKGO TEA. John Knutila, a sculptor friend who lives close by, was the first person to offer me a cup of this ancient tea. Made from the leaves of the ginkgo tree, the tea contains a naturally occurring chemical called a ginkgolide, which actually inhibits your body's production of platelet-activating factor (PAF). PAF encourages your body to produce the artery-clogging clots that can trigger a heart attack or stroke. It also relaxes the walls of blood vessels in the brain and heart so that clots are less likely to get stuck and cause a problem.

The increased blood flow created by this effect may also help prevent some of the memory loss that frequently occurs as we age. Also a help is the fact that ginkgo is a powerful tool that grabs hold of disease-causing molecules before they can cause damage that eventually leads to degenerative diseases like Alzheimer's.

How much ginkgo tea should you drink? That's hard to say. Most laboratory studies have been done with an extract made from ginkgo, rather than the tea itself. Your best bet is to start with one cup a day, see how you feel, then increase the amount as necessary.

One caveat: If you're taking anticlotting drugs such as aspirin, hold off on the tea until you've checked with your doctor. The tea could increase your medication's effects.

GINSENG TEA. For centuries in China the ginseng root has enjoyed a reputation for promoting health, sexuality, and longevity. That reputation has followed it to the United States, where the sale of various forms of ginseng now exceeds $11 million every year.

Unfortunately, although most of these forms of ginseng claim to be something of a miracle that will cure whatever ails you, only panax ginseng has received any real scientific support.

Panax ginseng, which is available in both Asian and American forms (*P. ginseng* and *P. quinquefolius*) contains ginsenosides—steroid-like compounds that can apparently boost athletic endurance, increase mental agility, boost immune system defenses, and reduce your risk of oral, stomach, colorectal, liver, lung, and ovarian cancers.

How ginseng works is not exactly understood, although scientists have demonstrated that the root increases blood flow and your body's ability to absorb and use the oxygen your blood carries.

But studies are contradictory and controversial. In some studies, the root's ginsenosides seem to raise blood pressure, while in others they seem to lower it. Sometimes it acts as a stimulant, while at other times it acts as a sedative. While scientists have no solid explanation for

---

GINKGO TEA

BEST FOR HELPING YOU:

Prevent heart attacks

Ward off strokes

Prevent memory loss

GINSENG TEA

BEST FOR HELPING YOU:

Increase mental agility

Boost immune system defenses

Reduce your risk of various cancers

Boost athletic endurance

---

these seemingly contradictory effects, some researchers suspect that ginseng is actually an "adaptogenic" herb—a kind of "smart" herb that raises blood pressure in people with low blood pressure and lowers blood pressure in people with high blood pressure.

Unfortunately, while scientists are trying to sort things out, many manufacturers aren't waiting for the facts. Instead, they're flooding the market with a plethora of ginseng and ginseng tea products that may or may not do a thing. Several years ago, a group of researchers analyzed 54 ginseng products and found that one-quarter of them had no ginseng at all. A more recent study found some improvement. Only 10 percent of the products tested had no ginseng—although, as the study director said at a recent meeting, in some cases there was so little ginseng it was as though the ginseng root had just been dipped in solution and removed. In other words, there was just enough ginseng in the product to justify the label's claim—but not enough to achieve any kind of therapeutic effect.

If you'd like to see how ginseng works for you, check out the tea section of your local health food store. To increase your chances of getting an effective product, look for a sealed package of the dried ginseng root and make sure the words *P. ginseng* or *P. quinquefolius* are listed under the ingredients.

Once you're ready for a cup of tea, all you have to do is bring eight ounces of water and three teaspoons of the dried root to a boil. Simmer, covered, for 45 minutes, then strain the tea. Let it cool for a minute or two, then sip. Experts say you can drink up to two or three cups a day.

Because ginseng may have such wide-ranging effects on the body, some vulnerable people should avoid it. They include pregnant women, infants, young children, and those with asthma, emotional problems, fevers, heart palpitations, headaches, high blood pressure, and insomnia. Ginseng may aggravate some of these conditions.

HOREHOUND TEA. The Food and Drug Administration says that, contrary to what

---

HOREHOUND TEA

BEST FOR HELPING YOU:

Loosen phlegm

TEA TIME: THAT AFTER-DINNER CUP MAY BLOCK CANCER

Serving a glass of iced tea at your next barbecue may not be a bad idea.

Studies have found that tea is able to block the formation of cancer-causing substances created by chemicals added to processed foods like hot dogs and bacon.

In one study, for example, 14 young men were divided into two groups and fed a breakfast that included sodium nitrate, a substance commonly used to preserve bacon, which can combine with other substances in the stomach to cause stomach cancer.

One group of men drank their tea—either green, black, or oolong—before eating breakfast, while the other group drank their tea afterward.

The result?

Although all tea prevented the formation of at least some of these cancer-causing compounds, the guys who drank their tea after a meal had the fewest.

our mothers and grandmothers may have thought, there's no evidence that horehound relieves coughs. That's why they banned it from cough remedies in 1989.

Some folks aren't convinced horehound is useless, however. They point to the fact that horehound contains marrubiin, a naturally occurring chemical that's released only when the herb is heated. The marrubiin apparently stimulates secretions that may loosen the phlegm that frequently drips down the back of your throat.

Will this stop your cough? You'll have to find out for yourself. You can still buy horehound tea in many health food stores, or you can grow it yourself in an herb jar like I do. When you want a cup of tea, just pour eight ounces of boiling water over a teaspoon of the dried leaves. Steep for 10 minutes, add a drop of honey to counter the herb's somewhat bitter taste, then sip. Since horehound does tend to irritate throat tissues, some doctors suggest you have no more than one cup a day.

LICORICE TEA. Licorice root is a naturally sweet herb that can soothe coughs and heal stomach ulcers. Some scientists say it's almost as effective as a heavy-duty prescription ulcer drug.

Since real licorice root contains glycyrrhizin, a substance that can raise blood pressure and cause water retention, stick with deglycyrrhizinated licorice—or DGL as it's usually listed on labels.

To make a cup of tea, steep one teaspoon of the dried root in four ounces of water for five minutes. Strain before you drink. Some doctors suggest you drink no more than one-half cup of licorice tea three times a day after meals. They also suggest that pregnant women and those who have high blood pressure, heart disease, or liver disease should avoid it.

MARSHMALLOW TEA. Marshmallow has absolutely nothing to do with those soft packages of store-bought candy puffs you toast over campfires. It's actually a tall plant that grows near a marsh with a root that produces a gooey mucilage that soothes sore throats and reduces coughs.

To make a tea, pour eight ounces of boiling water over two teaspoons of chopped marshmallow root and steep for 10 to 15 minutes. Sip three or four table-

LICORICE TEA

BEST FOR HELPING YOU:

Heal ulcers

Soothe coughs

MARSHMALLOW TEA

BEST FOR HELPING YOU:

Soothe sore throats

Reduce coughs

CAN TEA PREVENT ALZHEIMER'S?

Sure looks like it. A team of researchers at Newcastle University's Medicinal Plant Research Center have just discovered that green and black tea inhibit the activity of acetylcholinesterase, an enzyme associated with the development of Alzheimer's disease. The only other thing that does that, reported the researchers, are drugs used to slow the development of Alzheimer's such as Novartis' Exelon and Pfzer's Aricept.

spoons of tea every few hours, never exceeding eight ounces a day.

MEADOWSWEET TEA. Meadowsweet is an almond-scented herb that contains salicin, the active ingredient in aspirin. It reduces fever and relieves the aches and pains of arthritis and headache.

To make the tea, pour eight ounces of boiling water over one teaspoon of the dried herb and let it steep for 10 minutes. Strain before drinking. The tea can be used instead of aspirin, but using it in addition to aspirin could cause a toxic reaction. Those who are allergic to aspirin should avoid it, and, as with aspirin, children shouldn't take it unless directed by a physician.

PEPPERMINT TEA. The oil in peppermint tea increases the number of digestive enzymes in your gut and encourages the entire digestive system to function smoothly. It also reduces gas, soothes intestinal spasms, and kills a number of microorganisms that cause the intestinal irritation and diarrhea often associated with diverticulitis or irritable bowel syndrome.

Tea is the perfect method to release the oil's healing properties. Peppermint candies frequently do not contain enough of the herb's active ingredient, while peppermint oil contains so much that it can be toxic.

One caveat: Peppermint in any form can make young children feel as though they're choking. Reserve the tea for those over age 12.

ST. JOHN'S WORT TEA. Although the crushed leaves and flowers of this herb have been used to heal wounds for more than 2,000 years, modern scientists have just recently found that St. John's wort also contains a naturally occurring antidepressant that may help reduce the symptoms of mild depression. An extract of the herb is also being tested for its ability to fight viruses—including the virus that causes AIDS.

If you decide to try St. John's wort tea, check with your doctor first. Depression is a serious illness that should always be categorized and monitored by a doctor.

People with high blood pressure should not drink St. John's wort tea, nor should anyone who is taking medication of any kind. Those who do decide to drink the tea, experts say, should drink no more than three cups a day.

SLIPPERY ELM TEA. Until Dutch elm disease decimated elms throughout the northeastern United States, slippery elm was one of America's favorite home remedies. The bark secretes a sweet, soothing mucilage that can coat an irritated throat.

MEADOWSWEET TEA

BEST FOR HELPING YOU:

Reduce headache and arthritic pain

Relieve fever

PEPPERMINT TEA

BEST FOR HELPING YOU:

Reduce gas

Soothe intestinal cramps

Reduce symptoms of diverticulitis and irritable bowel syndrome

---

ST. JOHN'S WORT TEA

BEST FOR HELPING YOU:

Reverse mild depression

SLIPPERY ELM TEA

BEST FOR HELPING YOU:

Soothe an irritated throat

Although you can't really find many elms today, you can find imported slippery elm and slippery elm teas in health food stores. Simply pour eight ounces of boiling water over a single teaspoon of the bark, steep for a few minutes, and drink.

WILD CHERRY TEA. Wild cherry is better known as a flavoring agent in cough syrups, but since it contains benzaldehyde, a naturally occurring substance that can loosen phlegm, some people like to drink a cup of wild cherry tea in the morning.

One caveat: Wild cherry can be toxic. Do not give it to children, scientists caution, or drink more than three cups a day yourself. And to make sure you don't inadvertently give yourself too much of the active ingredient, stick to commercial varieties with standardized ingredients.

WILD CHERRY TEA
BEST FOR HELPING YOU:
Loosen phlegm

SLOW PROSTATE CANCER

Since prostate cancer generally progresses at such a slow rate, cancer researchers know that if they can slow it down even more, the cancer will cease to be a life-threatening disease. Now, a breakthrough study at UCLA's Center for Human Nutrition reveals that both black and green teas may significantly slow the progress of prostate cancer. In the study, 20 men who were scheduled to have their prostate removed because of cancer were asked to drink five cups a day of either black tea, green tea, or soda for five days prior to surgery. When cells from each man's prostate were subsequently examined under a microscope after surgery, researchers found a decrease in the numbers of new cancer cells in men who had consumed either the black or green tea. Cancer cells in men who drank soda proliferated at a faster rate. The bottom line? If you're a guy, tea should be your beverage of choice.

Refreshing Chamomile and Tonic with Lime

Chamomile Cubes

The next time you prepare hot chamomile tea, make some extra. When it cools, pour it into an empty ice cube tray. About 1½ cups of chamomile tea will fill an ice cube tray. When the cubes have frozen, add them to your favorite cold drinks or make the following:

Refreshing Chamomile and Tonic with Lime

Add the cubes to a tall glass, fill with tonic water, and add a wedge of lime.

INGREDIENTS

YIELD: 1 SERVING

4 chamomile ice cubes
1 cup tonic water
1 lime wedge

PER SERVING

Calories	879
Carbohydrates	23 g
Fat	0 g
Dietary fiber	0.3 g
Cholesterol	0 mg
Sodium	11 mg

Chicken Marinated in Black Tea

Served over Spinach and Mandarin Orange Sections

Brew the tea for at least 10 minutes. Add the cooled tea to a glass pan along with the chicken and the remaining ingredients. Cover and allow to marinate in the refrigerator about 2 hours or overnight.

Heat a nonstick pan over medium heat. Remove the chicken from the marinade and add to the hot pan. Cook until one side is browned and then turn to the other side and brown it. When the chicken is cooked through, remove the chicken to a clean plate and reserve, keeping it warm.

Strain the marinade and add the liquid to the heated pan. Bring to a boil and skim off any foam that forms. Boil the liquid down until it becomes thickened and dark, about 10 minutes. About ⅓ to ½ cup of a dark liquid will be left.

Slice the chicken. Serve over dark greens, spinach, or oak leaf lettuce with orange sections. Pour some of the tasty, rich liquid over the chicken slices.

INGREDIENTS

YIELD: 4 SERVINGS

2 cups brewed strong black tea
1 pound skinless, boneless chicken breast
2 teaspoons minced garlic
¼ cup coarsely chopped ginger root
1 stick cinnamon (2½ inches)
2 tablespoons honey
2 teaspoons soy sauce
10 ounces fresh cleaned and washed spinach
1 can (10 ounces) can mandarin oranges, drained

PER SERVING

Calories	239
Carbohydrates	19 g
Fat	7 g
Saturated fat	2 g
Dietary fiber	2g
Cholesterol	69 mg
Sodium	200 mg

Iced Ginger Tea (Homemade Ginger Ale)

*E*llen's recipe for ginger tea makes a great cup of tea, but I like to add two teaspoons of honey to it. Another way to drink it is to chill the tea and then make iced ginger ale from that.

Finely chop or shred the ginger, which can be done easily in a food processor or hand grater. Boil the water and add the ginger to the water. Cover and let steep for 10 minutes. Strain. Add the honey. More honey or sugar can be added to taste. Allow to come to room temperature.

To use, pour ½ cup into a glass. Add seltzer, a lemon slice, and ice. Stir and serve.

Any leftover must be refrigerated or the mixture will begin to ferment and you will have ginger beer.

INGREDIENTS

YIELD: 4 SERVINGS

4 teaspoons fresh grated ginger
2 cups water
4 teaspoons honey
2 cups seltzer water
Lemon slices
Ice

PER SERVING

Calories	23
Carbohydrates	6 g
Fat	0 g
Saturated fat	0 g
Dietary fiber	0 g
Cholesterol	0 mg
Sodium	25 mg

Fruit-Flavored Tea

*C*ommercially bottled tea favorites are the peach, mint and mango flavored teas, at least those are the ones I often see being consumed. You can make your own flavored teas by using tea to prepare your favorite frozen juice concentrates. The calories would be the same but would come from the fruit juice concentrates rather than from high fructose corn syrup, which is just sugar.

Instead of diluting fruit juices with three cans of water, use three cans of tea! Old Orchard makes a frozen grape kiwi strawberry frozen concentrate which can be diluted with tea to make a delicious beverage.

Combine the juice concentrate with the 3 cans of tea and mix well. Chill and serve.

INGREDIENTS

YIELD: 6 SERVINGS

12 ounces frozen fruit concentrate
36 ounces (1 qt + ¼ cup) tea

PER SERVING

Calories	115
Carbohydrates	29 g
Fat	0 g
Saturated fat	0 g
Dietary fiber	0 g
Cholesterol	0 mg
Sodium	5 mg

Refrigerator Iced Tea

*I*ced tea can be brewed in the refrigerator as well as in the sun. More tea in proportion to water is needed to prepare this method successfully.

Combine the water and tea in a glass pitcher or jar. Cover. Refrigerate for 8 or more hours. Remove bags. Serve.

INGREDIENTS

YIELD: 4 CUPS

1 quart cold water
5 tea bags

Sun Tea

A simple way to make brewed tea is to add the water and tea bags or leaves, green or black, to a glass container, cover and place in the sun for several hours. The resulting tea is not as bitter or strong as tea made with boiled water.

Add the water and tea bags to a glass container. Cover and place in the sun. Usually 3 to 4 hours is enough brewing time. After 5 hours, remove the bags and refrigerate the tea.

INGREDIENTS

YIELD: 8 CUPS

2 quarts cold water
5 tea bags

The Honey Jar

As titmice ate breakfast at the bird feeder and a woodchuck dove for cover under a crumbling log, 40-year-old Sari Harrar stepped into her backyard to introduce me to her bees.

Her face softened into a mellow smile as she moved around a shaded garden running wild with lilies, vines, and ferns and caught sight of the bees returning from an early morning pollen run. Slowly she followed the bees toward three stacks of white boxes that stood in the sun.

"Here they are," she said, an undercurrent of delight reflecting her affection for these tiny, energetic creatures. "What do you think?"

I looked past Sari at the meadows edging her backyard. Surrounded by sunshine, bees, titmice, and marauding woodchucks, it was hard to think at all. It was mid-June, and the Pennsylvania countryside was blooming. Clover covered the pastures, orchards were swollen with blossoms, wild roses tumbled over every stonewall, fence, and tangle of vines they could find, and the industrious garden clubs that exist in every Pennsylvania community had turned every town square into an English garden.

2

HONEY JAR

BEST FOR HELPING YOU:

Heal stomach ulcers

Protect your stomach from aspirin and other drugs

Kill bacteria that cause stomachaches

Kill bacteria that cause intestinal upset

Heal superficial cuts, scrapes, and burns

What did I think?

Sari's backyard looked like a miniature version of O'Hare. Thousands of bees from her three stacked box hives were winging out to millions of fragrant targets for miles around, then returning home so stuffed with nectar and orange and yellow pollen that they could barely follow a straight flight path.

The sight was amazing.

The entrance to each hive was located at the bottom of each stack of boxes. Little more than a foot-long slit with a landing board in front, the entrance was so narrow that bees could enter it only in small groups. The narrowness of the entrance allowed guard bees to effectively defend the hive from neighboring "robber" bees who would fly into a hive and steal its honey. But it also caused major traffic jams that stacked up pollen-heavy bees in hover patterns that extended ten feet or more around the hives.

Eventually, each bee would get its turn. One by one, they would touch down on the landing board, make their way past guard bees, dodge bees that were taking off, then lumber inside. There they'd climb over the honeycomb and empty a special sac in which they had stored the nectar they'd drawn from flowers and mixed with enzymes made from their own bodies. Together, nectar and enzymes became honey. Here and there a little of the pollen that had dusted their bodies would fall into individual cells, coloring the golden amber of the honey with microscopic dots of pale orange or muted yellow. Then they were off again.

What did I think?

I think that I'll never again slip a spoonful of honey into my tea without being aware that honey is the energy and essence of the bees themselves—an energy and essence that connects me, in a very real way, to the earth itself.

The Gift of 60,000 Bees

A bee lives for one golden month every summer. It beats each of its four wings 11,400 times a minute, visits thousands of flowers and produces one-twelfth—one-twelfth!—of a teaspoon of honey

---

HONEY BASICS

HOW TO BUY: Most of the 300 varieties of honey have antibacterial properties of one kind or another. But only two have been found to work against the ulcer-causing *Helicobacter pylori*—honeydew honey from the pine forests of central Europe and manuka honey from the manuka bush in New Zealand. Both are extremely difficult to find unless you live in either location. (See "The Honey Pot" for mail order sources, p. 23.)

Whichever honey you buy, reach for one that's in its natural state—it will be labeled "raw" honey—or one that has been cold-processed. Heat destroys an enzyme in honey that produces the natural form of hydrogen peroxide. And because blends of various honeys are frequently heated during processing, make sure any honey you buy is made from the nectar of a single plant—"orange blossom" honey, for example.

HOW TO STORE: Honey should be stored in air tight containers away from light and heat.

HOW TO USE: To treat superficial cuts and scrapes, clean the area thoroughly with a sterile salt solution three times a day, says University of Waikato researcher Nicolette Brady. "Apply honey directly and cover with an absorbent sterile dressing."

How much honey you should use is pretty much relative to the size of the cut. "I'm currently treating a small cut to my toe with a dab of manuka honey sufficient to cover the area covered with a Band-Aid," Brady told me.

Where chronic stomachaches and ulcers are concerned, no one is exactly sure how much honey it will take to kill the bacteria that cause them. But where scientists fear to tread, commercial enterprises generally rush in. And in this case, at least one honey packer suggests that a tablespoon of honey on a slice of bread three times a day with meals and once before bed will do the trick.

Whether or not it will is anybody's guess. But keep in mind that stomachaches can be the result of anything from last night's pizza to cancer. So any stomach pain should be evaluated by your family physician before you start soothing it with honey. Once you've done that, however, it probably wouldn't hurt to try some honey—if you can afford the calories and don't have to watch your sugar intake because of diabetes.

ONE OTHER CAVEAT: Honey should never be given to infants and children. It can sometimes contain a toxin that is harmless to healthy adults, but deadly to little guys.

---

over its entire lifespan. Knowing that, some mornings it feels a little wasteful, a little decadent, a little frivolous to drizzle the life-work of 36 bees—one tablespoon of honey—in my tea.

Yet when I think of all the ways that even that tablespoon of honey benefits me, I like to hope that the bees would think their sacrifice worthwhile. Because the gift of their lifework is not simply a pleasant-tasting tea. No, according to researchers it's also the energy to snap open your eyes every morning, a soothing unguent that will heal your cuts and scrapes without a scar, and protection against various microbes that may invade your stomach or gastrointestinal tract. It also heals ulcers that can devour the lining of your stomach or gut.

Although some of these uses are new discoveries, honey itself has been associated with healing for centuries. Primitive drawings on cave walls indicate that hunter/gatherers first tasted the honeybee's gift some 8,000 years ago. Since then it has been incorporated into religious rituals, mixed with milk to nourish newborns, and used to sustain vast armies as they traveled over rugged mountain passes and hot desert sands. Poultices of honey healed blisters, abscesses, and wounds on the skin's surface, while honey-based tonics were used to treat everything from croup to sore throats.

The advent of antibiotics and other modern drugs meant that honey—along with other folk medicine—was abandoned by modern doctors, but today many physicians are reconsidering the healing properties of honey.

A number of studies, particularly from the Honey Research Unit at the University of Waikato in Hamilton, New Zealand, have found that our ancestral honey lovers knew what they were doing.

For one thing, taken internally, honey protects the stomach from the assaults of various drugs, such as aspirin, that irritate its lining. Honey also effectively kills nine different species of bacteria—including *Helicobacter pylori*, the bacteria that burrows into the stomach's lining and causes chronic stomachaches and stomach ulcers. And used externally, honey kills staph—*Staphylococcus aureus*—a particularly deadly bacteria that lives on the skin just waiting to enter your body through some cut or abrasion.

How Honey Protects

Just how honey kills bacteria is not totally clear. Some species of bacteria simply can't grow in the acidic environment that honey creates. Other bacteria are susceptible to the hydrogen peroxide produced when honey is diluted by body fluids. And unlike the product you buy at the drug store, the hydrogen peroxide naturally produced by honey kills the bacteria without also harming the surrounding cells.

There are at least nine other naturally occurring chemicals in honey that kill bacteria as well. How much any or all of these chemicals contribute to honey's healing abilities is still a puzzle. What is known, however, is that when honey is swabbed on freshly cleaned cuts, burns, and ulcerated skin, the inflammation, pain, and swelling are reduced. Dead skin sloughs off without the need for the exquisitely painful scrubbing that nurses must frequently do to prevent infection, and bandages can be removed without sticking to the cut and ripping off new skin. As a result, healing is speeded up and scarring is minimized.

What is also known is that a series of laboratory studies have demonstrated that when manuka honey—a type of honey made from New Zealand's manuka bush—is added to the *Helicobacter pylori* that causes ulcers, the bacterium dies. And although no human studies have yet demonstrated that honey heals ulcers, scientists know from other work that once the bacterium is eradicated, the ulcers heal.

That's actually the major reason I use one tablespoon of honey in my tea every morning.

Several years ago, a two-month course of heavy-duty anti-inflammatory drugs for a back injury left me with a "sensitive" stomach. I couldn't drink orange juice, salad dressings gave me a stomachache, and my stomach just seemed to feel irritated and uncomfortable much of the time. My doctor thought I had an ulcer from the drugs and prescribed a popular prescription antacid.

Unfortunately, that fussy, uncomfortable feeling never went away—at least not until I started using honey. A month or so after I did, my stomach returned to normal. And today I can drink all the orange juice I like.

Until recently, most scientists believed that honey contained only a trace amount of nutrients and, for the most part, that's true. But in 1998, researchers at the University of Illinois found that darker-colored honeys are so loaded with an-tioxidants that they're comparing them to vitamin C!

A Taste of Wildflowers

If the only kind of honey you've ever eaten is some sticky mess in a supermarket squeeze bottle, you've missed out on one of the more sensual pleasures in life.

That's because the only taste supermarket blends have is sweet. And, yes, sweet is good. But species-specific honeys like orange blossom honey from citrus in Florida, or sage honey from shrubs and hives along the California coast, are even better. They tend to have distinct, fairy-light flavors and ethereal fragrances as well.

Try substituting first one and then another in your favorite honey-sweetened recipe. If you'd like to find a supplier near you for one type or honey or another, check your local Yellow Pages for a listing of "Beekeepers." In the meantime, here's a rundown of some of the honeys available in the United States:

ALFALFA. When summer comes to Utah, Nevada, Idaho, Oregon, and most of the western states, the alfalfa plant celebrates with a profusion of beautiful blue blooms. Local bees go into overtime working from dawn 'til dusk to produce pound after

---

SWEET SUBSTITUTIONS

Not only is honey a more healthful sweetener than sugar, it also helps breads and cookies retain moisture. Open a week-old container of cookies made with sugar and you're likely to find them dry and crumbly. Open a week-old container of cookies made with honey and they'll be as moist as the day you made them.

If you'd like to substitute honey for sugar in your favorite recipe, experts at the National Honey Board in Longmont, Colorado, suggest that you begin by replacing half the amount of sugar with honey. You should also cut the amount of liquid in your recipe by one-quarter, add half a teaspoon of baking soda per cup of honey, and reduce your oven temperature by 25 degrees to prevent over-browning.

pound of an almost white honey with a gentle flavor and aroma that lends itself to almost any use.

BASSWOOD. Every June, the basswood tree produces a luscious crop of cream-colored flowers from Canada to Texas. Local bees collect the flowers' nectar and turn it into a sharp, biting honey. The best way to use it? Try it with meat, poultry, or vegetables, says New York-based recipe developer Jane Charlton, author of *A Taste of Honey*.

BUCKWHEAT. Buckwheat honey has a dark, full-bodied flavor. It's a little strong for a lot of us, but among buckwheat pancake-lovers in Minnesota, New York, Ohio, Pennsylvania, Wisconsin, and eastern Canada, it has practically achieved cult status. Try it with heavily spiced cakes and breads, Charlton suggests.

CLOVER. Honey from one variety of clover or another is on almost every supermarket shelf in America. Its smooth, sweet taste has made it one of our favorite honeys, and its unobtrusive flavor makes it suitable for almost any use in which you want other flavors to predominate.

EUCALYPTUS. Let a spoonful of eucalyptus honey slide across your tongue and you'll understand why honey was once thought to be the food of gods. Found mostly in Australia and California, euca-lyptus honey has a bold flavor that likes to stand on its own. Use it to wake up bland teas and nondescript muffins.

FIREWEED. Fireweed produces three-foot-tall spikes of pink flowers that dot the open woods of California, Washington, the northwestern and Pacific states and Canada. It's a spectacular display that also draws local bees. They gather its nectar and make a light, distinctive honey that enhances the flavor of just about everything. Try it on meat, poultry, and vegetables.

ORANGE BLOSSOM. Orange blossom honey does not taste like oranges. Instead, it tastes the way orange blossoms smell— light, fresh, and delicate. One whiff of its mystical scent and I'm likely to close my eyes and image I've been transported to a white-sand beach on the Gulf of Mexico. A wonderful complement to fresh grapefruit or a fresh fruit salad.

TULIP POPLAR. Wherever the tulip poplar grows east of the Mississippi, local bees are sure to whip up a comb or two. A dark honey with a mild taste, this honey is a perfect complement to fruit.

TUPELO. If the state of Georgia had a taste, this would be it. It's the honey Peter Fonda's character made in the wonderful movie *Ulee's Gold*. Slow, thick, and full-bodied, tupelo honey was made to

---

THE HONEY POT

Most raw and cold-pressed honey is easily found in health food stores, local orchards, and from your friendly local beekeeper. But manuka honey is almost impossible to find. Here's one direct mail supplier who'll charge it to a major credit card and send it to your home:

W. L. and M. Bennett, Richards Road, R.D. 8, Hamilton, New Zealand

be licked from the honeycomb on a soft, southern night in May. Its mild, distinctive flavor floats across the tongue and enhances just about anything it touches. Use it in cakes, fruit, and other desserts.

WILDFLOWER. If you're a beekeeper and you don't know where your bees have been, chances are you'll call the honey they make "wildflower honey." And that's why every jar marked "wildflower honey" will taste different than the one you had before. Use milder-tasting varieties in cakes and fruit, Charlton suggests, and stronger flavors for meat, poultry, and vegetables.

WILL WILD HONEY DISAPPEAR?

It might. Because the pesticides that we unthinkingly dust on our roses, mist on our trees, and spray over our lawns are joining forces with a naturally occurring mite epidemic in hives that threatens the existence of every bee in the United States.

More than 25 percent of managed bee colonies in the country have been wiped out since 1990 alone. The state of Maine, which also counts on bees to pollinate its blueberries and cranberries, lost 80 percent of its hives in 1996. Michigan lost 60 percent. And Massachusetts lost 50 percent.

Experts say the situation is even worse among wild bees, since they have no one to guard them against man-made chemicals or nature's predators. As a result, reports Defenders of Wildlife, a nonprofit wildlife conservation group in Washington, D.C., wild honeybees are gone forever from many states.

If you're lucky enough to have wild bees visit your yard and garden, here's what you can do to help keep them healthy and on the job:

Pick bugs and other creatures off roses. Yeah, I know, it's an icky, never-ending job. But every morning from June through September, the first thing my husband and I do after our feet hit the floor is go outside and frisk all six lavender roses growing in the giant wood planters that line our deck. We'd like to have more roses, but we keep it to six because that's all we can care for without using pesticides or putting the roses under 24-hour surveillance. (Keep in mind that we live in the woods, and every winged or sap-sucking creature within 10 miles knows that our house is the place to be when they've got a yen for roses. They act as though the roses are pure candy!)

Use natural predators. Check with your local county extension service and find out which natural predators like to lunch on the kind of bugs munching on the plants surrounding your home or in the garden. Then import a few—the extension agent will know where to get them—and let nature take its course. If you're not sure where to find your extension service, just call your county's administrative offices. They'll be happy to tell you.

Squirt. If the bugs are biting when you're barbecuing out back or working in the yard, squirt a tiny amount of insecticide on your socks, shoes, shorts, shirts, collars, sleeves, and hats or scarves. There's no need to envelop your body in a killing mist to kill off a few gnats. Nor do you need to envelop your backyard in a poisonous "fog" to kill off a few mosquitoes. Besides, if those sprays and foggers are designed to kill an insect when it absorbs those chemicals, common sense should tell you that it's certainly not doing the cells in your body any good either.

Fresh Honey-Lime Dressing

*T*his is a wonderful dressing for a tossed green salad as well as for a mixed fruit salad or as a dip for fresh fruit. I always use fresh-squeezed lime juice and then I have lime to peel, chop and add. Because each honey has a different flavor, I usually taste the honey before adding it to the dressing. I prefer a milder flavor. For testing, I used wild raspberry honey from Moorland Apiaries in Littleton, New Hampshire.

Combine all ingredients in a jar or bowl and shake or whip with a wire whisk until well-combined. Serve immediately or refrigerate. Will keep for several days in the refrigerator.

INGREDIENTS

YIELD: 1 CUP

½ cup plain nonfat yogurt
¼ cup honey
¼ cup light mayonnaise
¼ teaspoon finely chopped lime peel
1 teaspoon Dijon mustard
¼ cup lime juice (juice of two limes)

PER TABLESPOON

Calories	34
Carbohydrates	6 g
Fat	1 g
Saturated fat	0 g
Dietary fiber	1 g
Cholesterol	0 mg
Sodium	42 mg

Honeyed Carrots

*B*ring about 1 cup of water to a boil in a 1-quart saucepan. Add the carrots, cover, lower the heat to medium-high, and cook for 10 minutes or until the carrots are tender. Drain and set aside.

In the same pan, add the honey, lemon juice, lemon rind, and mustard. Bring to a boil. Add the carrots back into the pan and combine well, making sure the carrots are coated with the honey sauce. Cover the pan, lower the heat to medium, and cook the carrots with the sauce for 3 minutes or until the carrots are heated through and covered with the sauce.

INGREDIENTS

YIELD: 4 SERVINGS (½ CUP)

2 cups chopped carrots (about 3 large)
2 tablespoons honey (your favorite)
1 tablespoon freshly squeezed lemon juice
   (about ½ lemon)
¼ teaspoon grated lemon rind
¼ teaspoon Dijon mustard

PER SERVING

Calories	57
Carbohydrates	0 g
Fat	0.1 g
Saturated fat	0 g
Dietary fiber	2 g
Cholesterol	0 mg
Sodium	27 mg

The Cookie Jar

Standing in her sunny kitchen a few miles from the rolling blue mountains of northeastern Pennsylvania, Priscilla Benner, M.D., is focused on the 10-quart mixing bowl on the counter between us.

Her blond hair, hastily pulled back into a ponytail, is sticking out in five directions at once. The baggy jeans she yanked on this morning show more than one souvenir of the batter we're mixing. Her lime-colored blouse has been splashed with water as we've rattled around in her cheerful country kitchen, rinsing bowls, spoons, and pans and talking about children.

But Priscilla Benner isn't the type to worry about how she looks. At 40-something, she's too busy raising five kids, running a thriving general practice, tending her edible weed garden, developing highly nutritious cookie recipes, and heading an international organization called MAMA—"Mujeres Amigas Miles Apart."

MAMA—the name is a deliberate blending of Spanish and English words meaning "Mothers and Friends Miles Apart"—is a woman-to-woman effort between the United States and Honduras

that "came along" in the Benner household on Thanksgiving, 1984.

MAMA is a nutrition education and feeding project in Honduras that has, through the efforts of Dr. Benner's women's church group in Pennsylvania and a sister group in San Pedro Sula, significantly altered the lives of hundreds of thousands of Honduran children every year for the past decade. It has saved the sight of thousands, enabled hundreds more to learn, and cut the pediatric mortality rate in at least one hospital by more than 50 percent.

How? Priscilla Benner will tell you that it was through love, determination, commitment, education—and her nutrient-dense cookies.

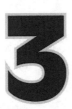

3

COOKIE JAR

BEST FOR HELPING YOU:

Fight anemia

Prevent constipation

Prevent heart disease

Prevent colon cancer

Build sound muscles

Build strong nerves

Cookies with a Purpose

As kids, friends of kids, neighbors, and her husband wander in and out of her kitchen on this hot August morning, Priscilla Benner offers me a cup of coffee, fires up her electric mixer, and shows me why the cookies are so important.

The Super Galletas, as they are called in Honduras, are high-protein, high-fat cookies spiked with vitamins. The cookies are made from soy meal that is 44 percent protein, defatted and heated to deactivate a protein-zapping enzyme which naturally occurs in soy. It also includes whole wheat flour, baking soda, salt, canola oil, sugar, molasses, whole eggs, vanilla, and—since most of the children don't have access to a balanced diet—a mix of powdered vitamins.

Nutritionally, each cookie has a full daily dose of vitamins and nearly a day's supply of iron. It also contains four grams of mostly "good" fat—meaning the kind of monounsaturated fat that builds the walls of your brain and not the saturated kind that lines the walls of your arteries—plus about 82 calories.

The cookies contain so much fat in order to help the children absorb the vitamins, and the high calories provide energy, says Dr. Benner. "And both are important if we want them to learn."

Education is a key component of MAMA's efforts. Supported by bike-a-thons, bowling parties, roller skating events, and an occasional food company's sponsorship of a "hole" in a miniature golf game near Dr. Benner's home in Pennsylvania, MAMA runs 17 preschools in four Honduran villages and an urban educational center that sponsors 200 women's nutrition "clubs" throughout the San Pedro Sula area.

Staffed by local women in Honduras, the organization also provides education-al seminars for local health officials, gives out about 500,000 vitamin A capsules—donated by a large pharmaceutical firm—to prevent nutritional blindness, works side by side with Habitat for Humanity to build new homes, and organizes groups of local women who bake Super Galletas for malnourished children at the preschools and local hospitals.

That's not bad for an organization that started 10 years ago with a group of Mennonite women who simply wanted to help other women and their children.

Fight Supermarket Nutri-trash

Although Dr. Benner's cookies were intended to correct nutritional deficiencies in Honduran children, they're also the perfect weapon with which to stave off the dietary deficiencies produced by a culture that pushes nutrient-lacking foods for its women and feeds its children sugary breakfast cereals, snack bags of fried fat, and six-packs of soft drinks—our own. (See "After-School Snacks," p. 216, and "Healing Snacks for Women," p. 219.)

They're also the perfect weapon to fight the nutri-trash now being sold in the cookie aisles of American supermarkets as a "healthy" alternative to traditional cookies.

Read a few cookie labels and you'll see

COOKIE BASICS

HOW TO BUY: Don't. Make them.

HOW TO STORE: Place cooled cookies into a container and cover with a tightly fitting lid. If you decide to freeze some for later, line a container with foil, then separate layers with additional sheets of foil. Seal container, then freeze.

HOW TO USE: Place cookie jar on your kitchen countertop for all to see. These are healthy cookies, so there's no reason to hide them away on the top shelf of your cupboard.

what I mean. Even the fat-free bar cookies allegedly made out of fruit look as if they're eight-tenths sugar, one-tenth preservatives and one-tenth a mixture of the cheapest fruits available.

Find that hard to believe when you're paying more than $3 a package? So did I—until one innovative nutrition scientist evaluated the claims of an "apple" cereal/cookie bar and found that you'd have to eat 70 of them to get the fruit equivalent of one apple.

Now, you and I know we haven't got time to bake cookies the three times a week it would take to keep cookie monsters off your back. But we're not talking Christmas cookies here. We're talking down-and-dirty basics. No rolling, no cutting, no decorating. Just mix, plop, bake, and eat whenever a nutritious mouthful is needed—before a run, after a workout, when a meeting runs over and cancels your lunch, or when hungry hoards threaten mutiny because their dinner's not on the table.

The kind of cookies I'm talking about take less than 15 minutes to make and another 15 to bake. And here's the clincher: if you use the right sweetener—honey—you can bake an entire week's cookie supply at once and they'll stay fresh all week...if they last that long.

You see, cookies made with sugar tend to dry out and crumble within hours of leaving the oven. But cookies made with honey don't. They stay moist. So instead of baking small batches every few days to keep something edible in the cookie jar, you can bake one giant batch Sunday afternoon, stuff them in the cookie jar, clamp down the lid, and know that they'll taste moist and fresh whenever you need them.

The Cookie Plot

If it sounds as though I'm pushing cookies, it's because I am. And it's not because of my own insatiable cookie appetite, which, in the interests of full disclosure, I herewith admit. No, I'm pushing cookies because I understand how people eat, how they should eat and how the common, ordinary cookie can help an entire generation make the transition from where we are to where we want to be.

Canadian nutritionist Louise Desaulniers, R.D., a nutritional consultant in Montreal, is the one who gave me the idea.

"I hate cookies," moaned Desaulniers into the phone when I called her for some suggestions on healthy cookie-making. "They're bad. They're full of fat and calories. And they teach people bad habits."

I know she's right. Cookies teach us to reach for rich-tasting baked goods when we're hungry instead of nutrient-dense fruits, nuts, and seeds.

So what does she suggest we do to give cookies a healthy boost?

"Experiment," urges Desaulniers. All cookies are made up of flour, fat, sweetener, and egg. So the trick is to alter each ingredient until the whole cookie does a nutritional one-eighty.

Just make sure you do it gradually, one ingredient at a time, cautions Desaulniers. That way you'll gradually recondition your family's taste buds to actually prefer a cookie that has less sugar, less fat, fewer calories, and a host of body-building nutrients. Here's how she suggests you do it:

Swap bad fat for good. Traditional cookie recipes call for butter, shortening, or melted margarine. All three are equally bad—butter because its saturated fat will trick your body into manufacturing excessive amounts of artery-clogging LDL cholesterol, shortening and margarine because their trans-fatty acids will do exactly the same. (See "Healthy Oils" for a complete discussion of oils, margarine, and butter.)

So replace butter, shortening, and margarine with a monounsaturated fat like olive, canola, sesame, or walnut oil. All four will actually lower LDL cholesterol and increase HDL cholesterol—the "good" cholesterol that vacuums LDL cholesterol out of your arteries and escorts it to the liver for disposal.

The mild flavors of olive and canola oil can replace butter or margarine without anyone being the wiser. Canola has the least flavor, although the cheaper brands of olive oil are fairly light-tasting as well. But both sesame and walnut oil have sharp, distinctive tastes that can overwhelm subtle flavors. So use them with discretion. If your favorite chocolate chip cookie recipe calls for a cup of butter, for example, try substituting three-quarters of a cup of canola oil and one-quarter cup of walnut oil. Not only will you avoid the saturated fat of butter, but the delicate flavor of walnuts will emerge without overpowering that rich, chocolate taste you crave. And the extra pennies you spend on walnut oil are easily made up by the pennies you don't spend on nuts.

Use fruit butters and yogurt. Once you've got the right fat in your cookie, it's time to cut it down. Because even if the fat you use is a good fat, it's still a fat. And in the amounts most cookie recipes call for, whatever fat you use is going to add too many calories—unless, of course, you play for the Dallas Cowboys.

So those of us who have yet to make the team should substitute a fruit butter—essentially boiled-down condensed fruit mixed with sugar and spices—or low-fat yogurt for some of the fat in our favorite cookie recipe. Either one will provide exactly the same moistness, texture, and feel as fat, with fewer calories. And it's an even exchange—one spoonful of oil out, one spoonful of fruit butter or yogurt in. Start with just a couple of spoonfuls, then work your way up to a half cup or so.

The swap also gives your recipes some versatility. You can, for example, opt for lemon yogurt rather than plain, thus introducing a fresh note that an otherwise bland cookie may have lacked. Or you can underscore a subtlety that may have been overlooked: substitute two tablespoons of peach yogurt for two tablespoons of oil, and even the plainest sugar cookie may make you think of mint juleps, shadowy kudzu vines, and soft, sultry nights along the Carolina coast.

The fruit butters are equally evocative. Pumpkin butter—which is technically a vegetable butter even though it's found with the jams and jellies at your local supermarket—adds the sweet note of a New England church supper after the fall harvest. And apple butter adds that spicy New York punch that makes you feel alive, awake, and ready to move.

Not all fruit butters add flavor, however. Prune butter, which is usually tucked away near the canned pie filling in your local supermarket, adds not so much a flavor as a feeling—that full, round feeling somewhere in the back of your mouth that makes you feel like a well-loved child. It's so mellow that anytime you want the flavors of other ingredients to predominate, prune butter is a good substitute for fat.

Mash some fruit. Using fruit purées to sweeten your cookie batter in place of all or some of a recipe's sugar allows you to add moisture and cut back on the amount of sugar you use. And that means serving up fewer empty calories and more of the vitamins, minerals, fiber, and phytochemicals that naturally come from fruit. (See "The Fruit Basket", p. 37.)

Experiment to determine how much sugar you can cut. Start by cutting the sugar in your cookie recipe by a half. Then toss a few peeled and cored fruits—apricots, peaches, pears, or mangos, for example—into your blender and purée. Pour enough of the puréed fruit into your cookie batter to equal half the amount of

---

MAMA'S COOKIES

Below is the recipe developed by Priscilla Benner, M.D., to fight malnutrition among Honduran children. It is usually prepared with a special vitamin pre-mix. To adapt the recipe for well-nourished families, swap two-thirds or more of the canola oil and sugar for a fruit butter or fruit purée (see above). Or leave it as is and make up a batch for your local food bank or homeless shelter.

Preheat oven to 350 degrees.

To make 240 cookies, mix the following in a 10-quart bowl and set aside:
12 cups of defatted 44% protein soy flakes (or meal)
6 cups whole wheat flour
4 teaspoons baking soda
2 teaspoons salt

Use an electric beater to whip together the following in a large bowl:
4 cups canola oil
4 cups sugar

Then add:
1 cup molasses
8 whole eggs
8 teaspoons vanilla

Beat the mixture until smooth. Add the dry ingredients and mix thoroughly with a heavy-duty wooden spoon.

Drop one large tablespoon of batter per cookie onto an ungreased cookie sheet, flatten with the bottom of a glass that has first been dipped in sugar, then bake at 350 degrees for 8 minutes.

Remove cookies from oven, cool slightly, then transfer to cooling racks. When cookies are completely cooled, you can either freeze them for later use or put them in a tightly covered cookie jar.

For further information about the MAMA project, contact Dr. Benner at P.O. Box 216, Pennsburg, PA 18073.

INGREDIENTS

YIELD: 240 COOKIES

12 cups of defatted 44% protein soy flakes (or meal)
6 cups whole wheat flour
4 teaspoons baking soda
2 teaspoons salt
4 cups canola oil
4 cups sugar
1 cup molasses
8 whole eggs
8 teaspoons vanilla

PER COOKIE

Calories	82
Carbohydrates	9 g
Fat	4 g
Saturated fat	1 g
Monounsaturated fat	3 g
Protein	4 g
Cholesterol	7 mg
Sodium	42 mg
Potassium	191 mg
Iron	11 mg
Calcium	22 mg
Phosphorus	57 mg

sugar your original recipe called for, and blend it in with a few swift strokes.

Not only are you swapping empty calories for nutrient-dense ones, you're also reducing total calories as well: since fruit is so much sweeter than sugar, you'll probably have to use less than an equivalent amount of calories to gain the same amount of sweetness.

Mix in some honey. Although Desaulniers doesn't see much difference between sugar and honey on a nutrient-by-nutrient basis, some cookie bakers prefer honey because its moistness prevents cookie-crumble and gives cookies an extended jar life. There are also several studies indicating that certain types of honey reduce the stomach bacteria that cause chronic stomachaches and even ulcers.

If you decide to use honey in place of sugar, honey experts at the National Honey Board in Longmont, Colorado, suggest you substitute honey for up to half the sugar your recipe calls for and adjust the recipe in three ways:

- Reduce any liquid in your recipe one-third cup for each cup of honey you use;
- Add half a teaspoon baking soda for each cup of honey;
- Reduce your oven temperature by 25 degrees to prevent over-browning.

Experiment with flours and seeds. Since 90 percent of the nutrients have been removed from all-purpose flour, it's the last flour you should use in a cookie—even when your recipe calls for it.

Instead, says Desaulniers, experiment with a variety of whole grain flours, each of which is bursting with vitamins, minerals, fiber, and other substances that foster health and prevent disease. Try:

- Whole wheat pastry flour, which gives you the cancer-fighting abilities of whole grain nutrition with a lighter texture than plain whole wheat flour.
- Rolled oats, which combine that comfortable old-fashioned tasty lumpiness with the cholesterol-lowering benefits of beta glucan, the substance in oatmeal that sops up artery-clogging cholesterol. Just 1½ ounces a day can drop your LDL cholesterol 14 percent. To turn oats into flour, just toss a cupful of rolled oats—not instant—into your blender and hit the "grind" button. (It's much cheaper than buying oat flour at your local health food store.)
- Flaxseed, which is the highest source of heart-healthy omega-3 fatty acids known to science—particularly the omega-3 known as alpha-linolenic acid. Studies show that less than one ounce of flaxseed a day can help prevent heart attacks by reducing the tendency of your blood to create artery-jamming blood clots. In a study at Harvard School of Public Health, for example, researchers found that people with higher intakes of alpha-linolenic acid cut their risk of heart disease in half. Flaxseed has also been found to inhibit all three stages of cancer development: initiation, tumor development, and spread. (See Anita's recipe for Cranberry-Chocolate Chip Cookies made with ground flaxseed and soy on page 36.)

One other flour you might try is the one Dr. Benner uses for her Honduran children: soy. Just drop by any pet supply or feed store—check the Yellow Pages under "Feed Dealers" for one nearby— and ask for a 44 percent protein, defatted soy meal. (City dwellers take note: there's a feed dealer in my Philadelphia Yellow Pages.) Soy flour will look like tiny flakes of yellow cereal. But it will work perfectly in your cookie batter and provide you with all the benefits of soy. Studies indicate that a single serving of soy every day on a regular basis can cut your risk of cancer in half, while swapping it for meat and dairy foods in your diet can drop your cholesterol levels 20 percent.

Grind nuts. Use a handful of nuts to increase your ability to fend off heart disease. Researchers at Loma Linda University in California found that those who ate a handful of nuts at least four times a week had half the number of heart attacks as those who did not.

Researchers aren't sure how nuts exert a protective effect. But they note that nuts do contain both a rich store of heart-healthy magnesium and a naturally occurring chemical that relaxes arteries. So if you eat nuts, your arteries are less likely to tighten up and choke off the supply of blood to your heart.

Toss one-third cup of almonds into your blender and hit the grind button, suggests Desaulniers. Then delete two or three tablespoons of flour from your recipe and add the nuts in their place. Since ground nuts will release their oil into the batter, you should also delete one or two tablespoons of any liquid in the recipe as well.

Spice things up. The more flavorful a cookie tastes, the less it needs to depend on sugar to please its audience. So add spices with a liberal hand, says Desaulniers. Begin with ½ teaspoon of spices your palate knows—cinnamon, ginger, allspice—then become more adventurous. And every time you add a new spice, remove a spoonful of sugar. Ten to one, no will notice the difference.

Add some zest. Pump up your cookies' nutrient power with a teaspoon of lemon or orange rind. Both will add a dramatic burst of fresh flavor and a hefty dose of cancer-fighting flavonoids. Just scrape the skin of an organically grown lemon or orange against a metal grater, gathering up—along with the skin—a teaspoon's-worth of the white stuff just under it. That white stuff is where the flavonoids are located. And once you've eaten cookies with grated orange or lemon rind, you'll never, ever allow yourself to use the bottled zest from your supermarket again. The difference is that great.

Buy super-charged eggs. Most recipes call for an egg or two to hold things together. You can use an egg substitute, of course, or simply replace each whole egg with two egg whites. But to get maximum nutritional impact, says Desaulniers, use one of the new eggs that contain omega-3 fatty acids. If you haven't seen them in your supermarket yet, keep your eyes peeled. They're on the way.

Decorate with dark chocolate. Yes—you read that right. Milk chocolate is enriched with so much added fat that two bites are enough to make most of us comatose. On the other hand, dark chocolate, which is not enriched, has far less fat and sugar. So it's the perfect way to give ourselves that feeling of decadent chocolate indulgence without the nasty consequences, such as obesity and artery-clogging cholesterol.

Dark chocolate still has quite a few calories, cautions Desaulniers, so you can't go hog wild. That's why you should buy the dark mini chocolate chips and sprinkle a few across the top, or melt a square of dark chocolate and drizzle a bit over the top. I guarantee—the minute that cookie hits your tastebuds, you'll be in chocolate heaven—without having to pay a price for your sins.

Apricot-Honey Oat Bar Cookies

*T*he recipe is modified from the National Honey Board in Longmont, Colorado. Instead of three tablespoons of margarine, I substituted two tablespoons of canola oil. I used one egg substitute instead of two egg whites, which tend to give a rubbery texture to a product. I also used whole wheat flour instead of wheat germ and white flour, since it has the wheat germ included in it.

Preheat oven to 325 F.

Spray an 8-inch square baking pan with nonstick spray.

Combine all the ingredients in a bowl. Pour mixture into prepared pan and smooth evenly. Bake for 25 minutes, or until center is firm and edges are lightly browned. Cool and cut into 16 squares.

INGREDIENTS

YIELD: 16 SQUARES

1½ cups old-fashioned rolled oats (uncooked)
½ cup finely chopped dried apricots
½ cup honey
¼ cup nonfat plain yogurt
¼ cup egg substitute
¼ cup whole wheat flour
2 tablespoons canola oil
½ teaspoon cinnamon
½ teaspoon vanilla
¼ teaspoon salt

PER SQUARE

Calories	104
Carbohydrates	19 g
Fat	3 g
Saturated fat	0.3 g
Dietary fiber	2 g
Cholesterol	0 mg
Sodium	48 mg

Cinnamon Applesauce-Raisin Cookies

*P*reheat the oven to 350 F.

Combine the flours, cinnamon, baking soda, allspice, salt, and flaxseed. In another bowl beat together the honey, egg substitute, and vanilla. Add the applesauce.

Combine the wet and dry mixtures. Finally add the raisins. Combine well.

Using about 2 tablespoons of dough, drop a cookie onto a nonstick sprayed baking sheet. Press the cookie flat with a glass or your hand.

Bake for 10 minutes.

INGREDIENTS

YIELD: 24 COOKIES

1¼ cups whole wheat flour
¼ cup low fat soy flour
1 teaspoon cinnamon
½ teaspoon baking soda
½ teaspoon allspice
¼ teaspoon salt
¼ cup milled flaxseed
¼ cup honey
¼ cup egg substitute
½ teaspoon vanilla
¼ cup applesauce, unsweetened
⅓ cup raisins

PER COOKIE

Calories	53
Carbohydrates	11 g
Fat	0.8 g
Saturated fat	0 g
Dietary fiber	1.4 g
Cholesterol	0 mg
Sodium	56 mg

Peanut Butter-Banana Chocolate Chip Cookies

Take the original crisscross decorated peanut butter cookie and make it lower in fat and higher in nutrients by adding dried milk, soy flour, and substituting mashed banana for the butter or margarine. Only ¼ cup of honey is used for the sweetener.

Preheat the oven to 350 F.

In a medium bowl mash the banana completely with a fork and add the peanut butter, honey, vanilla, and egg substitute. Combine the flour, baking soda, baking powder, salt, powdered milk and soy flour in another bowl. Add to the peanut butter mixture. Blend thoroughly. Stir in the chocolate chips. Drop about a tablespoon of batter per cookie onto a nonstick sprayed cookie sheet using two spoons. Flatten the dough with a well-floured fork in a crisscross pattern.

Bake for 8 to 10 minutes.

INGREDIENTS

YIELD: 36 COOKIES

½ cup mashed ripe banana (about 2 small bananas)
½ cup unsalted peanut butter
¼ cup honey
½ teaspoon vanilla
1 egg substitute
1¼ cups unbleached flour
¾ teaspoon baking soda
½ teaspoon baking powder
¼ teaspoon salt
2 tablespoons powdered nonfat milk
2 tablespoons low-fat soy flour
2 tablespoons chocolate mini chips

PER COOKIE

Calories	53
Carbohydrates	7 g
Fat	2 g
Saturated fat	0.4 g
Dietary fiber	0.5 g
Cholesterol	0 mg
Sodium	54 mg

Carrot-Oatmeal Drop Cookies

When honey is used in cookies, pick a mild honey so the honey flavor is not the only flavor that comes through. In these cookies, the lemon rind flavor is most powerful and the texture of the oats is memorable. I like a blueberry or raspberry honey for use in these cookies.

Preheat oven to 375 F.

In a medium bowl, combine the oil and honey. Beat in the egg substitute. Add the grated carrot and lemon rind.

In a small bowl, combine the flour and baking powder. Add the oats and mix well.

Add the oat mixture to the honey bowl. Mix well. Drop by the rounded tablespoonful onto a nonstick sprayed baking sheet.

Bake for 10 to 12 minutes or until the cookies are slightly browned on the edges.

INGREDIENTS

YIELD: 35 COOKIES

¼ cup canola oil
½ cup mild honey
¼ cup egg substitute
1 cup finely shredded or grated carrot (about 2 carrots)
2 teaspoons grated lemon rind
1 cup whole wheat flour
2 teaspoons baking powder
1 cup rolled oats

PER COOKIE

Calories	54
Carbohydrates	9 g
Fat	2 g
Saturated fat	0.2 g
Dietary fiber	0.8 g
Cholesterol	0 mg
Sodium	33 mg

Cranberry-Chocolate Chip Cookies

With Ground Flaxseed and Soy

These cookies, adapted from a recipe from the Flax Council of Canada, also have ground flax, soy flour, and oatmeal in them! These are powerful cookies. The margarine I used is the Promise stick with no trans fatty acids. I find when I use this margarine in a recipe that I have used before with a regular margarine or butter, I need to add more flour to make the recipe work.

The flax in the recipe was ground in an electric coffee grinder. Flax should be ground as needed. If there is any left over it should be stored in the refrigerator with any whole flaxseed so that the oil does not get rancid. Flaxseed oil oxidizes quickly if not stored properly. Always keep flax refrigerated and always buy from a store that keeps it refrigerated or frozen.

Preheat the oven to 350 F.

Combine the margarine, granulated sugar and brown sugar in a medium bowl and beat together until smooth. Beat in egg substitute and vanilla.

In another bowl, combine the flour, soy flour, oats, flaxseed, salt, baking powder, and baking soda. Add to the sugar mixture. Finally stir in the cranberries and chocolate chips.

Drop by the tablespoon onto an ungreased baking sheet. Bake for 10 minutes.

INGREDIENTS

YIELD: 36 COOKIES

½ cup trans fat–free stick margarine
½ cup granulated sugar
½ cup brown sugar
1 egg substitute
1 teaspoon vanilla
¾ cup unbleached flour
¼ cup soy flour
1 cup oats
¼ cup ground flaxseed
¼ teaspoon salt
½ teaspoon baking powder
½ teaspoon baking soda
½ cup dried cranberries
½ cup chocolate chips

PER COOKIE

Calories	86
Carbohydrates	13 g
Fat	3.6 g
Saturated fat	1 g
Dietary fiber	0.9 g
Cholesterol	0 mg
Sodium	59 mg

The Fruit Basket

A very smart dietitian once told me, "Put fruit in the crisper, and no one will eat it. Put it in a basket on the kitchen counter, and it will disappear overnight."

Hoards of hungry children and their parents have proven her right. And in those homes where fruit is stored seductively in the open, there is far less likely to be heart disease, lung cancer, digestive disease, chronic constipation, and a host of other ills.

A 17-year study of 11,000 men and women in the United Kingdom found, for example, that those who ate fresh fruit on a daily basis cut their risk of heart disease by 24 percent, their risk of stroke by 32 percent, their risk of lung cancer by 41 percent, and their risk of death due to any cause by 21 percent. A recent study from the Harvard School of Public Health in Boston recently questioned how effectively fruit prevented some cancers, but it confirmed the amazing fact that five or more servings a day of fruits (and veggies!) significantly reduced the risk of heart attack and stroke.

Find that hard to believe?

Then take a look at what sits in the fruit basket on my kitchen countertop—and read why it's there.

Apples: Health from the Orchard

One deep breath of the fresh, clean smell of apples inside Vermont's Apple Barn and visions of apples—cobbled, strudeled, sauced, and cidered—danced through my head. I simply breathed in deeply, tugged on my husband's sweater, and pointed toward the hundreds of wooden baskets overflowing with Macouns, McIntoshes, Courtlands, Galas, Northern Spies, and 30 other varieties.

The huge baskets had been stacked on double-sided wooden bleachers that ran down the middle of the barn from one end to the other. Macouns sat next to Mutsu, which sat next to Ida Reds, next to Paula Reds. A bakery selling—what else?—apple pie, apple muffins, apple cookies, apple bread, and even apple cider dough-

---

4

FRUIT BASKET

BEST FOR HELPING YOU:

Cut your risk of diabetes in half

Reduce your risk of a heart attack by 40 percent

Lower cholesterol by 20 percent

Build strong nerves and muscles

Speed "sluggish" digestion

Soothe the symptoms of celiac disease

Quell constipation

Prevent bowel impactions

Keep diverticulitis from acting up

Eliminate hot flashes

Prevent osteoporosis

Lower high blood pressure

---

nuts was strategically situated across from the door at one end, while a cash register surrounded by chrysanthemums stood at the other.

Subconsciously, I knew that the walls were lined with various other Vermont country products—the ubiquitous syrup, common crackers, fresh-roasted coffee, a summer's worth of jams, jellies, and butters—but all my apple-loving eyes saw were the baskets of fragrant fruit piled three tiers deep down the middle of the barn.

My husband just sighed, pulled out his Visa card and followed my fluttering hand.

"These?"

"And these?"

"These too?"

"And these…?"

The Apple Barn has been the last stop on our annual fall foliage pilgrimage through Vermont for the last 20 years. So my husband is well-trained. He knows that until visions of homemade apple sauce, baked apples, fresh apples, dried apples, and apple cobbler have stopped dancing around in my head, there will be no intelligent conversation in our house.

Tucked deep among the rolling green hills just a few miles southwest of Bennington, the Apple Barn contains the roadside market for Southern Vermont Orchards, a 300-acre orchard that was planted in 1912. Originally growing only a half dozen varieties, today the orchard

APPLE BASICS

HOW TO BUY: It takes two pounds of apples to make a nine-inch pie, one pound to make 4 ½ cups of sauce, and at least half a pound to fill one teenager. So whichever kind of apple you buy, buy a lot. Since bruised fruit decays quickly, look for bruise-free apples that are firm to the touch. Also look for freshly picked, organically grown fruit. If you can't find it, at least stay away from the shiny, wax-coated varieties. It's almost impossible to remove that coating, and the various pesticides and other agricultural chemicals that may have been applied to the fruit will be trapped under the coating and impossible for you to scrub off.

HOW TO STORE: Put a couple of apples in the fruit basket on your kitchen counter so they're readily available for healthy snacking. The rest should go into cold storage—either your refrigerator or a cold, preferably humid, cellar. If you store other produce nearby, make sure your apples are stored in a plastic bag. As part of their ripening process, they produce ethylene, a naturally occurring gas that will encourage other nearby fruits and vegetables to ripen as well.

HOW TO USE: Scrub with warm water before eating, cooking, or baking. Peel if the fruit is waxed, then rinse with cold water. The fastest way to slice and core apples is to use an inexpensive "apple slicer" that you can purchase at the supermarket. It's a circular steel device with steel spokes radiating out from a hole at its center. Place it over the top of a freshly scrubbed or peeled apple, push down, and the apple is sliced and cored in one motion. Once you have a bowl of apple wedges, you can eat them as a snack, sprinkle them with cinnamon and walnuts and serve them for dessert, add them to a salad, stir them into a rice pilaf, bake them into a pie (replacing the sugar in your recipe with a half-cup or so of boiled down apple cider), or turn them into sauce.

produces more than 30 different kinds of apples. And it has helped keep one generation after another of Vermonters healthy for more than 80 years.

Apple Barn manager Harry Diamond agrees. "Farming is tough," says the 30-something Vermonter. "I work from 5 A.M. until 11:30 P.M. seven days a week. And I don't know, but I think apples are one of the things that give me enough energy to keep going."

Apples Cut the Risk of Heart Disease and Cancer in Half

With 80 calories, no fat, a smidgen of potassium, and five grams of fiber, apples are, without a doubt, a good source of energy. But researchers have also found that they may prevent both heart disease and cancer as well.

In a study recently presented at the 16th International Congress of Nutrition in Montreal, for example, researchers from Finland's National Public Health Institute in Helsinki and the University of Kuopio reported that the more apples you eat, the less likely you are to develop lung cancer—even if you smoke.

Twenty-five years ago, the researchers asked nearly 10,000 men and women what they ate, then monitored their health for the next quarter century. And what they found was startling: those who ate apples cut their risk of lung cancer in half.

What's more, Belgian studies of 3,669 men and women have demonstrated that apples reduce the risk of colon and rectal cancer anywhere from 30 to 75 percent.

No one knows exactly how many ap-
ples it takes to reduce the risk of cancer or how apples work their anticancer magic. But researchers suspect that it may have something to do with the high flavonoid content of apples.

Flavonoids are strong antioxidants that neutralize cancer-causing molecules generated by anything from outdoor air pollution and cigarette smoke to your body's own metabolic processes. They do so by grabbing on to a free radical—literally a maverick molecule zinging around your body bent on trouble—then escorting it to your body's nearest exit for disposal.

Nabbing those free radicals not only prevents them from initiating a tumor somewhere in the body, it also prevents them from chemically changing the LDL cholesterol in your arteries. And that prevents the chemical process that leads to cholesterol being roughly spackled all over the walls of your coronary arteries—a redecorating job that narrows the arteries and sets the stage for a heart attack.

But flavonoids also do you another favor: they slow the build-up of red blood cells that can clump together and block that narrowed artery—an action that triggers either angina or a heart attack.

APPLES

BEST FOR HELPING YOU:

Lower cholesterol

Prevent heart disease, angina, and heart attacks

Prevent colon, lung, and rectal cancer

Prevent premature death

How Effective Are They?

One clue comes from the Zutphen Elderly Study, a study that looked at what caused chronic disease in a group of 805 Dutch men aged 65 to 84. Twenty years ago, the researchers conducting the study asked participants what they ate and checked the levels of flavonoids in their diet. Then the researchers monitored the men's flavonoid intake and health for the next five years.

They found that the more flavonoids in the diet, the less likely the men were to have the clogged coronary arteries of heart disease—or to have had a heart attack during the study period. In fact, the researchers reported, men who ate the most flavonoids—more than 30 milligrams a day—had about one-third the risk of heart disease as men who ate less.

Even if the men already had a number of risk factors for heart disease, they had far less chance of having a heart attack. And that means that even if they were fat, smoked cigarettes, had high blood pressure, forgot to eat a diet rich in other fruits and vegetables, had a high cholesterol level, drank coffee, and never looked a bowl of high-fiber cereal in the face—it simply didn't matter. Flavonoids made a serious difference in their health.

A second clue as to the effectiveness of both flavonoids and apples comes from another study by Finland's National Public Health Institute and the University of Kuopio. Researchers who conducted that study of more 5,000 men and women between the ages of 30 and 69 found that both flavonoids and apple intake were directly related to the number of deaths due to heart disease. When compared to men who ate the least number of apples, men who ate the most reduced their risk of premature death by 20 percent. Women who ate the most reduced their risk of premature death by 43 percent.

AMERICA'S FAVORITES

Americans love apples. They're harvested from late August through November, although many are stored and sold to us throughout the year. Somehow or another we manage to eat nearly 50 pounds apiece every year, either as fresh fruit out of hand, or as sauce, pies, or cider. And although there are more than 2,500 varieties produced here, 90 percent of the apples we eat are one of the following 15:

RANK	VARIETY	FLAVOR	BEST FOR...
1	Red Delicious	Sweet	Snacking
2	Golden Delicious	Sweet	Pie
3	Granny Smith	Tart	Snacking
4	Rome	Slightly sweet	Pie
5	Fuji	Sweet & spicy	Snacking
6	McIntosh	Sweet/tart	Sauce
7	Gala	Sweet	Snacking
8	Jonathan	Tart	Snacking
9	Empire	Sweet/tart	Snacking
10	York	Moderately tart	Snacking
11	Ida Red	Moderately tart	Snacking
12	Newtown Pippin	Slightly tart	Snacking
13	Cortland	Slightly tart	Snacking
14	R. I. Greening	Tart	Snacking
15	Northern Spy	Slightly tart	Pie

Which Apple Is Best?

In every study that demonstrates the connection between health and flavonoids, apples have been a key source of flavonoid content, particularly the flavonoid quercetin. In a recent study at Cornell University in New York, for example, lab animals fed apple-derived quercetin showed significantly less Alzheimer's-type brain damage as they aged than did animals who were not fed apples.

Unfortunately, no one yet knows which apples contain the most flavonoids in general or quercetin in particular—although apple industry representatives agree that it's a safe assumption that, in this case at least, there's no such thing as a bad apple.

So until research can give us a more definitive guideline, it's probably just as well to let your taste buds do the apple picking. Which apple do most of us choose?

The number one pick of Americans is the Red Delicious apple, reports the U.S. Apple Association in McLean, Virginia (see "America's Favorites"). Unfortunately, however, although the Red Delicious is a great snacking apple to leave in a bowl on the kitchen table, it's not a good apple for sauce or baking. It just kind of dries up and dies.

That's why I asked Apple Barn manger Harry Diamond, who has probably sampled more apples than I'll ever see in a lifetime, which apple is best for baking and sauce.

For baking, he likes the Northern Spy, a slightly tart apple that holds its shape through the baking process. As for sauce, "It all depends on where you were raised and what you're used to," says Diamond. "I grew up in the suburbs and ate Mott's. So I like a smooth creamy texture and a sweet/tart taste.

"When my wife and I first came here, we wanted to try every variety. So we picked one variety and made sauce, then picked another and made more. After a while, we just kept picking, making, and eating, and I didn't notice which apples we were using. Then one day she put some applesauce down in front of me and I said, 'Wow! What kind was that?'"

He chuckles. "It was made from a McIntosh—the most common apple in Vermont."

Naturally, I decided to put Harry's fa-

CHUG THAT CIDER!

A recent study at the French National Institute for Health and Medical Research reveals that apple peels are loaded with procyanidins, powerful antioxidants that impede cancer growth. What's more, in a subsequent study, researchers found that laboratory animals fed a mixture of water and apple had half the risk of developing colon cancer after being exposed to cancer-causing agents that normally would trigger the disease.

The best source of apple skins? Apple cider, suggested French researchers. Unlike other apple products, the whole apple—in fact, many whole apples—is used in its making.

Just don't forget to buy the organic kind. There's no point in eating something to prevent cancer and then buying the kind that might be contaminated with cancer-causing agrichemicals.

vorite to the test. So once back home, I took a few of the Apple Barn's McIntoshes, peeled, cored, and chopped until I had a bowlful of little apple bits. Then I added a splash of apple cider for sweetening and a (big) pinch of cinnamon, just as my friend Anita had taught me. (See Anita's recipe at the end of this chapter.) Unfortunately, I kept eating as I peeled, so preparing the apples took a lot longer than the 10 minutes she'd assured me it should. And, of course, I had to peel a little extra for the dogs—all three surrounded my legs as I worked and kept nudging me with their muzzles until they'd each gotten a few sweet spoonsful of mashed apples on which to nibble. (And, yes, vets approve of mashed apple for dogs—just not big chunks.)

Once everyone was satisfied and I'd washed my hands for the third time, I covered the sauce, shoved it into the microwave, and nuked it on high for three minutes. I stirred it once, re-covered it, nuked it for another three minutes, and it was ready for the table.

The result?

By the blissful look on my husband's face, I doubt he'll ever put canned applesauce on the grocery list again.

Bananas:
Band-Aids for a Bad Stomach

If my 87-year-old Aunt Gladys is any judge, bananas are God's gift to those who've been blessed with delicate stom-

achs, because on those days when everything else makes her throw up, she can eat bananas.

Studies say that my aunt's stomach is not alone in its appreciation of the banana's soothing properties. Not only do bananas coat the stomach's lining and protect it from various acidic insults—that extra-spicy salsa you ate just before bed, or even the aspirin you swallowed a few moments ago—they also seem to help lower blood pressure, inhibit the bacteria that cause chronic stomachaches and ulcers, protect against stroke, and even help prevent lung cancer.

In a study at the University of New South Wales in Australia, for example, researchers found that eating ripe bananas—so ripe that they're covered with tiny brown spots—apparently protects the stomach in two ways: It reduces the body's secretion of stomach acid and produces a substance that reinforces the stomach's lining so strongly that ulcer-causing bacteria can't penetrate. Normally, the bacteria bore their way through the stomach's protective lining and sets up housekeeping in the stomach wall. The banana somehow armor-plates that lining, and the bacteria—which are present in a large number of people—are unable to muscle their way through.

Researchers have found that bananas help the digestive tract a little lower down, as well: well-ripened bananas can frequently stop diarrhea in its tracks, while less ripe bananas—the ones with

BANANAS
BEST FOR HELPING YOU:
Soothe chronic stomachaches
Kill the bacteria that cause stomach ulcers
Prevent stroke
Lower blood pressure
Prevent lung cancer
Loosen up constipation
Slow diarrhea
Calm anxiety
Beat insomnia

the green tips—can frequently stop constipation. The carbohydrate content of unripened bananas is just different enough from that of ripened bananas to get your bowels moving when things seem to be stalled.

Bananas can also help you fight off more serious conditions. Researchers at the Regional Cancer Centre in Kerala, South India, have discovered that people who eat bananas regularly have significantly less lung cancer than those who don't. And in a study at the University of Naples in Italy, researchers found that adding four or five servings of a potassium-rich food such as bananas to the diet meant that most people could cut the amount of blood pressure medication they took in half.

And if that's not enough to put bananas in your fruit basket, a study of 859 men and women at the University of California at San Diego found that those who added a single serving of a potassium-rich food such as bananas to their diet lowered their risk of stroke by 40 percent!

Take Two Bananas and Call Me in the Morning

Although researchers know that bananas are a good source of potassium, fiber, and vitamin B6, they're just beginning to figure out all the things in bananas that make them such a healthy food.

One component some researchers are paying extra attention to, for instance, is the banana's carbohydrate content. That's because carbohydrate—what your mother might have called "starch"—has an indirect but significant effect on the brain. It's a major source of tryptophan, an amino acid that your brain uses to produce serotonin—a naturally occurring brain chemical that affects mood, appetite, learning, and memory.

Decrease the amount of serotonin that's available to your brain and you'll become cranky, irritable, hungry, and unable to concentrate long enough to learn—or remember what you've learned. Increase the amount of serotonin that's available and you'll become calm, sedate, satiated, and able to learn anything you please. It can also make you feel drowsy—which is why a carbohydrate-rich bedtime snack frequently seems to help you sleep.

BANANA BASICS

HOW TO BUY: Look for yellow bananas with a trace of green. Avoid bananas with split tops, blackened areas, or even brown freckles.

HOW TO SORE: On your kitchen countertop. At room temperature, they'll continue ripening. Brown spots are your signal that bananas are ripe.

HOW TO USE: Peel and eat. Bananas are the original convenience food—and with biodegradable packaging to boot. Eat those with a tinge of green to prevent or alleviate minor constipation; eat the ones with brown spots to boost serotonin and to prevent ulcers and other digestive problems. Use the over-ripe ones that have turned black to add flavor and moistness to baked goods. Squeeze the contents into a heavy-duty storage bag or plastic container and toss it into your freezer. It'll make the best banana bread you've ever eaten.

It doesn't take much carbohydrate to increase serotonin, either. Researchers say one or two ripe bananas eaten by themselves can do the trick.

The key phrase here is "eaten by themselves." Unfortunately, if you eat bananas with other foods, particularly a protein-loaded food like milk, turkey, or cheese, your brain will preferentially select chemicals produced by the protein to make you more alert. But if you eat the bananas by themselves, your brain will select chemicals produced by the banana's carbohydrate component and flood your circuits with sleep-inducing serotonin.

Grapes: Nature's Most Powerful Antioxidant?

University of Illinois researcher John Pezzuto fiddles with the mike attached to his lapel, shuffles a few papers on the lectern in front of him, and glances at the small group of elite scientists from around the country who have come to a small conference center just north of Chicago to pick his inventive brain.

A tall man who always manages to look a little rumpled, Dr. Pezzuto begins to explain just how it was that, while the rest of us were using grapes to garnish a fresh fruit platter or add a burst of flavor to a Waldorf salad, he and his research group were systematically taking the grapes apart, examining their molecular structure, and discovering that they contained resveratrol, a naturally occurring substance that may turn out to be the

most powerful antioxidant on the planet.

In laboratory tests of more than 6,700 substances, Dr. Pezzuto and his crew found that resveratrol, found predominantly in the skins and seeds of grapes, is one of only a handful of substances that naturally block cancer at all three stages of its development—when it invades, when it grows, and when it spreads.

Resveratrol actually detoxifies cancer-causing agents by stimulating your body's natural defense systems—specifically its phase II enzymes—to neutralize the agents before they can damage any cells, says Dr. Pezzuto, who is director of collaborative research in the pharmaceutical sciences at the University of Illinois. And if any of those agents manage to get by, the resveratrol circulating in your body after the cancer invaded can still eliminate the cancer by tossing a molecular monkey wrench into the chemical process by which tumors grow and spread.

In fact, when Dr. Pezzuto and his team exposed laboratory mice to a substance that frequently causes cancer, they found that mice that had adequate amounts of resveratrol were less than half as likely to develop any tumors. And those that did develop tumors had two-thirds fewer than mice that lacked resveratrol's protection.

GRAPES

BEST FOR HELPING YOU:

Prevent arthritis

Maintain a healthy weight

Prevent diabetes

Control blood pressure

Prevent heart disease

Maintain a healthy cholesterol level

Prevent heart attacks

Stop the initiation, development, and spread of cancer

Grape Protection

In addition to its amazing ability to prevent cancer from getting a foothold, resveratrol has two other significant characteristics: One, it can inhibit the tendency of red blood cells to clump together and form the kind of artery-blocking blood clot that can lead to a heart attack; and, two, it can cause the heart's arteries to relax even when you're under stress—a protective safeguard that may allow existing clots to pass through your heart without blocking an artery and shutting down your whole cardiovascular system.

This effect is so pronounced, in fact, that some researchers suspect it's responsible for what has come to be called the "French Paradox"—the ability of many who live in France to consume huge amounts of fat and still have relatively little heart disease. Since many of these same people also regularly consume red wine, say researchers, the wine's resveratrol may be preventing the heart attacks that would naturally follow from such a high-fat lifestyle.

Dr. Pezzuto's not so sure. There are other heart-healthy components of red wine that may be contributing to its effects on your health, he points out, although it certainly has a substantial amount of resveratrol.

Researchers are still debating exactly how much resveratrol it takes to produce a therapeutic effect. A study at the University of Wisconsin found that people who drank a five-ounce glass of purple grape juice twice a day reduced their tendency to form artery-clogging blood clots by 60 percent. So that gives us a clue.

To prevent cancer, however, you may need to eat or drink a hundred times that amount, says Dr. Pezzuto. "But keep in mind that there's a dose-response relationship between resveratrol and cancer," he adds. So no matter how many grapes or glasses of grape juice you're drinking, each one is still a bullet fired at cancer.

GRAPES BASICS

HOW TO BUY: Red grapes have far more resveratrol than white, says Dr. Pezzuto. Look for plump red grapes that are firmly attached to flexible stems. Fresh grapes will still have a white, powdery "bloom," and the grapes themselves should be firm, but not hard. Avoid soft grapes and grapes that have a whitened-out area around the stem.

You should also avoid giant pyramids of grapes stacked in markets. Grapes are too thin-skinned for this kind of treatment, experts say. Instead, look for grapes that are stacked no more than two bunches deep.

Fortunately, various varieties are available pretty much year round from California and Arizona.

HOW TO STORE: On the kitchen counter where they'll be eaten quickly. If any are left over after a day or two, move them to the refrigerator and put them on that night's dessert menu.

HOW TO USE: Nibble on them for snacks, or cut them in half and toss a bunch into yogurt or a fresh fruit salad. One caveat: Do not give to children under the age of two. They can choke on small foods.

Peaches: The Super Source of an Anti-Aging Nutrient

It's a good thing peaches ripen during the warmer months, because the only way to eat a ripe peach is outdoors, wearing minimal clothes, beside a large body of water.

Especially if you have kids. Then nobody minds the sweet, sticky juice of a truly ripe peach dripping off chins, cheeks, and hands. You just eat the peach, fling the pit, and dunk as much of yourself as needed.

But eating peaches is much more than fun in the sun—it also appears to be a sweet-tasting way to keep your body young and healthy. That's because peaches contain a hefty dose of glutathione, a powerful antioxidant that sinks its teeth into deranged molecules generated by cigarette smoke, stress, air pollution, sunlight, and other substances that can damage DNA, the body's cellular blueprint. And once damaged, your DNA can trigger many of the diseases we associate with aging: heart disease, high blood pressure, Alzheimer's, and cancer.

No one knows how well glutathione protects DNA. But a study at the University of Michigan indicates that it may be pretty powerful stuff. The Michigan researchers checked blood levels of glutathione in 33 people over the age of 60, then compared those levels to the number of health problems reported by study participants. They found that the more glutathione people had, the fewer health prob-

---

PEACHES

BEST FOR HELPING YOU:

Prevent Alzheimer's

Prevent arthritis

Prevent diabetes

Prevent heart disease

Prevent high blood pressure

PEACH BASICS

HOW TO BUY: Use your nose. Sniff out yellow or cream-colored peaches that smell as though you're standing in an orchard full of peach blossoms. Ripe or just-about-ripe peaches will also feel slightly soft.

Avoid peaches that are hard or have a tinge of green. Both are indications that the fruit was picked too early and will never reach peak sweetness.

You should also try to buy your peaches from a local orchard that still grows old varieties such as the fragrant white peach. Many of the newer varieties have been bred for a longer shelf life in the supermarket, and they just don't have that great peach taste.

HOW TO STORE: On your kitchen counter. Although peaches do not get any sweeter once they've left the tree, they will soften a bit more if left at room temperature. If, by some miracle, they are not grabbed out of your fruit basket within a day or two, move them to the fridge. The cold will hold them at that level of ripeness for a couple of more days.

HOW TO USE: Morning, noon, and night. Try them sliced over cereal, whole in your lunch bag, halved on the grill, quartered in a mulled wine, puréed over poultry, chopped into a salad, topped with vanilla yogurt, layered in a pie, or baked in a cobbler.

---

lems they reported. Conversely, they also found that the less glutathione people had, the more likely they were to report arthritis, diabetes, and heart disease.

The researchers don't know what's going on yet, although they did note that study participants with plenty of glutathione on guard in their bodies had lower blood pressure, lower cholesterol, and a healthier weight than those who didn't—and that alone is reason enough to keep these fragrant fruits around all summer long.

Pears: A Practically Perfect Source of Fiber

Pears are an endangered species in my house—whenever one reaches peak ripeness in the fruit basket on my counter, it always disappears. The problem is so pervasive that I actually didn't eat one fresh pear last year. I'd buy a couple from my local farmers market, stick them in the basket to ripen, and—hello?—where'd they go?

I guess I should be content since that meant the rest of my family was getting a good shot of fiber—nearly five grams per pear, or about one-seventh the amount researchers say we need every day to help prevent colon cancer, constipation, diabetes, heart disease, and high cholesterol.

Pears help protect against a particularly broad range of diseases because they contain several different types of fiber. Their insoluble fiber is the kind that scrubs down the intestines, mops up potentially carcinogenic bile acids generated by your own body, and traps other cancer-causing agents as well. It also relieves constipation and prevents hemorrhoids.

The lignin and pectin fiber in pears sops up cholesterol, thus lowering cholesterol levels and helping prevent heart disease. In fact, pears, which contain roughly 700 milligrams of pectin, are a great source of this particular fiber.

Pears are also a low-calorie source of boron, a mineral that researchers suspect is important in promoting bone health and mental agility. The nutrient apparently keeps bones strong by preventing the loss of calcium and potassium—a necessity for those at risk of osteoporosis. Equally important, a study by researchers at the U.S. Department of Agriculture indicates that increasing boron in the diet increases mental alertness.

That's not, of course, why my family eats them. They eat them because of their meltingly sweet taste.

And I would, too, if they'd let me.

PEARS
BEST FOR HELPING YOU:
Prevent colon cancer
Prevent or relieve constipation
Prevent diabetes
Lower high cholesterol
Prevent heart disease
Strengthen bones

Tropical Fruit: The Most Nutritious Fruit on the Planet

Just the sight of a peachy-melony mango, a pile of earthy brown kiwi, a juicy papaya, or a bright yellow guava sitting on my kitchen counter is enough to kick my immune system into high gear. And not just because of the hard-wiring between mind and body that influences health.

No, the main reason is that each and every bite of any of these fruits will significantly reduce my chances of both heart disease and cancer.

Take kiwi, for instance. According to Paul LaChance, Ph.D., director of the Neutraceuticals Institute at Rutgers University in New Jersey and a pioneer in food science, kiwi is the most nutritious fruit you can buy.

Dr. LaChance looked at the nutrient density of 27 of the most popular fruits sold in the United States and compared it to that of the kiwi. Then, since obesity is a health problem that affects more than 40 percent of those of us over age 30, Dr. LaChance factored in the number of calories each fruit contained, the number of calories each fruit used as it moved through the digestive system, plugged all the data into his computer, and came up with a list of the most nutritious fruit on the planet.

Heading the list was that plain, brown, hairy little fruit we call the kiwi.

Kiwi gives us the most nutrients for the least calories of any fruit we can buy, says Dr. LaChance. It contains twice the vitamin C of an orange, plus a wide range of phytochemicals that boost your body's ability to neutralize cancer-causing agents. Those phytochemicals—lutein, ellagic acid, flavonoids, and anthocyanins—are all powerful antioxidants with the ability to prevent cancer from taking hold. And three of them—lutein, flavonoids, and anthocyanins—also help maintain the strong veins and capillaries necessary for a healthy cardiovascular system.

PEAR BASICS

HOW TO BUY: Look for pears that are hard and green. Pears don't ripen on the tree, they ripen after they're picked. So a freshly picked pear is one that's as hard as a rock and as green as the day it was born.

Bartlett pears reach market in July, and the "ABCs"—Anjou, Bosc, and Comice—arrive in October. I generally look for the Comice. It's the sweetest pear available. You may have to look for it in farmers markets and gourmet shops rather than your supermarket, however, because much of the crop is snapped up for use in fancy gift baskets.

If the only pear you're used to looking for is the Bartlett with its space-capsule shape, you may not recognize the Comice when it appears. It has a squat shape and dull green skin that will yellow and take on a very light blush as it ripens.

Don't worry about marks on the skin—they don't affect taste or nutrition.

HOW TO STORE: On your kitchen counter. As the pears ripen, their starch will convert to sugar. So the more time they spend at room temperature, the sweeter and softer they'll be. If they're not snapped up at peak ripeness, however, move them to the fridge. They'll stay at peak flavor for at least another day, maybe two.

NEVER seal pears in a plastic bag. They need to breathe just like you. And if you interfere with their respiration, they'll reward you by turning brown at the core.

HOW TO USE: Unless you've managed to find organically grown pears, peel the skin before you eat. Yes, the skin contains a small amount of vitamin C, but not enough for you to consider them a good source.

I personally have never been able to resist eating a pear out of my hand long enough to use it any other way. Rumor has it, however, that sautéed in fruit juice and sprinkled with cinnamon, nutmeg, and cloves, pears make a hauntingly delicious side dish or desert. And my friend Denise loves to use them in fruit bread.

To reduce your risk of heart disease even further, kiwi also contains arginine, an amino acid that may widen arteries as it prevents cholesterol and other arterial debris from clogging them. Plus it contains a trace of inositol, a naturally occurring sugar that may help correct some of the chemical imbalance that occurs in depression and help in stabilizing diabetes.

What's more, kiwi also contains a small amount of both potassium and magnesium to help keep your blood pressure on an even keel; no fat; few calories; and 2.6 grams of fiber to help control cholesterol.

Triple Vitamin C Protection

Right behind kiwi on Dr. LaChance's "most nutritious" list is papaya, a sweet fruit with triple the RDA of vitamin C in just half a single fruit. It also has 2.6 grams of fiber, no fat, few calories and a smidgen of potassium and heart-healthy folate.

Fifth on Dr. LaChance's list are mangoes, a fragrant fruit that has taken the United States by storm. Widely consumed throughout the world, mangoes were hard to find in U.S. supermarkets until about five years ago. Since then, American consumption of the mango has quadrupled, and the fruit has become a common sight in local supermarkets. Containing a small amount of beta carotene and cryptoxanthin to keep your heart strong, mangoes also contain half a day's supply of the RDA for vitamin C, plus a small amount of vitamins A, E, and B6. They have no fat, few calories, and 2.1 grams of fiber.

TROPICAL FRUIT

BEST FOR HELPING YOU:

Build strong veins and capillaries

Stabilize diabetes

Fight depression

Reduce heart disease

Prevent cancer

Lower cholesterol

Lower blood pressure

Guava do not appear on Dr. LaChance's list, but they frequently appear on my kitchen counter. Guava contain nearly three times the RDA for vitamin C in a single serving, plus a small amount of potassium, vitamin A, vitamin B6, and niacin. They also contain a hefty 4.9 grams of colon-scrubbing fiber.

All these nutrients combine to help my family fight colon cancer, high cholesterol, high blood pressure, and heart disease. In a study at the Heart Research Laboratory in India, researchers found that people with high blood pressure who ate 16 ounces of guava a day for 12 weeks significantly lowered their risk of heart disease. Their cholesterol dropped 27 points, their triglyceride levels fell by nearly 9 percent, and their blood pressure plummeted 11 to 13 points.

That's not bad for a little yellow ball. You may not want to add an entire pound to your diet every day, but every ounce you toss on your cereal, in your yogurt, or over a salad will load the health scales in your favor.

The Healthy Hibachi

Maybe I spent too many years in California as a child, but nothing makes me happier than barbecuing chicken on a tabletop hibachi while the hot summer sun slowly melts into a fiery horizon. Put a barbecue fork in my right hand and a glass of raspberry iced tea in the other, and I'm a complete woman.

But in recent years my enjoyment has been tainted by concerns about the

HOW TO BUY: Kiwi, papaya, mangoes, and guava should all have a sweet, delicate scent and yield slightly to gentle pressure from your fingers.

Kiwi, which is grown in California from November through May and in New Zealand from June through October, should look fuzzy and plump.

Papayas, which are picked all year round, should be at least one-half to two-thirds yellow or yellow-orange.

Mangoes, which are available from Florida between May and August, should have a red or orange-yellow blush.

Guava, available from Florida and California between September and January, should also carry a bright yellow blush.

Actually, the more color in the skins of papayas, mangoes, and guava, the riper the fruit.

HOW TO STORE: On the kitchen counter. Most tropical fruits have been transported from their native habitats at cool temperatures. Assuming that you know your market's produce delivery schedule and were able to buy them the same day they were put on the shelf, it will take several days for your fruit to fully ripen at room temperature. So leave them out where their exotic shapes and textures will catch your eye and turn on your taste buds as the fruit reaches peak ripeness.

Should the fruit happen to ripen faster than you can eat it—a rare occurrence in most homes—either toss it into the blender and make your family a tropical fruit shake or slice it into a tongue-tingling fresh fruit salad.

If you really want to hold tropical fruit for a few more days, just pop each fruit into an individual plastic storage bag and store them in the refrigerator. Most varieties will last at least a few days longer, although their flavor may not be as intense.

HOW TO USE: Kiwi, believe it or not, can be eaten with the skin. And since that's the more nutritious way, that's what Dr. LaChance suggests. Just de-fuzz the kiwi by gently scraping it with a vegetable peeler. Then wash the plump brown fruit and slice. Its jade-green flesh and circular seed accents make it an attractive topping for high-nutrient, low-fat fruit "pizzas"—giant cookies baked in a 10-inch round pizza pan and topped with a smear of low-fat vanilla pudding and a heap of fresh fruit.

Mangoes are just as versatile—once you get rid of the thick pit and tough skin. The easiest way seems to be the slash-'n'-peel method: Hold the mango in one hand while you take a fruit knife in the other and carefully score the mango with four vertical slashes. Peel the skin off each quarter, cut through the fruit along each slash line, then insert your knife under the fruit and work it free from the pit beneath. It takes a tad more work than I usually have time for, but the mango's incredible vitamin A content and sweet flavor make it a welcome weekend topping for Sunday morning waffles.

Papaya and guava are even easier. You can remove the guava seeds if you like, but otherwise just slice and eat—or chop and add to the mangoes on top of your waffles.

healthfulness of eating food that's been exposed to smoke. The problem is that smoke causes the formation of nitrates on whatever you're grilling. And nitrates, when ingested, turn into chemicals that can cause stomach cancer. It may not happen every time, but it happens often enough that barbecuing had become a once-in-a-while treat.

But my time at the grill may be increasing because researchers have found that kiwi can block the process that turns nitrates into deadly chemicals. Two studies conducted in China, one in conjunction with the Massachusetts Institute of Technology in the United States and the other with Wexham Park Hospital in the United Kingdom, have found that the ascorbic acid and a powerful nitrite-scavenging compound—3-hydroxy-2-pyranone—in kiwi prevent the formation of 96 to 98 percent of the cancer-causing agents triggered by combining nitrates and smoke.

So how can you use kiwi at your next barbecue?

One way is to use puréed kiwi as a marinade. Loosely based on a recipe by Tim Hartog at Elroy's Restaurant in San Francisco, this is what works for me:

Defuzz three or four kiwi by scraping them lightly with a vegetable peeler, slice them into a blender, add whatever spices you like—a tablespoon each of ginger and chopped garlic with a splash of soy sauce is good—plus a quarter cup of olive oil. Purée, then pour into a rectangular baking dish and add however many pieces of chicken you need. Marinate in the refrigerator for 30 minutes, turning the chicken once. Then toss the chicken on your grill and trash any leftover marinade.

When grilled to your satisfaction, serve the chicken on a bed of rice—topped with a jumble of fresh-cut kiwi.

The Breadbox

The late October sun had finally swept the surrounding hills free of frost when Betty and T. Lyle Ferderber, along with their Labrador, Jetta, led me up the dirt road toward their mill.

We had just finished a lunch of Betty's homemade onion soup, fresh-picked greens, Amish cheese, and stone-ground bread at the Ferderbers' 200-year-old farmhouse, a busy home full of muddy sneakers, active kids, sweet-faced dogs, and working cats.

Nestled in the foothills of the Allegheny Mountains, not 25 miles north of Pittsburgh, the farmhouse is at the center of an 80-acre organic farm that is planted with soft wheat, corn, oats, and hay. Most of the oats and hay go to horses the Ferderbers board in their barn. But the wheat and corn—plus whole truckloads of organically grown blue corn from Nebraska, hard wheat from North Dakota, and buckwheat, soy, and rye from neighboring farms—are ground at the mill, then sold through the family store up the road.

"T," as family and friends call the 40-year-old organic farmer and miller, is passionate about what he does. As we walk toward the mill, he talks intensely about the nature and character of soil, the morality of giving back to the land that sustains his family, and the responsibility of feeding thousands of people who depend on him for flours that will provide the energy and substance of their lives. It's a lot to grasp in a single conversation. But as I look out over the fields around me and listen to T, I begin to understand how what he does affects the nutritional quality of what I put in my breadbox.

5

BREADBOX

BEST FOR HELPING YOU:

Prevent cancer

Prevent diabetes

Prevent heart disease

The Whole Grain Pharmacy

I came to the Ferderbers' farm because one study after another has found that the more fiber-rich whole grain foods we eat, the less likely we are to get heart disease, diabetes, or cancer.

A study of nearly 22,000 Finnish men found, for example, that those who ate little more than 10 grams of whole grain fiber a day—most of it from three slices a day of whole grain rye bread—had reduced their risk of death from heart disease by 17 percent. Those who ate 35 grams reduced their risk by nearly one-third.

Another study, this one of about 65,000 nurses in the United States, found that those who ate the most fiber-rich whole grains had less than half the risk of developing diabetes as those who ate the least.

And when 15 studies were recently analyzed by researchers at the University of

Minnesota, the researchers found that the more gut-scrubbing whole grains study participants ate, the less likely they were to get stomach, colon, or rectal cancer.

I don't need to be hit over the head to get the message, especially not when researchers are also telling us just what health-building nutrients whole grains contain: a whole slew of vitamins and minerals—vitamin E, zinc, selenium, magnesium, manganese, iron, and copper—that help nerves and muscles function even as they protect cells from damaging free radicals that age the body and trigger disease.

But emerging technology is also giving researchers a glimpse into a whole new world of substances that may prove even more potent: the phytochemicals. In particular, researchers have found that whole grains contain caffeic acid, ferulic acid, flavonoids, lignins, phytic acid, saponins, and tocotrienols.

Most of these naturally occurring chemicals seem to act as powerful antioxidants that block one phase or another of a disease.

Tocotrienols, for instance, are potent antioxidants that help prevent dietary cholesterol from changing into a form that will attach itself to artery walls. Some researchers even think tocotrienols are 50 percent more powerful than vitamin E.

Saponins grab hold of cholesterol that's roaming your arteries and toss it to the liver for disposal—then may even turn around and increase the number of infection- and cancer-fighting natural killer cells available to your immune system. Lignins prevent cancer from spreading. And some flavonoids in whole grains prevent red blood cells from sticking together and blocking an

---

BREAD BASICS

HOW TO BUY: Buy only freshly milled, whole grain flours. Stone-ground flour is the best because all three nutrient-dense layers of the grain are ground into the flour at once. Their exposure to nutrient-robbing heat generated by the grinding is minimal. Other whole grain flours are usually made by putting the grain through a series of heat-generating rollers and sifters which split the grain into its component parts. The components are brought back together just before the flour is bagged so that they can be labeled "whole wheat."

Some experts don't seem to see much difference between the two methods, but others feel that less processing makes it more likely that the grain's nutrients will retain their heath-promoting abilities. And no one has any idea how either process affects the grain's phytochemicals. At this point, most phytochemicals seem to be heat stable.

HOW TO STORE: Because whole grains contain vitamin E and other healthy oils, whole grain flours can go rancid if left in a warm place. So store them in a cool cupboard or pantry if you're planning on using them within a month. If you need to keep them longer, store them in a tightly sealed container in the freezer.

HOW TO USE: Mix and match. Each whole grain flour produces a distinctly flavored bread, but the flavor can be significantly altered by mixing one flour with another. Cornmeal, rye, and wheat can produce a sophisticated brown bread that will stand up well to a plate of spicy baked beans, while barley and wheat can create a lightly nuanced loaf that serves as a delicate backdrop for a low-fat cheese.

artery, while others trigger the body's natural cancer-fighting enzymes.

That's a pretty powerful pharmacy contained in just one slice of bread. Unfortunately, there are a lot of manufacturers turning out flours, breads, and other grain products that may not deliver these health benefits. They strip the grain of its most nutrient-dense elements to extend its shelf life, then label their products in such a way as to mislead us into thinking we're getting one thing when we're getting another. The problem is so pervasive, it's a national scandal.

A perfect example is whole wheat bread. Walk down the bread aisle at your local supermarket and you'll find "wheat" bread, "cracked wheat" bread, "made with whole wheat" bread, "stoned wheat" bread, "wheatberry" bread, "multigrain" bread, and "12- 9- or 7-grain" bread, among others. None of these are probably the real thing. Only the breads labeled "whole grain" or "whole wheat" will—by law—give you the entire package of vitamins, minerals, fiber, antioxidants, and other phytochemicals that you expect in the bread you buy.

The other "wheat" breads are more than likely made from refined grains with a dash of cheap wood or vegetable fiber instead. And because they're so unhealthful, federal standards require that manufacturers "enrich" their products with a handful of synthetic vitamins. Unfortunately, there is as yet no provision for restoring vitamin E or those powerful phytochemicals that keep heart disease and cancer out of your life.

A Lesson from the Mill

To understand how whole grain breads can help you prevent disease—and why most of the bread at your supermarket just doesn't do it—take a look at the grain's anatomy, then visit a miller like T.

Structurally, all grains are pretty much alike. A single wheat grain is simply a seed that has four layers—a hard outer husk, an inner covering of bran, a core called the endosperm, and a tiny embryo called the germ.

The germ makes up only 3 percent of the seed, yet it's the most concentrated source of nutrients in the grain. It contains iron, magnesium, polyunsaturated fats, potassium, protein, zinc, vitamin E, and the B vitamins folate, thiamin, riboflavin, and pyridoxine. The bran, which accounts for about 15 percent of the seed, contains copper, manganese, and selenium, all of which are components of antioxidant enzymes that boost your body's defenses against cancer and heart disease—plus 75 percent of the grain's fiber. The endosperm, which represents roughly 80 percent of the seed, contains a tiny amount of protein, a large amount of starch, and about 25 percent of the grain's fiber.

What happens to these layers during milling?

That's what I had come to find out. So while Jetta the dog waits patiently outside with Fester, the mill's highly skilled rodent patrol, Betty and T escort me inside the mill.

The mill feels cool after we've walked through the bright autumn sun. It's divided into two huge two-story rooms scented with the light, sweet smell of freshly milled grain. All around the entry, sacks of organic grains are stacked shoulder-high on wooden pallets waiting to be milled, while over on a table by a window, sacks of flour are being measured into coarse brown paper bags.

I walk across the flour-silted floor to meet Brian, who is carefully scooping freshly milled flour into a bag, and Eric, who is actually doing today's milling. Tall, wearing white coveralls and coated with a fine white mist of flour that turns his short brown beard and smiling face a frosty white, Eric is running the modern equivalent of the grist mill: a surprisingly small machine that grinds the organically grown grain into flour.

Encased in a steel housing no higher than my hips, one stone about the size of a large bicycle wheel endlessly turns, slowly grinding the grain Eric has loaded into the hopper against a second, fixed stone. Once the bran, germ, and endosperm are crushed into flour, a fan beside the stones pulls the fresh flour out of the grinding chamber, keeping it cool and preserving the flour's valuable nutrients, then drops it into a heavy-duty brown bag that Eric has tied to one end.

When it's full, the bag is passed over to Brian in the next room, who will weigh it, saddle-stitch it across the top, then label and date it. This is the method that produces stone-ground whole grain flour.

Now compare this to high-tech milling in which grain is put through 14 sets of high-speed steel rollers and an increasingly finer meshed series of sifters. The process, including the heat it generates, causes the grain to split into its component parts. Hull, bran, and germ are then sifted out of the flour. The manufacturer can sell the bran and germ separately—and charge you a pretty penny for it to boot—and at the same time extend the shelf-life of the flour. The remaining flour—basically the endosperm—has lost 75 percent of its fiber and 80 percent of its vitamins and minerals.

That's what we eat when we buy a loaf of "white," "wheat," or "oat" bread.

Unfortunately, on any given day, this is exactly what 61 percent of us do. Some of us are confused by the misleading la-

THE GRANARY

Whole grain breads and flours are available from most supermarkets and health-food stores. Not all are stone-ground, however, and even fewer are ground from organically grown grains. If you prefer to use flours that are both, here are three suppliers who will ship their flours directly to your door:

Arrowhead Mills
Box 2059, Hereford, TX 79045
806-364-0730

T. Lyle Ferderber
Frankferd Farms Foods
717 Saxonburg Blvd., Saxonburg, PA 16056
412-352-9500

Wysong Organic Foods
1880 N. Eastman, Midland, MI 48640
800-748-0233

bels, while others don't like to pay the extra dime or quarter a loaf of whole grain bread will usually cost. Still others simply prefer the airy, lightweight bread that refined grains produce. And there are at least a few of us who just don't see what all the fuss is about. They'll pick up whatever's on sale.

Well, I like a good sale, too. But not when it's my health that will ultimately pay the price. So either my husband picks up a loaf of whole wheat bread when he does the food shopping—or I bake.

Bake Your Own Healthy Loaf

Although I once kneaded, turned, prodded, patted, and punched down dough in the centuries-old way of nurturing women, there's no way today that you or I can spend half a day wrestling with a loaf of bread. But with breadmaking machines flooding the market at increasingly reasonable prices, there's no reason why we have to.

Simply buy the machine, dump in a cup or so of warm water, measure in about three cups of flour, add a dash of salt, a pinch of yeast, and a splash of oil. That's it. The breadmaker mixes, kneads, punches, shapes, and bakes the bread. And if you were smart enough to get a bread machine with a timer, you can punch a few buttons, go to bed, and wake up to the heavenly smell of freshly baked bread.

Making your own bread gives you all kinds of nutritional options. If someone in your family is prone to heart disease, for example, you can turn out loaf after loaf of whole grain rye bread that's similar to the rye bread used in the Finnish heart study. It's impossible to find in a store, so making it yourself is the only way you can get it.

Other health problems can also be prevented, managed, or solved by regularly serving whole grain bread. If someone in your family has diverticulitis—a thinning and pouching of the bowel wall that affects some 40 percent of our older folks—you can bake up a loaf of whole wheat bread to kind of ease things through the gut. And if anybody's got chronic constipation, regular servings of barley bread will help them get things moving.

To help you decide which flours to keep on hand, here's a roundup of some of the more nutritious whole grain flours—along with the reasons they belong in your kitchen:

Barley lowers cholesterol. Barley flour is one of my favorites. It bakes up into a sweet, fresh-tasting bread that I can get into even the fussiest eaters. It's a good source of fiber and chromium, a mineral that helps regulate blood sugar levels, plus it contains tocotrienol and beta-glucan, both of which are known to lower cholesterol. In a study at Texas A&M University in College Station, researchers found that 30 days on a diet rich in whole grain barley flour was enough to drop the elevated cholesterol levels of both men and women by 6 percent. What's more, a study of 22,000 men in Finland showed that eating as little as three grams a day—that's less than an ounce—of the beta-glucan in barley reduced the men's risk of death from heart disease by 27 percent.

Barley also has a slew of vitamins and minerals—folate, iron, magnesium, niacin, phosphorus, thiamin, and zinc—but its most spectacular contribution to human health may be its effect on the bowel. In a second Texas A&M study, researchers asked 22 volunteers to supplement their normally low-fat, low-cholesterol diet with 30 grams of barley flour a day. That's roughly one ounce, or a couple of slices of bread a day.

A similar group ate the same diet, but without the barley flour. Five days later the researchers compared the bowel health of each group. And what they discovered was that those who regularly ate barley flour decreased the amount of time it took food to work its way through the digestive tract by a whopping eight hours.

Now, that may sound like a pretty simple thing to you and me. But to some of the older folks in my family who suffer from a "sluggish" gastrointestinal tract—a common condition among those past age 60—decreasing the transit time from one end of the tract to the other by eight hours means less bloating, less abdominal discomfort, less constipation. and less chance of an impaction—a blockage caused by a large, rock-hard stool.

If you'd like to bake a loaf of barley bread, pick up a bag of whole hulled barley flour at your local health food store. Ignore flours made from pot, scotch, or pearled barley. They're overprocessed and not nearly as nutritious as whole barley. And if you can't find whole barley flour locally, contact one the suppliers listed in "The Granary" on page 56.

Buckwheat beats diabetes. Buckwheat isn't really a grain, but I'm going to pretend that I don't know that. In fact, I'm going to pretend that I never heard that

---

FROM THE MILLER'S KITCHEN: BETTY'S EVERYDAY BREAD

Betty Ferderber sits at the kitchen table in her sunny farmhouse kitchen, long blond hair falling over her shoulders as she reaches down to stroke Mother, the stray calico cat who came to stay.

I had just told Betty how much I envied her pantry full of just-canned salsas, pickles, relishes, jams, and jellies, and the freezer overflowing with home-grown broccoli and cauliflower.

How did she manage to get it all done, I asked—especially when she works every day in the family farm store and is still a hands-on mom to an active teenager?

"Well, I don't bake bread as much as I used to," she confesses with a guilty smile.

Bread? She bakes bread as well?

It took me about half a second to stop feeling like an underachiever and ask for her favorite recipe. Here it is:

If you're using a breadmaker, follow the manufacturer's instructions. But if you don't have one, or if you suddenly find the time to develop a half-day relationship with a loaf of bread, mix the ingredients together by hand.

To begin, dissolve 2 tablespoons of honey and the yeast into 2 cups of lukewarm water and set aside for 10 minutes. Then, in a large bowl, mix 4 cups of

INGREDIENTS

YIELD: 4 LOAVES

½ cup plus 2 tablespoons honey
4 tablespoons dried yeast
½ cup unrefined corn oil
4 teaspoons salt
(about) 5 pounds organic whole wheat flour
6 cups warm water

lukewarm water into ½ cup honey, ½ cup unrefined corn oil, and 4 teaspoons salt.

Add the yeast mixture to the bowl, then gradually stir in the 5 pounds of flour. When the dough feels as though it's so stiff you can't stir any longer, turn your dough

---

it's actually first cousin to a rhubarb plant and, as such, is really a vegetable.

The reason I'm going to play this little game is that, scientific classification notwithstanding, buckwheat is rarely used for anything but making buckwheat flour. And the clincher is that it's sold in the "baking" section of your supermarket with both flour and pancake mixes.

Buckwheat has a strong, nutlike flavor that you either love or hate. It contains the antioxidant rutin, a naturally occurring substance that may help prevent heart disease, and two components of fiber, or starch—amylopectin and amylose—that may help those with diabetes keep their blood sugar on an even keel.

In a study at the University of Oklahoma, for example, researchers found that people who regularly ate a buckwheat pancake with each meal were able to reduce the sharp, after-meal blood sugar rise that, over time, can lead to kidney disease and blindness.

It's also a good wheat flour substitute for those who have wheat allergies or celiac disease, a condition in which the gluten in wheat tears up their insides.

If you'd like to try baking with buckwheat flour, look for the kind made from

out onto a lightly floured surface and flatten into a circle. Flour your hands, then knead the dough by pushing against it with the palms of your hands. As the dough begins to resist your efforts, turn it counter-clockwise a quarter circle. Grab the edge of the dough farthest away from you and fold it toward you over the rest of the dough. Knead again, then turn and fold the dough. Repeat kneading, turning, and folding until the dough begins to feel stiff—about 10 minutes.

To see if you've added enough flour, pick up a ball of dough and lift it above the bowl with your hand palm-side-up. Wait a few seconds, then turn your hand palm-side-down. If the dough sticks to your hand for a second or two, put it back in the crock and add more flour. But if it drops onto the table or countertop without sticking, then shape the kneaded dough into a ball, place it in an oiled bowl, and leave it in a warm place to rise.

When the dough has doubled in bulk—it takes about one hour in a sunny kitchen—punch it down and divide it into four equal parts.

Put one part on a lightly floured surface and flatten it with your hands into a square. Fold the left edge of the dough in toward the center of your square; then fold the right edge in to meet it. It should look like a rectangle. Now, grasp one of the longer sides of the rectangle with both hands and roll it into a nice, tight cylinder. Place the cylinder into a well-oiled bread pan.

Repeat the folding and rolling for each of the other three parts of the dough, then let them rise undisturbed for no longer than 45 minutes.

When the timer goes off, pop them in the oven at 350 degrees and bake for 35 to 45 minutes. The loaves are done when you knock on the pan and hear a hollow thud.

Cool on wire racks, then freeze three of the loaves for future use and put one on the table with a pot of strawberry jam.

It'll be gone before the oven cools.

hulled whole groats. Unroasted white groats will have the mildest flavor; roasted groats are an acquired taste.

Corn cuts heart attack risk. Cornmeal, which is made from the only grain that actually originated in the United States, is an integral part of many North and South American cuisines. In South Carolina, where my Aunt Ellen lives, for example, no barbecue is complete without the sunny yellow presence of cornbread.

Its primary contribution to your health is twofold: It contains phytosterols—naturally occurring plant substances that may inhibit your body's tendency to absorb cholesterol from the foods you eat—and it's one of the best sources of fiber on the planet. Two tablespoons of the bran contained in cornmeal has a whopping 7.9 grams of fiber—roughly one-quarter of your daily nutritional needs.

Researchers have found that the bran itself has a powerful effect on cholesterol. In a study at Georgetown University Hospital in Washington, DC, those participants who added 17 to 34 grams of corn bran—barely more than an ounce—to their usual daily diet saw their cholesterol levels plummet 20 percent within 12 weeks. What's more, their triglyceride levels, which are considered a marker for heart disease by most doctors, fell an amazing 31 percent. Given the fact that the American Heart Association reports that high triglycerides triple your risk of a heart attack, including corn bran in your diet on a regular basis is clearly the way to go.

Unfortunately, corn flour doesn't contain any corn bran. Nor do most of the pre-packaged cornbread mixes you see in the market. Only whole grain, unsifted cornmeal contains both the bran and the germ. So check package labels and make sure that's what you buy.

If you haven't made whole grain cornbread before, you might be surprised by how easily it falls apart or how heavy it is—especially as compared to the lightweight cornbread that's served at many restaurants. Healthy cornbread is heavy because cornmeal lacks the gluten that makes wheat breads rise. That makes it a good choice for those with celiac disease, since it's the gluten in wheat flour that gets their insides in an uproar. But if the crumby texture or heaviness of whole grain cornbread makes in politically unacceptable in your house, just combine it with whole wheat flour in a ratio of one part cornmeal to four parts whole wheat. You can gradually increase the cornmeal as your family realizes that what your cornbread's gained in weight, it's also gained in taste.

To weight the scales in your favor, substitute an unrefined corn oil for whatever fat your cornbread recipe calls for. As Betty Ferderber pointed out to me, unrefined corn oil makes everything it's in taste like fresh-picked corn. And it's available at most health food stores.

Oats lower cholesterol, high blood pressure, and diabetes risk. If you'd like to be as healthy as a horse, maybe you should start eating like one—in substance if not amount. Oats and hulled whole oat flour are not only loaded with heart-healthy flavonoids, saponins, tocotrienols, and the cancer-fighting caffeic and ferulic acids, they also contain betaglucan, a gummy fiber that glues itself to artery-clogging LDL cholesterol and escorts it out of the body. A study of 156 people at the Chicago Center for Clinical Research found that in just six weeks those who ate 56 grams of oat bran—the amount found in about a bowlful of oatmeal—reduced their LDL cholesterol by nearly 16 percent.

That's not bad for horse feed.

But whole oats also have an effect on two other risk factors for heart disease—high blood pressure and diabetes. Researchers in China found that 100 grams—about 3½ ounces—of oats every day reduced blood pressure three points in three days among a large group of people. And in a study at the University of Alberta in Canada, another team of researchers found that middle-aged men with diabetes were better able to control their blood sugar when eating oat bread. What's more, they also reduced their ratio of bad to good cholesterol by 24 percent. So eating oats and oat products can lower blood pressure, control blood sugar, and lower cholesterol.

It's studies like these that have fueled an explosion of oat products at your supermarket. Unfortunately, most of the bread products seem to be more air than substance. Many are mostly refined wheat plus a few tablespoons of oat flour.

Check the label and you'll find on most breads that oat flour is listed halfway through the list of ingredients—about four ingredients down from wheat flour and about two ingredients above the additives that increase the bread's shelf life. Since industry standards require that ingredients be listed in descending order of their amount in a product, you can get a pretty good idea of exactly how much "real oat goodness" is in the loaf.

Not all manufacturers who mix other flours into their oat flour are deliberately trying to mislead you, however. Since oat flour has no gluten to make it rise, they're simply trying to lighten their loaves by mixing it with a flour that does rise. In fact, all by itself, oat flour tends to sink down in the bowl until it resembles a lumpy tan rock.

You can avoid the rock problem and still get more "oat goodness" by using the bread manufacturers' own strategy, albeit with a more nutritious twist: mix the oat flour with another whole grain flour.

Start with a 1 to 3 ratio. If your recipe calls for three cups of flour, for instance, try making that two cups of whole wheat and one of oat flour. If you like the way the finished loaf looks and tastes, next time you bake, try increasing the proportion of oat flour. In fact, do that every time you bake until the difference in taste becomes apparent; then cut back if necessary.

Rye reduces heart disease and hot flashes. Rye bread is a staple in northern Europe, Russia, and Finland where researchers have found that eating about three slices of whole grain rye bread reduces the risk of death from heart disease by 17 percent.

But there's one thing you should know before you run out and buy whole grain rye flour: the rye bread eaten in Finland is very different from the rye bread you may have eaten at your local deli. Rather than a smooth-textured bread with a light beige color, it's dark, dense, and flavorful. And rather than giving you a touch of fiber and a lot of calories, bread made from whole grain rye flour is rich in fiber, rutin, saponins, phytic acid, and even phytoestrogens—plant estrogens that may help reduce hot flashes and prevent osteoporosis during menopause. It even contains more B vitamins, iron, and protein than whole wheat.

If you'd like to make real rye bread a part of your diet, start by baking a bread that uses half whole wheat flour and half rye flour. Gradually add more rye and less wheat as you become accustomed to the taste.

Wheat strengthens your heart. There are several different forms of whole wheat grains, and each of them seems to be just as nutritious and healthful as the others. So are the flours into which they're ground. Each contains a good amount of protein, B vitamins, vitamin E, iron, magnesium, potassium, and the powerful antioxidant selenium. Wheat is also a natural source of ferulic acid and tocotrienols, both of which help protect you from cancer and heart disease.

In a series of studies over the years, researchers have found that whole wheat fiber grabs hold of a variety of cancer-causing substances in the gut and lugs them out. And in a study at Loma Linda University in California, researchers compared the incidence of heart attacks in people who regularly ate white bread with those who ate whole wheat. The result? Those who ate whole wheat bread had reduced their risk of a heart attack by 40 percent.

As my dad used to say after he said grace: "Praise the Lord and pass the ammunition—hand me the bread."

Pineapple-Sweet Potato Bread

This is a sweet quick bread that would be good with tea.

Preheat the oven to 350 F.

Peel and cube the sweet potatoes. Boil until tender, drain, and mash.

Combine the oil and sugar. Beat in the eggs one at a time. Beat in the mashed sweet potatoes and pineapple with juice.

In a separate bowl, combine the flour, soda, baking powder, cinnamon and allspice. Add the dry ingredients to the liquid mixtures and mix just until combined well.

Spoon half of the batter into each of two 9-inch x 5-inch nonstick sprayed bread pans. Bake for 45 minutes or until golden brown and a toothpick inserted in the center comes out clean.

NOTE: This bread can also be prepared with half whole wheat and half all-purpose flour. Chopped walnuts and/or raisins can be added.

INGREDIENTS

YIELD: 20 SLICES

2 sweet potatoes
    (about 1 pound)
½ cup canola oil
2 cups sugar
¾ cup egg substitute or 3 eggs
1 can (8 ounces) crushed pineapple in juice
3½ cups unbleached flour
2 teaspoons baking soda
½ teaspoon baking powder
1½ teaspoons cinnamon
1 teaspoon allspice

PER SLICE

Calories	234
Carbohydrates	45 g
Fat	5 g
Saturated fat	0.5 g
Dietary fiber	1.4 g
Cholesterol	0.2 mg
Sodium	160 mg

Flax Prairie Bread

(Prepared in the bread machine)

The recipe for this bread was adapted from a recipe from the Flax Council of Canada that contained more salt and more sunflower and poppy seeds. It's probably called Prairie Bread because it's made from grains and seeds that grow on the prairie. A warning: This bread rose more than any bread I have ever seen—I thought it was going to emerge from the bread machine like something from an old *I Love Lucy* episode!

Measure ingredients and place in bread machine in order recommended by manufacturer. Select whole wheat cycle with light crust.

When completed, remove bread and allow to cool.

INGREDIENTS

YIELD: A LARGE LOAF (1½ LBS.)

1¼ cups water
1 teaspoon salt
2 tablespoons canola oil
2 tablespoons honey
2 cups bread flour
1¼ cups whole wheat bread flour
⅓ cup whole flaxseed
2 teaspoons yeast

PER SLICE

Calories	124
Carbohydrates	22 g
Fat	3.2 g
Saturated fat	0.2 g
Monounsaturated fat	1 g
Protein	4 g
Dietary fiber	0 g
Cholesterol	0 mg
Sodium	147 mg

Harvest Pumpkin Wheat and Soy Bread

*T*his recipe uses a good amount of soy flour, which adds protein and fiber to the bread, plus a great supply of isoflavones.

The soy flour used here was a full-fat soy flour, but the fat can be cut by using a defatted soy flour. Defatted soy flour can be purchased mail order from Great Valley Mills, 1774 County Line Road, Barto, PA 19504. Telephone 1-800-688-6455 and fax 610-754-6490.

Preheat oven to 350 F.

Combine the flours with the cinnamon, baking soda, baking powder, cloves and nutmeg.

In a separate bowl, cream the margarine and add the sugar. Beat until light. Add the eggs and beat until light. Add the pumpkin and the water. Then add the dry ingredients and combine well. Pour the batter into a greased 9-inch by 5-inch loaf pan.

Bake for 65 to 75 minutes. Remove the bread from the pan and allow to cool on a wire rack.

INGREDIENTS

YIELD: 12 SERVINGS

1 cup whole wheat flour
⅔ cup soy flour*
2 teaspoons cinnamon
½ teaspoon baking soda
½ teaspoon baking powder
½ teaspoon ground cloves
¼ teaspoon ground nutmeg
¼ cup trans fat–free stick margarine
1 cup sugar
2 egg substitutes or eggs, slightly beaten
¾ cup puréed pumpkin
2 tablespoons water

PER SERVING

Calories	161
Carbohydrates	27 g
Fat	5 g
Polyunsaturated fat	2 g
Dietary fiber	2.4 g
Cholesterol	0 mg
Sodium	114 mg

*NOTE: You can substitute all wheat instead of using the soy, but if you do, omit the two tablespoons of water. (Soy soaks up moisture so when using it, extra water must be added.) The temperature should also be raised to 375°F so the bread will bake faster. When using soy, the temperature is lowered slightly because soy browns easier and faster than whole wheat.

Flaxseed Hamburger Rolls

(Prepared in the bread machine)

*O*ther seeds can be substituted for the flaxseed; for example, sesame, caraway, or poppy seeds.

Measure ingredients and place in bread machine in order recommended by manufacturer. Select dough cycle. This cycle should take about 1½ hours, and the dough will have gone through the first rising.

Spray two baking sheets with nonstick spray. Open the machine and punch down the dough. With oiled hands, remove the dough from the machine. Shape the dough into 12 hamburger rolls and place them on the prepared baking sheets. Cover the rolls with plastic wrap and allow to rise in a warm place until doubled in bulk, about 30 minutes to 1 hour.

Set the oven to 350 F and when preheated, place the rolls in the oven and bake for 20 to 25 minutes or until the rolls are golden brown on top. Remove and cool for several minutes. With a metal spatula, remove from the pan and cool on a wire rack.

INGREDIENTS

YIELD: 12 ROLLS

1¼ cups water
1 teaspoon salt
2 tablespoons canola oil
2 tablespoons honey
2 cups white bread flour
1¼ cups whole wheat bread flour
⅓ cup whole flaxseed
2 teaspoons yeast

PER ROLL

Calories	165
Carbohydrates	29 g
Fat	4 g
Saturated fat	0.25 g
Dietary fiber	4 g
Cholesterol	0 mg
Sodium	196 mg

Barley Bread

(Prepared in the bread machine)

Add ingredients to bread machine following manufacturer's directions. Use regular setting and light crust.

When bread is completed, remove from pan and allow to cool.

INGREDIENTS

YIELD: 1 LOAF (1½ LBS.)

6 to 7 ounces water
1 teaspoon salt
2 tablespoons canola oil
2 tablespoons honey
2¼ cups bread flour
1 cup barley flour
2 tablespoons nonfat milk powder
½ cup cooked hulled barley
2 teaspoons dry yeast

PER ROLL

Calories	153
Carbohydrates	29 g
Fat	3 g
Saturated fat	0.3 g
Dietary fiber	2 g
Cholesterol	0.13 mg
Sodium	198 mg

Cranberry-Oatmeal Bread

(Prepared in the bread machine)

Add ingredients in order suggested by manufacturer. Bake at whole wheat setting with a light crust.

When bread is completed, remove from the pan and allow to cool.

INGREDIENTS

YIELD: 1 LOAF (1½ LBS.)

9 to 11 ounces water
1 teaspoon salt
2 tablespoons canola oil
2 tablespoons honey
½ cup rolled oats
2 cups bread flour
1½ cups whole wheat bread flour
½ cup oat flour
2 tablespoons nonfat powdered milk
2 teaspoons dried yeast
½ cup craisins or dried sweetened cranberries

PER ROLL

Calories	217
Carbohydrates	40 g
Fat	3.4 g
Saturated fat	0.3 g
Dietary fiber	4 g
Cholesterol	0.13 mg
Sodium	199 mg

The Refrigerator

While the refrigerators of my childhood were likely to be short, white, electricity-guzzling models full of whole milk, butter, cheese, meat, and chocolate cake, today my refrigerator is more likely to be a tall, color-coordinated, and energy-efficient model stuffed with fresh fruits, vegetables, juices, low-fat milk, and yogurt.

Why such a radical change? One reason is that what was in my family refrigerator when I was a child left me with a weight problem that will probably follow me to my grave. Another is the overwhelming numbers of scientific studies clearly demonstrating that the more antioxidant-rich fresh fruits, vegetables, and low-fat dairy foods we eat, the less likely we are to develop osteoporosis, heart disease, high blood pressure, diabetes, high cholesterol, and a whole alphabet's worth of different cancers.

Bruce Ames, Ph.D., a brilliant researcher at the University of California at Berkeley who has led much of the pioneering research on antioxidants, estimates that the one-quarter of the American population that eats the fewest fruits and vegetables has twice the incidence of cancer as those who eat the most. A diet deficient in antioxidant-rich fruits and vegetables causes the same damage to your cellular DNA as radiation, says Dr. Ames. And because fruits and vegetables are also a major source of folate, a B vitamin that is responsible for repairing the DNA that tells your body how to make new cells, a diet deficient in fruits and vegetables also prevents your body from using the mechanisms God gave us to heal it.

In a study at the University of New York at Buffalo, researchers looked at the diets of 297 women over age 40 who had been diagnosed with breast cancer. Then they looked at the diets of similar premenopausal women who didn't have breast cancer. After comparing the two groups, there was one inescapable conclusion: The women without breast cancer were far more likely to eat a diet rich in fresh fruits and vegetables. In fact, concluded the researchers, women who loaded their diets with fruits and vegetables reduced their risk of breast cancer by nearly half!

Studies evaluating the effects of fruits and vegetables on heart disease have had similar results. A study of more than 50,000 men conducted at Harvard University found that those who ate the most fruits and vegetables had 41 percent few-

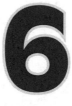

6

REFRIGERATOR

BEST FOR HELPING YOU:

Prevent cancer

Beat diabetes

Lower high cholesterol

Prevent heart disease

Strengthen bones

er heart attacks than those who ate the least.

What's more, a diet rich in fruits and vegetables also reduces the risk factors that trigger heart disease in the first place. Another Harvard study found that the more fruit a group of men ate, the less likely they were to develop high blood pressure. And a study at St. Michael's Hospital in Toronto found that when two groups of people are put on exactly the same low-fat diet, the group that also eats plenty of fruits and vegetables will lower their cholesterol an additional 34 to 49 percent! If you eat a low-fat diet, then get frustrated when your cholesterol levels plateau before they get to a healthy level, this study offers clear evidence that eating more fruits and vegetables is your solution.

The effects of fruits and vegetables on stroke risk are even more pronounced. In another Harvard study—this one involving over 800 men and lasting more than 20 years—researchers found that those who ate the most fruits and vegetables had 59 percent fewer strokes than those who ate the least. The effect was so significant that researchers could actually calculate the effects of every bite: for every serving of fruits and vegetables a man ate, he reduced his risk of stroke 7 percent.

But knowing that fruits and vegetables could make the difference between health and disease still wasn't enough to get them in my refrigerator on a regular basis. And in that I'm not alone. Federal surveys say that only half of all Americans eat a minimum of five fruits and vegetables a day. Two out of four don't eat the recommended three servings of vegetables a day, while three out of four don't eat the recommended two servings of fruit. Particularly disturbing is the fact that less than half of us eat any fruit at all on any given day.

What finally screwed my head on straight was the desire to nurture my wonderful baby-growing body during pregnancy. That, plus the seductive photos and imaginative recipes splashed throughout such magazines as *Eating Well*, *Cooking Light*, and *Prevention*—the latter the grandmother of all health magazines and my alma mater as a writer.

But getting fresh fruits and vegetables into my refrigerator was still only half the battle. What actually got them onto my plate and into my mouth was the handful of chefs up and down the West Coast who fell in love with the fresh fruits and vegetables on their doorstep and shared that love with the rest of us.

These chefs—Alice Waters and her associates at Chez Panisse in Berkeley, California, in particular—taught me and an entire world how the excitement of texture, vibrant color, and the subtleties of flavor could ignite a passion for healthy foods that were, without a doubt, what God intended us to eat.

That's not to say that, should you stop by my kitchen in Vermont, you won't find chocolate in the fridge. Old habits die hard, and the battle of the bulge rumbles on. But the chocolate is more likely to be a bottle of Hershey's fat-free chocolate syrup that I drizzle and drip rather than guzzle. And, unlike the refrigerators of my childhood, this one's stuffed with every fruit and vegetable in season. Late winter mesclun from the coldframe gives way to spring peas and broccoli, followed by a summer of strawberries, cherries, raspberries, blueberries, corn, cantaloupe, honeydew, watermelon—the list goes on and on. If I can't pluck it from the rich earth myself, I'll get it at a roadside stand, local market, or, during the winter, the canned and frozen sections of a supermarket.

The point, as the following pages illustrate, is that my refrigerator holds almost all the elements of good health and long life.

I hope yours does, too.

Apricots

These sugar-kissed little balls of sunshine are packed with two carotenoids that have been shown to help prevent heart disease, cancer, and macular degeneration, a vision problem that is a leading cause of blindness in elderly people.

In a study of more than 90,000 nurses, researchers found that those who ate the most carotenoids were 25 percent less likely to develop heart disease than those who ate the least. Men may benefit even more, researchers say. A study of 1,379 men in Europe indicates that those who ate the most lycopenes, one of the two carotenoids in apricots, were half as likely to have a heart attack as those who ate the least.

What's more, a Harvard University study of 1,271 people over age 88 found that those who ate the most fruits with a high carotenoid level reduced their risk of cancer by a third.

Apricots are also a good source of potassium to help keep blood pressure down and muscles working well. And just three of the tiny fruits will supply you with nearly half the daily amount of vitamin A your body needs to

---

APRICOTS

BEST FOR HELPING YOU:

Prevent macular degeneration

Maintain healthy muscles

Keep blood pressure healthy

Fight cancer

Prevent heart disease

Keep viruses at bay

APRICOT BASICS

HOW TO BUY: Apricot season runs from May through August, so that's the time to load up. Look for firm apricots that are dark yellow or yellow-orange. Avoid any that are dull, soft, or bruised.

Stick to fresh apricots if you can, or apricots canned in fruit juice if you can't. Avoid canned apricots packed in syrup—they have twice the calories and half the carotenoids of fresh. Dried apricots are a good option when fresh ones are not available. A single 3-ounce serving has a whopping 1,300 milligrams of potassium. One caveat: Dried apricots are definitely only for high-energy kids who are spending all their time running around (See "After-School Snacks" on page 216). A single serving has 238 calories—more than most of us adults can afford.

HOW TO STORE: Fresh apricots are fragile. Pop them into a plastic bag, seal it, and place it gently in your refrigerator. Eat within a day or two.

HOW TO USE: Rinse apricots in cold water, dip them in boiling water for 20 seconds, then slip their skins off with a fruit knife and remove the pits. Chop them into yogurt, cookie batters, and hot oatmeal, or serve them cold with a sprinkling of lemon juice and cinnamon. You can also poach them with cinnamon and cloves—just a pinch!—for a delightful dessert. Just keep the poaching time short since heat tends to reduce both nutrients and flavor.

keep vision sharp and strengthen cell walls against viruses.

Artichokes: A Natural Weapon against Liver Disease

Although shoppers under the age of 12 may beg their parents to let them play with those "little green hand grenades in the produce aisle," ten to one eating them for dinner is not what's on their agenda. And that's a shame, because artichokes contain silymarin, a naturally occurring antioxidant that seems to have an amazing ability to keep your liver healthy.

The liver, of course, is responsible for detoxifying and disposing of toxic substances that have insinuated their way into your body and converting all food into the chemicals your body needs to live. It also regulates blood clotting, monitors and maintains the appropriate blood levels of any drugs you may be taking, cleans your blood and gets rid of any waste products, maintains hormone balance, removes bacteria from the bloodstream, produces several immune system helpers, and controls the production and elimination of cholesterol. It's an amazing organ that can be damaged by alcohol, drugs, and the hepatitis virus.

Preliminary studies indicate that silymarin has a protective effect on the liver. In studies with problem drinkers, for example, those who took a concentrated form of silymarin were less likely to die than those who didn't. In other studies, when patients admitted to a hospital for a variety of liver diseases and infections were given silymarin, liver function improved significantly more than in a group of people who were not given silymarin.

How much silymarin do you need to protect your liver? Scientists don't know.

ARTICHOKES

BEST FOR HELPING YOU:

Heal your liver

Prevent cancer

ARTICHOKE BASICS

HOW TO BUY: Look for heavy, unblemished artichokes with an even green color and leaves that squeak against each other when they're pulled. The best artichokes come from California in the spring. Baby artichokes come from the same plant as their big sisters, just farther down on the stem.

HOW TO STORE: Sprinkle with water, seal in a plastic bag and refrigerate. Artichokes will keep for up to a week.

HOW TO USE: Rinse well, cut off the stem so the artichoke will sit upright, then trim off the top third. Use a melon-baller to scrape out the fuzzy center stuff and discard it.

If you're planning to stuff the artichokes with chicken salad or some other mixture, snuggle the artichoke in a dish of crushed ice, then stuff and serve.

If you're planning to stir-fry, sauté, or drop parts of the artichoke into a casserole, however, bend back the outer petals until they snap off near the base. Toss them in the compost or garbage disposal. The petals that remain on the artichoke heart are what you're after. Pull them off and stir-fry, sauté, or bake to your heart's content.

The petals also make an excellent "chip" for your favorite dip.

What they do know, however, is that eating a varied diet that includes a good source of silymarin like artichokes in it is an excellent way to tilt the odds in your favor.

Plus, artichokes have an extra special blessing: They are one of the most potent cancer-fighters on the planet. According to a study a the USDA's Arkansas Children's Nutrition Center in Little Rock, artichokes have more antioxidants in them than almost any other vegetable measured.

Asparagus: The Vegetable that Keeps You Young

The first fresh, earthy breath of spring has no sooner drifted through my kitchen window than I'm pestering local farmers to see if they've got any asparagus. The tall, graceful spears are available for such a short time where I live that I find myself waiting for them through those late winter weeks as impatiently as a child waits to be let out of school.

My craving for this elegant vegetable is not solely due to its sweetly earthy taste. It's also be-

---

ASPARAGUS

BEST FOR HELPING YOU:

Conserve muscle

Maintain a healthy weight

Reduce cholesterol

Lower blood pressure

Prevent cancer

Fight heart disease

Ward off arthritis

ASPARAGUS BASICS

HOW TO BUY: Look for thin, tender spears with tightly closed tips and straight stalks. Buy only from merchants who know enough to keep the asparagus upright on beds of ice, under refrigeration or standing in several inches of cold water. Asparagus that are tossed on a produce counter at room temperature will lack the nutrients and flavor of their cool counterparts. Avoid canned asparagus. It has fewer nutrients and sometimes seems to pick up a bitter taste.

HOW TO STORE: Wrap the stalks in a damp cloth, seal in a plastic bag and place in the bottom of your refrigerator. Use the day you buy it—the next day at the latest.

HOW TO USE: Fill your kitchen sink with cold water, then drop in the asparagus. Swish it around so that any sand caught in its tips will float out. Dry with a towel, pick up each spear individually and break it in two. The spear will break naturally at the point where the stalk becomes woody. Compost the woody part, and use only the upper spear and tips.

Everybody has their own favorite way of preparing asparagus. Mine is to drizzle the spears with a little olive oil, add a splash or two of water, cover and microwave for a few minutes until the asparagus are bright green. My sister-in-law Jamie likes to set them upright in a pot of boiling water and steam the spears for three to five minutes. Other friends like to chop the asparagus into one-inch pieces, then drop them into a hot frying pan with a tablespoon of sesame oil and stir-fry for three or four minutes. However you choose to prepare it, as long as you respect its need to get from field to table in just a few days, asparagus will provide you with the full flavor of spring.

cause asparagus is a great source of folate, a B vitamin that your body uses to repair the DNA in cells that have been damaged by everything from your own metabolic processes to the deadly chemicals in a friend's cigarette smoke or the PCBs you may have been exposed to. If your body doesn't have enough folate to repair its DNA, you're more susceptible to cancer and, if you're pregnant, your child is at risk for a serious birth defect called spina bifida, in which the spine is deformed.

You're also more susceptible to heart disease. That's because folate is one of the B vitamins that helps reduce the amount of homocysteine in your body, a substance it manufactures from high protein sources like meat. Since high levels of homocysteine are associated with high levels of heart disease, I'm very happy to eat anything that will keep them low.

I also look forward to the spring asparagus because it contains a good shot of muscle-maintaining potassium, and because it's the richest food source of glutathione, a naturally occurring chemical that can protect me—and you—from many of the diseases associated with old age—particularly arthritis, diabetes, and heart disease. In one study, for example, researchers looked at 33 people over age 60 and found that those who ate the most glutathione-rich vegetables such as asparagus had lower cholesterol, lower blood pressure, and healthier weights than those who ate the least. They also had fewer minor illnesses and were significantly less likely to have arthritis, diabetes, or heart disease.

That's why several pounds of glowing green spears of asparagus, glistening with the sprinkle of olive oil in which they were steamed, are the featured vegetable on my table every spring when the family gathers at Easter. In one way, the spears are there because I want to serve food that will give my 91-year-old father- and mother-in-law the nutrients they need to stay with us for a few more years. In another, it's because, when I'm 91, I want to be here with my kids and grandkids, too.

Asparagus is my prayer that I will be.

AVOCADOS

BEST FOR HELPING YOU:

Stimulate a sluggish digestive tract

Prevent constipation

Gain weight healthfully

Prevent heart disease

Reduce the "bad" LDL cholesterol

Increase the "good" HDL cholesterol

Avocados: A Miracle for Elderly Lightweights

Reclaimed from California by the rest of the world, fresh avocados are able to provide us with a rich source of monounsaturated fat—the only type of fat that actually helps us prevent heart disease and stroke. (See "Healthy Oils" on page 242 for a detailed discussion of various fats.)

In a Mexican study, for example, researchers put two groups of people on low-fat diets. The diets were pretty much the same, except that one of the groups ate avocados while the other did not. And that made a big difference. When researchers compared each group's results, they found that both groups lowered the artery-clogging LDL cholesterol that can set you up for a heart attack. But only the low-fat diet plus avocado also lowered triglycerides, a particularly nasty type of blood fat that doctors use as a marker for heart disease. It also raised HDL cholesterol, the good kind that "kidnaps" LDL cholesterol and takes it for a ride—the kind from which it never returns.

But here's the catch: This wonderful gift from the California coast has so many calories (731 per fruit!) and so much fat (30 grams!) that, no matter how great it is, very few people can afford to avail themselves of its virtues.

I certainly can't—one avocado would use up nearly half the number of calories and two-thirds the amount of fat that are optimally in my daily diet.

But avocados are nothing less than a miracle fruit for one of my aunts. At 81, this woman was at a healthy weight for most of her life. But once she passed 75, keeping her weight up has been a fight that's left both of us feeling grumpy. The problem is a fussy digestive tract. As with many older folks, it no longer allows her to eat the rich ice creams and butter-

creamy mashed potatoes of her youth. The Golden Guernsey whole milk she used to drink now gives her cramps, and so do her favorite fried foods. The result is that in the last six years she's slipped from a healthy 120 pounds to a scary 91.

I'm terrified that she'll just melt into a pile of skin and bones and disappear. But because those first 75 years of a high-fat diet have clogged her arteries and led to a couple of mini-strokes—transient ischemic attacks that frequently foreshadow a major stroke—we can't just indiscriminately start feeding her high-calorie, high-fat foods. Instead, we have to find high-calorie sources of food with lots of monounsaturated fat to lower that artery-clogging cholesterol. In short, we need to find something that will fatten her up without making her arteries worse.

The perfect food? The avocado. And its added benefits are a nice chunk of po-

AVOCADO BASICS

HOW TO BUY: If you're looking for the high-calorie, high-fat fruit described above, look for a California avocado. If you'd love to eat avocados but can't take their calories or fat, buy the ones shipped from Florida. They have nearly two-thirds the calories and half the fat of their West Coast cousins.

To get the most bang for your buck, look for an avocado that yields to gentle pressure. That means it's ripe and ready to go. If you want to hold the avocado for a few days, pick one that's firm.

HOW TO STORE: Ripe avocados will stay fresh in your refrigerator for four days or so. Unripe avocados should be left out at room temperature until they become soft, then transferred to the refrigerator.

HOW TO USE: Rinse well and dry. Then run a knife lengthwise around the fruit and twist. The two halves will separate and you can insert a spoon under the pit to lift it out. Place each half cut-side down and slip off the peel, then sprinkle with lemon juice to prevent discoloration. The remaining fruit is highly versatile. You can mash it and spread it on bread as a substitute for bad-fat mayonnaise—it's particularly good with turkey sandwiches, a nice, easy-on-the-tummy entrée that older folks frequently like. Or you can add some chicken broth and yogurt, then puree it in the blender for a cold soup. Or you can just eat it out of hand. The only thing you don't want to do is cook it. Cooked avocado has a bitter flavor that no one seems to like.

tassium to keep a lid on her blood pressure, plus a whopping dose of fiber to prevent the sluggishness and constipation that frequently plagues an elderly digestive tract. In fact, at 10 grams of fiber per avocado, this incredible fruit packs more of a wallop than the densest bran muffin you can buy.

Berries: The All-Around Top Choice

Berry season starts in June around my neck of the woods with big, luscious strawberries that taste as good as they look. Generally I start visiting berry farms by June 5, buying a pint here and a pint there to see who's got the best. Then I get out the canning jars, buy new lids, lay in a supply of fruit pectin, and wait for a week of hot sun to intensify the flavor of the berries.

Once I'm sure the berries are ready, I send my son over to this year's se-lected berry farm. He collects basket after basket of freshly picked berries still sprinkled with morning dew, loads them in the Subaru, and hauls them home.

The moment they arrive on my kitchen counter is the official opening of berry season. Strawberries in early June are followed by raspberries and blackberries later in the month; blueberries arrive in July and cranberries in September. And during this brief four-month period, I will serve berries by themselves bursting with flavor, berries dipped in sugar, berry breakfast shakes, berry pancakes, berry bread, berry parfait desserts, berry and yogurt whipped pies and—to the delight of my son and his college roommates—berries drizzled with and dipped in chocolate.

If I sound like a berry nut, it's because I am. The sweet, puckery taste of a berry fresh from its bush, plant, or vine is heaven. The warm aroma makes me feel as mellow as if I

BERRIES

BEST FOR HELPING YOU:

Discourage varicose veins

Overcome poor circulation in those with diabetes

Strengthen blood vessels

Prevent cancer

Fight heart disease

Control bladder infections

Clear up constipation

Improve memory

THE PIE SAFE: A FOUR-BERRY FOURTH OF JULY PIE

This pie is absolute berry madness. And it's so simple you'll make it over and over again during berry season.

Prepare one nine-inch graham cracker pie crust according to directions on the side of a box of graham cracker crumbs. Bake as directed, then set aside to cool.

Wash and hull 1 cup each of strawberries, raspberries, blackberries, and blueberries. Drain the berries well, then quarter the strawberries. Place all berries in a glass or ceramic bowl, sprinkle with 1 tablespoon fresh lemon juice and about ½ cup granulated sugar. Mix and set aside for 30 minutes.

Heat ½ cup of strawberry jam—preferably your own—until it turns into a shiny liquid, about 20 seconds in the microwave.

Now, take the pie crust, dump the berries in and drizzle with jam. Let sit in the refrigerator until filling thickens, then serve with a tablespoon of vanilla yogurt on top.

were dozing in a freshly mown field. And the deep, bold colors tell me the berry is bursting with anthocyanins, a naturally occurring substance that is one of the most powerful cancer-fighting substances on the planet. Plus it helps strengthen capillary walls, which may prevent varicose veins and some of the circulation problems that occur in those with diabetes.

There is probably nothing more healthful I can do for myself than eat a handful of berries. In a study at Tufts University in Boston, USDA researchers who were studying the ability of more than 40 different fruits and vegetables to neutralize the free radicals frequently involved in triggering cancer found that three of the top five cancer-fighting fruits and vegetables were berries: blueberries took top honors followed by blackberries and strawberries.

Now this sounds fabulous, but researchers don't really know how much therapeutic power berries have. So the Tufts researchers launched a second study to find out. They asked eight elderly women to drink a special beverage made from strawberries. The beverage was equivalent to only eight ounces of fresh strawberries, but it boosted the women's ability to neutralize cancer-causing free radicals by a whopping 20 percent. Just think— a pint of common, ordinary strawberries that you can buy at a roadside stand did what even the most expensive prescription drug at your local pharmacy can't: it increased the body's ability to fight cancer by one-fifth!

Blueberries may be even more potent. Even though their therapeutic power hasn't been tested on people, when researchers have gone nose to nose and berry to berry in the lab, blueberries have shown they have twice the anticancer power of strawberries.

There's just no way to lose with any kind of berry. As a group, berries contain large amounts of ellagic acid, another naturally occurring cancer fighter. They also

---

BERRY BASICS

HOW TO BUY: Buy fresh and in season. Every day away from the bush, plant, or vine on which they grew is a loss of flavor and nutrition—especially vitamin C, which all berries have to some degree. Look for plump, firm, deeply colored berries and avoid anything soft, wrinkled, or leaking juice.

Strawberries should have their green caps attached, with little or no green or white around the top. Both signal unripe fruit that will never reach full flavor or maturity. Blackberries and raspberries should not have their caps intact, nor should they have a touch of green, since both indicate immaturity as well. Blueberries should be nearly black with a white frost on their skins; cranberries, the simple folk in berrydom, need only be firm and red to give you all of which they're capable.

HOW TO STORE: Unwashed, in a moisture-proof container in your refrigerator.

HOW TO USE: Rinse the berries thoroughly in cold running water just before you use them. Then drop them in your morning oatmeal, toss them in the blender with a pint of low-fat yogurt, drop them into a pancake batter, sprinkle with flour and fold into a cake, use in a fruit salad, pop them into a pie or roll them into a bread. There is no way that berries don't taste berry, berry good!

contain between two and seven grams of insoluble fiber, the kind that further lowers your risk of colon cancer.

Individually, blackberries contain salicylic acid, an aspirin-like substance that reduces your body's production of artery-clogging clots. Cranberries and blueberries contain a substance that prevents bacteria from adhering to bladder walls and causing a urinary tract infection. Cranberries also seem able to interfere with the ability of breast cancer cells to replicate and spread. And strawberries contain a good shot of potassium to keep your blood pressure healthy.

The point is, berries can help you stay clear of cancer, heart disease, high cholesterol, diabetes, constipation, high blood pressure, and bladder infections. They're absolutely amazing. And if they're not on my table fresh, then you can bet I have some in the freezer.

One caveat: People who are allergic to aspirin, those who have diverticular disease, and those who have had bladder stones should check with their family physician before adding any type of berry to their menu. In some cases, berries can cause a flare-up of these problems.

Cantaloupe: A Sweet Source of Carotenoids

Slice up a chilled cantaloupe on a hot summer's day, stick it in front of a bunch of hot kids, and they'll have eaten an entire day's supply of vitamin A within two minutes.

That's because cantaloupe is both delicious and nutritious. A single serving has not only half a day's supply of the vision-sharpening vitamin A, but a full day's supply of vitamin C, 25 percent of the potassium you need to keep blood pressure at healthy levels, and a smidgen of fiber to keep your digestive tract moving along.

Most of the vitamin A in cantaloupe is available as beta carotene, a substance that, in foods, has been associated with a reduced risk of cancer. A study of 1,271

CANTALOUPE

BEST FOR HELPING YOU:

Avoid cataracts

Lower high blood pressure

Prevent cancer

CANTALOUPE BASICS

HOW TO BUY: What Americans call "cantaloupe" is really the European muskmelon. So look for cantaloupes in the States and muskmelons abroad. But whatever its name, keep in mind that the riper the melon, the more nutrients it contains. Ripe melons are intoxicatingly fragrant with a nice creamy yellow under the netting of their rind—not green, which indicates a lack of maturity. And the blossom end—the one with the nickel-sized circle—gives when you press it. Cantaloupes peak in July, so that's the most economical time of year to serve them.

HOW TO STORE: In the refrigerator for four or five days.

HOW TO USE: Fresh from the fridge. Wash the outer rind well, cut the melon in half, then scoop out the seeds. After that it's a matter of personal choice. Scoop out the sweet, moist flesh with a spoon, or slice each half for eating out of hand. You can also cube the melon and mix it with other melons like honeydew and watermelon.

---

people over age 65 found, for example, that those who ate the most carotene-containing fruits and vegetables reduced their risk of death due to cancer by an amazing 30 percent.

A second study at Harvard, this one of more than 50,000 nurses, found that those who got the most carotenoids, of which beta carotene is one, were 39 percent less likely to develop cataracts than nurses who got the least. And a third Harvard study found that men who ate fruits and veggies rich in vitamin A reduced their risk of duodenal ulcer by 54 percent.

Given the fact that most young people spend serious amounts of time either in the sun or at the computer—both of which practically suck vitamin A out of the eyeball—it may not be a bad idea to throw them a couple of melon balls whenever you can. Then maybe they'll still be able to see at age 60.

CELERY

BEST FOR HELPING YOU:

Reverse the constriction of diseased arteries

Lower blood pressure

CHILE PEPPERS

BEST FOR HELPING YOU:

Get rid of a stuffy nose

Drain an achy sinus

Protect your stomach from alcohol

Relieve pain from arthritis, diabetes, shingles, and phantom limbs

Aid digestion

Prevent heart disease

Prevent stroke

Lower cholesterol

Celery: Keeping Your Arteries in Shape

You may think of celery as something cute to stick in the dip, but it's also a super-crunchy way to help your arteries stay healthy. That's because celery contains 3-n-butyl phthalide, a naturally occurring chemical that relaxes constricted blood vessels. It also reduces the amounts of various artery-constricting hormones released by your body when it's under stress. Since constricted arteries raise blood pressure, the tongue-twisting 3-n-butyl phthalide actually helps your blood pressure stay low when you're stressed out. And given the stresses placed on most of us these days, that makes celery a must on everyone's plate.

Chile Peppers: Nature's Decongestant

Thanks to my son, the Culinary Adventurer, I finally tried hot peppers about ten years after ev-

CELERY BASICS

HOW TO BUY: Look for long, green, stiff stalks with perky leaves attached. Leave anything soft at the market.

HOW TO STORE: Sprinkle with water, wrap in plastic, and toss in your refrigerator's crisper.

HOW TO USE: Rinse thoroughly then use as a "shovel" for dip or salsa. Or chop into a salad to give it extra crunch. Celery pieces can also be used in a wide variety of soups and tomato sauces without much nutrient loss.

eryone else on the planet had been smitten with their fiery bite. And, just like everyone else, once I'd been "burnt," I couldn't stay away from the fire.

Now every restaurant meal becomes an opportunity to explore the peppers of a different culture, every family gathering becomes an opportunity to try out a recipe with a new pepper, and every visit to our local cantina becomes a chance to up the temperature gauge on my plate another notch.

"Ah!" I cry as I take a bite and the sweat beads on my forehead. "Yeth!" I enthuse as my seared tongue tries to regain its movement. I may not be the most dignified diner in the restaurant, as my husband has occasionally pointed out, but one thing's for sure: I've got the best-draining sinuses in the room.

The reason? Capsaicin, a naturally occurring plant chemical in peppers, seems to liquefy everything in my head but my brain and eyeballs. It unstuffs my nose, clears out my sinuses, sweats clean my pores, and clears the back of my throat—

something that only a doctor with a 12-syllable subspecialty had previously been able to do.

But I also like to eat peppers because studies show that they aid digestion, cut cholesterol, and "thin" your blood so that the artery-blocking blood clots that trigger heart attacks and strokes are less likely to form. What's more, preliminary studies in India indicate that peppers may also reduce a substance involved in triggering arthritic pain by 88 percent.

As if that's not enough to ask of any one nutrient, capsaicin will protect your stomach lining from the irritating effects of alcohol and acidic foods—a particular benefit around the holidays when someone accidentally overindulges in one or the other.

Mixed into a cream that's sold under the trade name Zostrix, capsaicin is also a topical pain reliever. Spread over an arthritic joint, on shingles, across a psoriatic plaque, on a nerve-damaged diabetic foot, or even over the area from which a limb has been amputated, the cream forces

CHILE BASICS

HOW TO BUY: Fresh or dried, hot peppers should be glossy, with a smooth skin. Pick Anaheim peppers for a mild bite, jalapeño for a taste of fire, and habañeros for an experience that strips the taste buds from your tongue.

HOW TO STORE: Fresh hot peppers should be wrapped, unwashed, in paper towels and placed in the refrigerator. They'll last for three weeks. Dried hot peppers should be kept in an sealed container at room temperature.

HOW TO USE: First, pull on a pair of plastic or rubber gloves. Then rinse the pepper under cold running water. If you want the full blast of a fresh pepper's heat, leave the seeds and interior ribs intact. Otherwise, take them out. Score the pepper with a knife, drop it into whatever you're cooking, then remove it before you serve.

For dried hot peppers, either pulverize them and add to the pot before cooking, or cut them into small pieces, soak in warm water for 30 minutes, then add peppers and water to whatever you're cooking.

Either way, peppers turn any dish to which they're added into something hot. Very hot.

nerves in the area to cough up all their substance P, a neurochemical that transmits pain messages to the brain. Fortunately, once nerves have cleared out their supply of substance P, they can't seem to make any more—at least not as long as you continue to rub the area with capsaicin.

The cream is so effective that in a study at the Geisinger Clinical Oncology Program in Danville, Pennsylvania, it cut post-surgical pain among cancer patients in half.

Unfortunately, the capsaicin in peppers is likely to take your skin off if you try smearing a homemade paste directly on your body. So if you'd like to try it as a topical pain reliever, check with your doctor first. He or she can help you figure out the appropriate strength and dosage of Zostrix.

Citrus: A Power Punch against Breast Cancer and Heart Disease

With all the researchers gathered around the giant poster on one side of the room in Montreal, it was hard to see what all the hubbub was about. But little by little, as each researcher finished reading, stepped away from the poster shaking his head and talking excitedly to one colleague or another in any one of the half dozen languages around me, I moved in a little closer. Finally I found myself right in front of the poster, next to a slim woman with light hair.

The woman was Najla Guthrie, Ph.D., a researcher at the University of Western Ontario's Centre for Human Nutrition in

---

CITRUS

BEST FOR HELPING YOU:

Prevent breast cancer

Lower cholesterol

Fight off heart disease

Prevent kidney stones

Lower blood pressure

Relax stiffened arteries

Stabilize blood sugar

Reduce the risk of colon cancer

Canada. And all the excitement spreading around the conference room full of scientists was due to a couple of studies she and her colleague Elzbieta Kurowska, Ph.D., had done on orange and grapefruit juice. Together, these women had demonstrated that orange and grapefruit juice could prevent breast cancer and lower cholesterol levels 43 and 32 percent respectively.

As I read first one and then the other study, factually laid out step by step on the giant posters, I could hardly believe what I was seeing.

In one study, Dr. Guthrie had given mice orange juice, grapefruit juice, or a supplement containing hesperidin and naringin—two naturally occurring substances in citrus—in place of their normal drinking water. The mice were genetically bred to develop breast cancer and Dr. Guthrie wanted to see whether the juices or the supplement might be able to prevent tumors once the process had been triggered.

The results? When cancer cells were injected directly into the breast tissue of each mouse, the mice that drank orange juice or grapefruit juice had half the tumors of the mice that drank regular water, says Dr. Guthrie.

They also had lower cholesterol levels. But the experiment hadn't been set up to evaluate cholesterol, so Dr. Kurowska did a separate study. Using rabbits fed a cholesterol-inducing diet, Dr. Kurowska found that, when compared to rabbits given plain water, rabbits that drank grapefruit juice had cholesterol levels that were

32 percent lower, and rabbits that drank orange juice had cholesterol levels that were 43 percent lower.

What's particularly interesting is that when animals were given supplements containing two flavonoids that were thought to be responsible for what was going on, the supplements didn't work as well as the whole juice.

"We're not completely sure what caused these effects," says Dr. Guthrie. It could be the liminoids or flavonoids in the juices—both of which are potent antioxidants. It could also be an as-yet undiscovered constituent of the whole fruit. Or it could even be a kind of synergy among the plant's constituents.

Clearly, more research is needed before scientists can say just how much juice a woman might need to get the same effects as lab animals, says Dr. Guthrie. "But I drink a glass of grapefruit juice every morning—and I'm glad that I always have."

The Fuss over Vitamin C

Aside from their potent ability to prevent cancer and high cholesterol, most citrus fruits also provide at least a day's supply of vitamin C, a decent amount of potassium, and a good shot of both soluble fiber—the kind that helps those with diabetes stabilize their blood sugar levels—and insoluble fiber, the kind that helps prevent constipation and colon cancer. Oranges, for example have about seven grams of fiber, while half a grapefruit has about six.

CITRUS BASICS

HOW TO BUY: Although most of us tend to reach for the biggest, orangy-est orange we can find, we may frequently be disappointed when the fruit is not as sweet as we expect. That's because the color of an orange has little to do with its sweetness. Oranges grown in Florida, for instance, are frequently greenish when ripe simply because the orange is exposed to warm temperatures day and night. Or sometimes it simply reverts to green when it sits ripely on the tree. Oranges grown in California and Arizona are usually a deep orange, but simply because they're exposed to warm days and cool nights.

To find the sweetest oranges, look for the smallest one with a green tinge. If you want lots of juice, pick a thin-skinned orange; if you want lots of flesh, pick a larger orange with a thicker skin. Other than that, don't worry about it. Since state laws govern when an orange is considered mature, an unripe orange rarely gets to market.

The same is pretty much true for grapefruit. Look for round, smooth, heavy globes and don't worry about whether or not they're ripe—they are.

HOW TO STORE: Oranges can be stored either in the refrigerator or on the countertop for up to two weeks. Grapefruit can be stored on the countertop for up to a week, then in the refrigerator for up to six weeks.

HOW TO USE: Fresh is best. Oranges can be rinsed, peeled with your fingers and eaten out of hand. Grapefruit should be rinsed, then cut in half and served with a drizzle of honey or a sprinkling of brown sugar. You might also like to scrape grapefruit sections out of the half shell, toss them with nuts, berries, and other fruits, then return the mixture to its shell.

What's more, a study at the University of Texas Southwestern Medical Center has found that orange juice may help prevent kidney stones, one of the most painful conditions—next to childbirth—that humans experience. The researchers first suspected a connection because orange juice contains two of the same constituents as the stone-fighting drug potassium citrate. To test their idea, the researchers asked 11 men with kidney stones to try three different regimens for three weeks. For the first week, the men were given potassium citrate. For the second, they were given a placebo. And for the third week, the men were given orange juice—about 400 milliliters three times a day.

When researchers compared urine samples from each week, they discovered that orange juice produced some of the same chemical effects as the potassium citrate. It didn't do quite as good a job as the drug, but it did do well enough that the researchers think it can help those with kidney stones who, for one reason or another, can't take the drug.

Orange juice and oranges have one more benefit that those with heart disease should seriously consider: The vitamin C they contain can actually lower blood pressure, increase the amount of HDL cholesterol, the kind that cleans clogged arteries, and relax the stiffened arteries that contribute to a heart attack.

In a study at the Medical College of Georgia, researchers found that the less ascorbic acid—the chemical name for vitamin C—you have, the higher your blood pressure is likely to be.

A second study, this one with more than 800 men and women done at the USDA's Human Nutrition Research Center in Beltsville, Maryland, found that the more vitamin C the study subjects had circulating in their bloodstream, the more HDL cholesterol was on the job to sweep up the LDL cholesterol that clogs arteries and sets you up for a heart attack.

And a third study, conducted by researchers from both Boston University Medical Center and Harvard Medical School, found that large amounts of ascorbic acid actually reverse some bad chemistry that can lead to a heart attack in people who already have heart disease. Specifically, the ascorbic acid restores normal functioning to the insides of disease-stiffened arteries. That allows them to relax and get bigger whenever a blood clot wanders through. The result is that the clot keeps on moving rather than getting stuck in the coronary artery and causing a heart attack.

How much ascorbic acid or vitamin C do you need? Although federal guidelines recommend only about 60 mg a day—the amount found in one small orange—most of the studies cited above found the kind of benefits they did with larger amounts. To get the same higher HDL levels as in the USDA study, you'd have to take up to 215 mg a day if you're a woman and 345 mg a day if you're a man—that's four to six servings of citrus.

There are two points here to remember: 1) You need more than a single serving of citrus a day to gain many of its benefits; 2) In several studies, eating the whole fruit or drinking a glass of its juice confers health benefits, while taking a supplement containing some of the orange's constituents does not.

Corn: Munch Your Risk of Colorectal Cancer in Half

Munching on the first ear of Silver Queen fresh from my neighbor's field is one of summer's special moments. The corn is rarely more than an hour or two from the sunburned fields, so each bite causes the kernels' smooth white skins to burst open with an audible pop. In fact, once I've placed a giant platter of steaming cobs on the picnic table—in those few moments of summer peace at twilight when the hummingbirds zip in for a last drink at the feeder, the barn swallows dip and dart over a field, and the bats fly overhead wondering if the cat's too big for an airlift back to their nursery—the contented sound of corn crunching and crickets is all you'll ever hear.

Canned or frozen corn never quite lives up to expectations nurtured by the rich flavor of field-ripened corn, so I generally stick to buying corn fresh and in season. And that means that from mid-July to the end of August, anyone who stops by our house around dinnertime is likely to sit down to a steaming feast of those pale, earthy cobs. As long as they don't slather the corn with butter, it also means that they're likely to leave the table a little healthier than when they arrived.

CORN

BEST FOR HELPING YOU:

Prevent colorectal cancer

For one thing, studies show that people who eat corn are less likely to develop colorectal cancer. In a study at the University of Hawaii Cancer Research Center in Honolulu, for example, researchers asked more than 1,100 men and women with colon or rectal cancer what they ate, then asked another 1,100 similar folks without cancer the same thing. When the researchers compared the diets of the two groups, they found that those who ate the most fiber from vegetables like corn were the least likely to have cancer. In actual numbers, men who ate the most fiber from vegetables like corn cut their risk of colorectal cancer by 40 percent. Women cut their risk in half.

The reason for this dramatic advantage among vegetable lovers in general and corn munchers in particular is still a mystery. The researchers found a protective effect for corn over and above its fiber content, so that made them suspect an as-yet-unidentified plant chemical at work. Although it will take a lot more re-

---

CORN BASICS

HOW TO BUY: Fresh. From the farm or from a refrigerated display at your market. Corn loses nearly half its natural sweetness within a day of being picked, so the closer you are to where it's grown and the colder it's kept before you buy it, the better. Look for deep green husks with damp, shining gold corn silk at the top. Pull back on one of the leaves just an inch or two and look for small kernels that look ready to pop. Large kernels at the end mean its over-ripe; dry brown corn silk means it probably hasn't got a nutrient left in its ear.

HOW TO STORE: Leave the husks on, drop the ears into a plastic bag, and place the corn in the refrigerator until it's time to shuck.

Whole books have debated this point, but the best way to preserve both flavor and nutrients seems to be a quick warming. Bring a pot of water to the boil, drop in a teaspoon of sugar, then drop in the ears. Shut off the heat and let it sit for five minutes. Serve promptly and forget about the traditional butter bath. With corn this fresh, you won't need it.

search before scientists can say exactly what's going on, one group of substances they're considering is protease inhibitors, naturally occurring chemicals that help your body fight off cancer.

But don't feel you have to wait for the final verdict. Whenever you're lucky enough to get next to fresh corn, feel free to stuff yourself silly.

Crunchy Crucifers: The Green Revolution

Not too long ago, crucifers were those stinky green vegetables you left behind with childhood. Today they're a major part of the green revolution that has overtaken American cuisine—and liable to pop up on your plate wherever you go.

And well they should. Broccoli, brussels sprouts, cabbage, cauliflower, kale, and mustard greens all contain two ingredients that, between them, provide one of the most effective anticancer arsenals on the planet. One nutrient is sulforaphane, a $12 word for a naturally occurring substance that boosts your body's defenses by increasing the number of enzymes that detoxify cancer-causing agents that slip into the body. The second nutrient is indol-3-carbinol, a substance that lowers levels of estrogens that feed certain types of cancers—specifically, breast, prostate, ovarian, and colon.

How effective are these nutrients? In a study at the Johns Hopkins Institutions, where researchers first identified sulforaphane, scientists exposed 145 laboratory animals to a cancer-causing agent. Some of the animals had not received any protective treatments, while others had received high doses of sulforaphane. Yet when scientists compared the two groups a couple of months later, nearly 70 percent of the unprotected animals had cancer, while only 26 percent of those given sulforaphane had a single tumor. The bottom line? Researchers are still puzzling it out, but it looks as though sulforaphane practically tripled the animals' ability to protect themselves from cancer.

Not bad for the constituent of a vegetable many of us used to sneak to the dog.

But as exciting as this new research is, let's not lose sight of all the other good nutrients in crucifers. Aside from its spectacular anticancer compounds, broccoli also has one-third of the vitamin A and folate you need to keep vision sharp and your body's DNA repair crew on the job every day. Brussels sprouts have nearly one-quarter the amount of

CRUNCHY CRUCIFERS

BEST FOR HELPING YOU:

Prevent cancer

Lower cholesterol

Maintain sharp vision

Repair damaged DNA

NO-STINK SPROUTS!

Even if you hated brussels sprouts as a kid, give 'em a second chance. New varieties developed by growers have less of the taste that made every red-blooded American kid think of running away from home. And many sprouts are now shipped under refrigeration—which means they're less likely to develop that bitter taste.

KIDS' FAVORITE FRUITS & VEGGIES

Tired of struggling to get your kids to eat more fresh fruits and veggies? A food industry survey reveals that these are the ones kids like best:

1. Bananas
2. Apples
3. Grapes
4. Oranges
5. Plums

6. Carrots
7. Lettuce
8. Tomatoes
9. Broccoli

CRUCIFEROUS BASICS

HOW TO BUY: As far as broccoli's concerned, do the opposite of what nutritionists have been telling you for years. Instead of looking for broccoli that's bright green and crisp, look for broccoli that's beginning to yellow, suggests John Pezzuto, Ph.D., director of the program in collaborative research in the pharmaceutical sciences at the University of Illinois. That tells you that the plant is under stress and will make as many protective nutrients as it can—including the ones that protect you from cancer. (Plants aren't selfless—they make those protective chemicals to protect themselves.)

As for brussels sprouts, forget trying to maximize nutrition and reach for the greenest ones you can find. Unfortunately, old brussels sprouts smell so bad that it's unlikely anyone entering your home will ever stay long enough to benefit from the extra protection they generate in their stressed state. (See Anita's "Brussels Sprouts in Garlic Butter" recipe on page 113 for a stinkless and yummy side dish featuring you-know-what.)

Cabbage heads should be heavy, with tightly furled leaves; cauliflower should have compact heads that are totally white. Mustard greens and kale should be small with fine stems and crisp green leaves.

All six crucifers should be bought only from refrigerated cases. Crucifers left at room temperature for any length of time will develop a bitter taste.

HOW TO STORE: Unwashed, in the refrigerator's crisper. First wrap greens in damp paper towels, drop them in a plastic bag and seal it before you place them in the crisper. Cauliflower, cabbage, brussels sprouts, and broccoli should go in an unsealed plastic bag.

HOW TO USE: Raw. Lightly steamed at the most. That's because a study at the University of Illinois found that cooking, storage, and freezing all destroyed anywhere from half to all the protective nutrients in broccoli. And until somebody proves differently, you can assume that the same thing happens with all the other crucifers.

Wash all crucifers before use and trim any stems. Cut into pieces for use in salads, or to steam rapidly in a small amount of water. The faster you steam crucifers, the fewer nutrients you lose, the more color you retain, and the less chance you have of developing a strong flavor.

folate you need, plus five grams of fiber to help keep cholesterol levels down. Cabbage has a touch of vitamin C and a dash of folate, while mustard greens have a quarter of the vitamin A and folate you need every day. And kale has a tiny smorgasbord of nutrients that includes vitamins A and C, calcium, iron, magnesium, and potassium.

Leafy Greens: Graze for All You're Worth

If you do nothing else to live a healthy life, try adding a plate full of leafy greens to your diet every day. No matter what goes wrong with your body, ten to one the variety of vitamins, minerals and neutraceuticals on that plate will give you enough ammunition to fight back—particularly against heart disease and cancer.

In a study of 70,000 nurses at Harvard Medical School, for example, researchers found that those who ate foods rich in folate and other B vitamins—all found abundantly in leafy greens—were half as likely to develop heart disease as those who didn't. What's more, a British study of some 11,000 health-conscious people found that after 17 years those who ate the most raw salad—yep, including leafy greens—were 26 percent less likely to have died from heart disease than those who went straight to the main course.

Where does such amazing protection come from? Greens offer a smorgasbord of nutritional warriors that attack disease on six different fronts. Here's how researchers tell us they do it:

LEAFY GREENS

BEST FOR HELPING YOU:

Maintain a steady heartbeat

Prevent heart disease

Prevent cancer

Keep your vision sharp

GREEN BASICS

HOW TO BUY: Crisp, green and fresh off the farm. If you shop at a supermarket, find out which days produce are delivered and be there. Buy only from refrigerated displays. Buy prewashed, precut bags of mixed greens only when you're bored and want to try a new mix of greens. Nutritionists are still arguing the matter, but it looks as though prewashed greens might not have quite the nutritional punch as greens left the way they were harvested.

HOW TO STORE: Wrapped and in your refrigerator for no more than a couple of days.

HOW TO USE: Swish in a sinkful of cold water, shake dry, remove stems where necessary, and tear or slice into bite-sized bits. The minute greens are cut, they start to lose nutrients, so keep preparation time as close to meal time as possible.

Serve greens raw. Cooking destroys the antioxidant lutein, a potent anticancer compound found in many greens. If you really must serve a hot green, you'll loose the least nutrients by washing the leaves in cold water, then—without drying—putting them in a covered dish and microwaving them according to manufacturer's directions. The water from their bath will steam the greens in seconds.

- Antioxidants like the carotenoid lutein in the leaves zap maverick molecules released by everyday air pollution, cigarette smoke, and normal body processes before they can cause trouble that leads to heart disease, cancer, arthritis, high cholesterol, and macular degeneration, the leading cause of blindness in elderly people.
- Indole-3-carbinols in leafy greens like arugula boost the numbers of your body's natural enzyme defense force to repel any carcinogen that tries to set up shop.
- Isothiocyanates in spicy greens like watercress also zap cancer-causing agents.
- Omega-3 fatty acids in purslane help chill the inflammatory process involved in a number of diseases including arthritis. They also help prevent artery-clogging blood clots from forming, a process that frequently leads to a heart attack or stroke.
- The folate in such heavy hitters as chicory, turnip greens, romaine and even iceberg lettuce literally counteract the heart disease-causing homocystein produced by your body whenever you eat protein.

Each green brings a unique group of vitamins, minerals and neutraceuticals to your plate. Chicory, in addition to its folate, for example, also has four grams of fiber plus nearly 10 percent of the magnesium and potassium you need every day to keep your heart beating in an even rhythm. It also contains nearly a third of the vitamin A you need to keep your vision sharp long into the future.

Beet greens, in addition to the antioxidant lutein, contain 2.1 grams of fiber, one-third the amount of vitamin A you need, plus a sprinkling of calcium, folate, iron, magnesium, potassium, riboflavin, and thiamine. Like folate, riboflavin and thiamine are also involved in helping your body neutralize homocystein.

Mustard greens, which add a nice tang to any salad mix, contain small amounts

---

MAKE YOUR OWN MINI-GREENHOUSE FOR GREENS!

Professional grower Connie Chipman of Bradford, Vermont, doesn't understand why everyone doesn't grow their own greens throughout the year.

"It's so easy," Chipman says in exasperation, "and you don't need a fancy greenhouse." Just grab a couple of old lawn chairs from the garage or basement. Pull off and recycle the plastic webbing, then twist the back and seat—each now a large, perfect square of aluminum pipe—apart from the rest of the chair. Stand the two squares on end, push them into the ground about four feet apart, and cover with heavy-duty clear plastic. (Tip: The cheap plastic drop cloths you find at paint centers everywhere are perfect.) Shovel dirt over the plastic's edges on three sides to weight it down. After your seeds are planted, weight the plastic's fourth side with rocks so that you have easy access.

The mini-greenhouse is great for growing broccoli, lettuces, radishes, and mini-carrots, says Chipman. You can even grow radishes and carrots all winter long. Just sow the seeds in September and cover with hay after they sprout. Then whenever you want some fresh carrots, just dig and enjoy!

of calcium, fiber, and folate, plus vitamins A and C.

Lamb's-quarters, which many people grow themselves, are a virtual multivitamin and mineral plant. In addition to nearly two grams of fiber, each serving contains a whopping 90 percent of your daily vitamin A requirement, 15 percent of the calcium you need to build strong bones, plus decent amounts of vitamin C, folate, magnesium, riboflavin, and thiamine.

Swiss chard, which is first cousin to a beet green, has nearly two grams of fiber plus 28 percent of a day's worth of vitamin A, 22 percent of the magnesium, and 20 percent of the iron, plus a small amount of calcium, potassium, and vitamin C.

The point is that although every leafy green is packed with nutritional warriors to protect your body from major problems like heart disease and cancer, each green is also nothing less than a tiny energy pump of nutrients able to keep cells, muscles, and organs running at peak efficiency.

Graze on a mixed variety of these babies, and you'll have every ounce of nutrition you need to live long and prosper.

Milk: Low-Fat Works Miracles

Unless you're into scarfing down a can full of sardines or football-shaped supplements every day, milk is your best bet to get the bone-building calcium you need to help protect against osteoporosis. It also contains lactoferrin, an amazing little protein that protects the body during

---

THE BROCCOLI ALTERNATIVE

Everybody likes the cancer-fighting nutrients in broccoli, but not everybody likes the taste.

What can you do? Eat broccoli sprouts instead. The sprouts have a mild, nutty taste that goes particularly well on a turkey sandwich with tomato, greens, and a low-fat vinaigrette. Yet they contain 10 to 100 times more of the anticancer nutrients than mature broccoli. What's more, while the amount of anticancer nutrients in mature broccoli varies widely from one plant to the next, the amount of anticancer nutrients in broccoli sprouts only varies between two levels: high and higher.

Broccoli sprouts are just beginning to appear in markets, but you can easily grow your own. Just buy some organic seeds and grab a one-quart, wide-mouthed canning jar out of your cupboard. Rinse the seeds, then soak them overnight in a jar two-thirds full of water. Any kind of water is fine as long as it's not chlorinated. The next morning, drain the seeds and rinse them with fresh water. Cover the top of your jar with an old (but clean) piece of cheesecloth and stick the jar on the kitchen counter out of the way and out of the light. As the seeds begin to sprout, rinse them twice a day, making sure to hold them upside-down over the sink to drain so that no water is actually left in the jar between rinsings. In three days your sprouts will have a rich earthy taste and you'll have a potent cancer fighter.

One caveat: Seeds intended for planting are frequently treated with chemicals. So make sure that any seeds you buy are organic and intended for your mouth, not the earth. If you have trouble getting them where you live, call Seeds of Change at 505-438-8080. They're a mail order company that specializes in organic seeds.

life-or-death moments when you have a severe infection, and it contains a sprinkling of vitamins and minerals that build sound muscles and nerves.

It can also protect you from stroke. A 22-year study of more than 3,000 middle-aged men at the Honolulu Heart Program found that men who drank two cups of milk a day cut their risk of stroke in half—a benefit not extended to those who passed up milk and tried to get their calcium from supplements.

And milk can apparently protect you from kidney stones as well. In a study at Harvard School of Public Health, researchers asked more than 45,000 men between the ages of 40 and 75 about the amount of calcium they got from food. Four years later, they took a look at who had had kidney stones and who had not. Significantly, they found that those who ingested the most calcium-rich food had reduced their risk of kidney stones by 44 percent.

But keep in mind that there is a vast difference between the health benefits of whole milk and low-fat milk—as evidenced by the people of Finland. Twenty-five years ago, the Finns were dying of heart attacks in unprecedented numbers. Scientists got busy with a public education campaign about the differences between whole milk and low-fat milk and, over time, the Finns began drinking low-fat milk and eating low-fat margarines. When researchers tallied up the results, they found that these simple dietary changes had cut the number of those dying of heart attacks in half.

Why such a difference? Just switching to lower-fat versions of milk and margarine significantly reduced the amount of saturated fat in Finnish diets, researchers explain. And since saturated fat is the raw material from which the body makes most of the cholesterol that clogs arteries, that one simple change knocked cholesterol levels down, and tuned an entire nation's hearts to a healthier beat.

On average, a study of more than 27,000 Finnish men and women found

MILK

BEST FOR HELPING YOU:

Fight off life-threatening infections

Prevent kidney stones

Prevent osteoporosis

Prevent stroke

MILK BASICS

HOW TO BUY: Buy low-fat or fat-free milk for adults; check with your family physician or pediatrician about which milk your child should drink. Keep in mind that children need some fat in their diet to absorb fat-soluble vitamins. Milk may or may not be a good source of that fat—especially since there's some concern among researchers that cow's milk can trigger non-insulin dependent diabetes when given to susceptible babies.

HOW TO STORE: In the fridge.

HOW TO USE: Straight up, over cereal, or whirled with fruit in the blender into a fruit smoothie. People who would like to drink fat-free milk but don't like the thin texture may find that adding a tablespoon of powdered fat-free milk to a glass of fat-free milk turns it into a totally acceptable beverage.

that individual cholesterol levels fell from 262 mg/dL to 228 mg/dL for men; and from 259 mg/dL to 212 mg/dL for women. Collectively, researchers found that the percentage of men between the ages of 30 and 59 with high cholesterol levels dropped from 15 percent to 3 percent. The percentage of women with high cholesterol fell from 16 percent to 2 percent.

Such a dramatic change makes sense when you realize that whole milk is 3.25 percent fat—or a whopping eight grams of fat per serving. Low-fat milk contains 1 percent fat with 2.5 grams of fat per serving, and skim milk is fat free. Now think

about drinking four glasses of milk a day, which is what most of us need to get our daily allotment of bone-building calcium and vitamin D. If we drink whole milk, that's 32 grams of fat a day—and nearly 22 grams of it is pure, artery-clogging saturated fat!

Very few of us have arteries that can withstand the onslaught of 32 grams of fat every day—especially not in addition to the fat that we get in the rest of our food. But 10 grams of fat from low-fat milk, especially when you consider its protective effects, is definitely more affordable. And for those of us who need to watch our weight, skim milk—with all the nutrients and only a trace of fat—is the best deal around.

Unfortunately, USDA surveys indicate that 25 percent of Americans between the ages of 20 and 50 are not drinking any milk at all.

Mushrooms: Fragile Fungi with the Power to Boost Your Immune System

Nurtured by crumbling logs and moist woods, "'Shrooms"—as fungiophiles call them—have been used to heal for nearly 4,000 years in the East. Those of us who live in the West haven't used them for anywhere near that long, but as East and West continue to open their markets and minds to one another, the most potent of these mushrooms—enoki, maitake, and shiitake—are finding their way into our homes and hearts.

Enoki are a mild-flavored white mushroom frequently used as a visual counterpoint to a bed of mixed greens in Japanese restaurants. Not well studied in Western terms, some doctors think that enoki contain a cancer-fighting compound called flammulin, which may strengthen the immune system.

Maitake mushrooms have a little more flavor and probably a lot more healing power than their enoki cousins. A study at Gunma University School of Health Sciences in Japan found that something in the maitake mushroom reduced the rate of bladder cancer in laboratory mice by 46 percent. Other studies at Tokyo University of Pharmacy and Life Science show that eating maitake mushrooms actually activates several immune system cells that protect you from cancer-causing agents. Generally sold in large, flavorful strips, maitake mushrooms are used in Japan to enhance the effects of chemotherapy, protect the liver, and fight hepatitis B.

Shiitake mushrooms—my favorites—have a deep, smoky flavor that complements chicken, pork, or shrimp in particular. Laboratory studies show that they contain eritadenine, a naturally occurring substance that lowers cholesterol, and lentinan, a related substance that seems to block the formation of cancer-causing agents commonly found in many fruits and vegetables. Lentinan may also stimulate natural killer cells and macrophages, which are two key players in your immune system that are known to attack and kill tumor cells.

Other studies indicate that lignins—a major constituent of dietary fiber—in shiitake mushrooms may protect the body from cold sores and herpes infections, while they also discourage HIV cells from maturing and growing up to damage the body's T-cells.

More research is necessary before doctors start saying, "Take two mushrooms and call me in the morning." But it looks as though those who regularly incorporate 'shrooms into their diet are giving their bodies a healthful boost.

MUSHROOMS

BEST FOR HELPING YOU:

Enhance cancer treatment

Increase immune system cells

Fight viruses that cause cold sores and HIV

Protect your liver

Fight hepatitis B

Lower cholesterol

Prevent cancer

Okra: Power Pods with Digestive Punch

Despite attempts by northern bigots at character assassination, okra is not slimy. Cooked right—i.e., by my Aunt Ellen—okra is a crisp vegetable with a sharp taste that adds a bite of reality to anything in which it's mixed. It also has so much fiber that it helps prevent diverticulitis, chronic constipation, irritable bowel syndrome, and high cholesterol.

In a study at Harvard School of Public Health, for example, researchers asked more than 47,000 men about their dietary habits, then, for the next four years, checked on what they ate. After adjusting their figures for everything under the sun—age, dietary fat, and physical exercise, for example—researchers found that those with diets rich in vegetable fiber—yes, the kind found in okra—were 42 percent less likely to develop diverticular disease than those who ate very little.

MUSHROOM BASICS

HOW TO BUY: Dried or fresh. Fresh mushrooms should be blemish-free with a dry, unwrinkled surface. Dried mushrooms should be professionally packaged and labeled—not scooped out of a dusty basket and tossed in a paper bag. Nor should they be harvested from your backyard. Do not ever, ever pick mushrooms on your own. What you don't know can kill you.

HOW TO STORE: Fresh mushrooms should be stored, unwashed, in a paper bag in your refrigerator. They'll stay fresh for up to five days. Dried mushrooms should be stored either in their original packaging or in a glass jar. Keep them away from light and humidity.

HOW TO USE: Anything that grows in the woods has a microbe factory hanging on to its gills. So let mushrooms soak in a sink of warm water for 10 minutes, then swish them around to loosen any soil. Rinse each mushroom individually under cold running water.

All fungi contain natural toxins that are destroyed by heat. So always cook mushrooms before eating, even if you're using them in a salad. Mushrooms are fabulous added to everything you cook—stir fries, pasta dishes, vegetable medleys, baked chicken, and just about anything you can think of.

Dried mushrooms must be reconstituted before use. To do so, soak in warm water for 15 minutes, then discard the liquid. You'll lose some of the nutrients, but there are many more from which to benefit.

A second study, this one at the University of Kentucky, found that those who increased their fiber consumption by only five grams a day were able to reduce their cholesterol levels by an incredible 13 percent. Okra has about 5½ grams of fiber per serving.

Okra also contains 6,800 units of the carotenoid lutein, which fights macular degeneration in older folks, plus 88 micromilligrams of folate—a nice chunk to help your body fight off heart disease, cancer, and some potentially life-threatening birth defects that strike in the earliest moments of pregnancy.

Onions: Living, Breathing Heart Builders

Onions deserve far more than a perch on top of your hamburger. They contain more than 25 different compounds—most of which seem determined to keep your cardiovascular system and respiratory tract in peak condition—that should earn them a more prominent place on your plate.

One compound is prostaglandin A-2, a naturally occurring substance that helps reduce your blood pressure. Another is quercetin, an antioxidant that prevents LDL cholesterol from damaging your arteries, vacuums up excess iron from your blood, and slows the buildup of platelets in your bloodstream that can clump together to trigger a heart attack. A third compound is actually a whole family of compounds that give onions their stink. The same constituents that cause the stink also enable these compounds to increase the HDL cholesterol that removes LDL cholesterol from your bloodstream and decrease triglycerides, which are nasty little fat molecules in your blood that doctors use as a marker for heart disease.

OKRA

BEST FOR HELPING YOU:

Prevent diverticulitis

Fight chronic constipation

Soothe an irritable bowel

Lower high cholesterol

OKRA BASICS

HOW TO BUY: Look for fresh pods not more than three inches long. Longer ones tend to be tough and stringy. Frozen okra works in soups, stews, and gumbos.

HOW TO STORE: Au natural. Bag it and pop it in the fridge.

HOW TO COOK: Wash first. Then decide whether you're using the okra in a salad, as a side dish or to thicken a soup, stew, or gumbo.

If you're using it for a salad, microwave the pods whole with a tablespoon of water in a covered dish for three or four minutes. Cool in the refrigerator, then slice into cartwheels and toss into your salad.

If you're using okra for a side dish, sauté either tiny whole pods or sliced larger ones quickly in a little canola oil either alone or mixed with chopped onions, garlic, and tomato. Serve hot.

Or if you're using okra to thicken a soup, stew or gumbo, cut it up and drop into the pot and simmer.

The rule of thumb is: Cut it into pieces if you want the slimy stuff (some people like it); use small, whole pods if you don't.

What's more, they also tend to smother inflammation throughout the body, particularly in your respiratory tract where it may be the result of allergies or asthma.

How effective are onions?

A study by the National Public Health Institute in Finland may give us a clue. Researchers there asked more than 5,000 women and men between the ages of 30 and 69 what they ate, then monitored their diet and health for the next 20 years. And, of course, they kept track of who died. Amazingly, the researchers found that women who ate the most onions were half as likely to have died of heart disease as those who ate the least. Men didn't have quite as good a result—but 26 percent were less likely to die.

Some researchers also feel that onions protect against cancer. In one study, for example, researchers at the University of Limburg in the Netherlands monitored more than 3,000 men and women between the ages of 55 and 69 over a three-year period, then studied what everyone had eaten. They found that those who consumed at least half an onion a day had half the risk

ONIONS

BEST FOR HELPING YOU:

Prevent death from heart disease

Lower cholesterol

Smother respiratory inflammation

OKRA: A NEW TWIST ON A TRADITION FROM THE OLD SOUTH

The traditional way to cook okra is to slice it, roll it in cornmeal and fry it in bacon grease in a big old black skillet you inherited from your mama who, of course, got it from her mama before her.

Unfortunately, this absolutely meltingly scrumptious way of preparing okra is one of the reasons that the South has traditionally had more heart disease and stroke than many other areas of the country. Frying creates a slew of free radicals that damage your arteries, and your body turns the saturated fat in bacon grease into cholesterol that will travel those arteries looking for any cells the free radicals have damaged. When the cholesterol finds a damaged cell, it tries to repair the damage by spackling itself over the area. The result is a narrowed and stiffened artery that will reduce blood flow to your heart and brain. So after the grease squad gets done with its repair job, all it would take to trigger a heart attack or a stroke would be a wandering blood clot that hit that narrowed patch of artery and got stuck.

That's why, as fabulous as okra fried in bacon grease tastes, I just don't make it. Instead, I take a half-pound of okra, wash it, slice it, roll it in organically grown cornmeal, then quickly sauté it with a handful of crisp, already cooked and drained bacon bits in just a tablespoon or two of canola oil.

The result is a crunchier okra that honors its Southern heritage, but pledges its allegiance to the more health-conscious cuisine of the New South.

of stomach cancer as those who ate less. In fact, the effect was so strong that it looks as though every bite of onion decreased the risk of stomach cancer.

But laboratory studies by the same researchers have also found that onions do not protect against cancer of the breast, colon, or lung. And at least two laboratory studies at the Osaka City University Medical School in Japan have found that several of the sulfur compounds in onions may, in fact, promote the growth of cancer in certain organs, particularly the liver.

Nobody's sure exactly what's going on, but the Japanese researchers cautioned that onions may protect some organs, while actually stimulating tumor growth in others.

The bottom line? Researchers are back at their test tubes trying to find it. But until they get it figured out, common sense suggests that those who are at risk for heart disease should feel free to chomp down as many onions as they like. Those who have cancer, have a genetic predisposition or family history of cancer, or smoke should talk to their doctors before loading up.

Radishes: A Healthy Garnish that Fights Cancer

Although generally thought of more as a garnish for summer salads, radishes actually contain isothiocyanates, protease inhibitors, kaempferol, dithiolthiones, and vitamin C—all of which seem to play important roles in reducing your risk of cancer.

Their content shouldn't be surprising when you consider that they're charter members of the cruciferae family—a family in which such notable progeny as broccoli and cabbage have been found to be powerful anticancer agents.

No studies have yet proven the radish's firepower at the table, but with cousins like these you can pretty well assume that it's a great idea to include them at your family gatherings.

ONION BASICS

HOW TO BUY: Look for firm, fresh onions with dry, papery skins. Avoid sweet onions, which have fewer of the healthy sulfur compounds than their more pungent cousins. Also avoid any onions that are tinged with green or any that have started to sprout. Feel free to buy fresh leeks, shallots, scallions, and chives as well. All contain the same heart-healthy compounds.

HOW TO STORE: Unwrapped, in your refrigerator's crisper. Leave enough room between each onion for air to circulate.

HOW TO USE: Most of the health-enhancing compounds an onion possesses are found in the papery skin and outer rings. So try to find recipes like soups and stews that will allow you to use the whole onion, skin and all. Just rinse the onion under cold running water, quarter it, and toss all four quarters into the pot. Cover and simmer with other veggies according to recipe directions.

Shellfish: A Fabulous Replacement for Meat

The one thing you can count on when I come to town is that if there's a Red Lobster, Crab Trap, or local Seafood Shanty, that's where we'll have dinner.

Shellfish is my passion. And although dipping any part of a lobster, crab, clam, or scallop in pure butter is likely to instill bliss, I generally prefer to tug the sweet, delicate meat from its shell and slurp it down au natural. That way I can sense all the flavor subtleties of the sea as the shellfish slides over my taste buds.

Avoiding traditional additives like butter and cream sauces is, of course, the key to using shellfish healthfully. Fresh from its shell, any shellfish is the perfect alternative to meat. It's low in calories, low in fat, and—despite popular belief—low in cholesterol. (Years ago, nutritionists made the mistake of measuring a particular kind of fat as cholesterol. Newer analytical methods have corrected the error.)

A single three-ounce serving of steamed blue crab contains an amazing 17 grams of muscle-building protein, three times the amount of vitamin B12 you need for steady nerves, a whopping 34 micromilligrams of heart-healthy selenium, more than 10 percent of the folate you need to repair damaged DNA, and 25 percent of the amount of zinc you need to run three major body systems: the immune system, nervous system, and endocrine system.

Unfortunately, there's a bit of a catch: 362 calories, 2 grams of mostly good fat, and 85 milligrams of cholesterol.

Lobster does almost as well. A 3½-ounce serving of cooked lobster contains 21 grams of protein, 25 percent of the zinc, and all the vitamin B12 you need for an entire day, plus 13 percent

---

RADISHES

BEST FOR HELPING YOU:

Reduce your risk of cancer

SHELLFISH

BEST FOR HELPING YOU:

Maintain your immune system

Build muscle

Build strong nerves

Stay at a healthy weight

RADISH BASICS

HOW TO BUY: Radishes comes in a variety of shapes and colors. Generally, they should all be hard and solid, with a smooth, unblemished surface and perky green leaves. If you're buying red radishes, reach for the smallest. Larger ones are likely to have a mealy texture inside.

HOW TO STORE: Remove the tops and use in a salad the day you bring them home. Store the radish globes in plastic bags, punch a couple of holes in the bags, then toss in the crisper. Use as soon as possible.

HOW TO USE: Scrub well, then slice off the root and stem ends. Do NOT peel. Much of a radish's nutritional goodness is found in its skin. Use radishes much as you would any other vegetable: Microwave them, covered, with a tablespoon of water, for two or three minutes or stir-fry them with other vegetables in a colorful vegetable medley.

of the magnesium you need to keep your blood pressure on an even keel and prevent kidney stones. The price tag for this delicious treat is even less than for crab: 98 calories, a trace of fat, and 72 milligrams of cholesterol. (But we won't talk about real price tags here—unless you're in Maine, lobster's pretty pricey.)

But my nominee for healthiest shellfish of them all is the lowly clam. A single 3½-ounce serving of steamed clams has 26 grams of protein, nearly five times the daily amount of vitamin B12 you need to run your nervous system, close to a two-day supply of iron, 31 percent of the riboflavin your body needs to use many of the nutrients you eat, and 25 percent of the zinc you need to power the immune, nervous, and endocrine systems.

The cost? A meager 148 calories, 2 grams of mostly good fat, and 67 grams of cholesterol. And with 112 milligrams of sodium, clams have far less sodium than most of their shellfish brethren.

Shellfish is a particularly important source of zinc for older folks. A study at the University of Pavia in Italy found that although the elderly are frequently deficient in this mineral, increased amounts of dietary zinc can help zip up an aging immune system.

SHELLFISH BASICS

HOW TO BUY: Fresh—and preferably from a local fishmonger rather than a supermarket. Fishmongers are specialists who know what's good from where and when. In my experience, supermarket folks rarely seem to know more than the price per pound.

From November through May, look for fresh stone crab claws from Florida. Mid-May, check for the incredibly sweet soft-shell crab fresh from the Atlantic. Midwinter, Alaskan crab legs are at peak, although you'll likely only find them frozen. Fresh lobster off the coast of Maine is available from January through June. Fresh sea scallops are harvested off-shore all year-round, while the tiny bay scallops are available fresh only in the fall. Oysters and clams are available year-round, although you may want to avoid them during the warm-water months. (Because both clams and oysters filter at least 15 gallons of water a day through their shells, many people in populated shore areas prefer not to eat them in warm months when bacteria counts in water are high.)

In general, you should use your eyes and your nose. Clams, oysters, and mussels should have tightly closed shells. Crabs and lobster should be moving. Scallops should smell sweet and have a healthy sheen. Healthy scallop colors range from pink to beige. (Avoid any that are pure white—it may indicate that they have been soaked in water to up their weight.)

Other shellfish, like shrimp, are available year-round in a frozen state.

HOW TO STORE: Fresh shellfish should be covered with damp paper towels and placed in the refrigerator as soon as you buy them—particularly if they're live. Don't place them in any type of bag or in water. They'll die. And the healthiest shellfish is the one who's kept happy right up until the moment he dies.

HOW TO USE: As a replacement for meat as often as you can afford it.

Spinach:
A Triple-Threat Green

Whether it's a crinkly Savoy or a generic flat-leaved variety, spinach leaves are rich in heart-healthy folic acid and cancer-fighting carotenoids. Raw, it contains more than 10,000 units of the carotenoid lutein, a powerful antioxidant which accumulates in the eye to prevent macular degeneration—the leading cause of blindness in older folks. Cooked, it contains even more—12,600 units in a single serving. And that makes it one of the best sources on the planet.

A single serving of spinach also contains nearly 50 percent of the amount of folate you need to repair free radical damage to your body's DNA and help keep heart disease at bay. A recent study at the Harvard School of Public Health in Boston reveals that one single serving a day of green leafy vegetables reduces the risk of a heart attack or stroke by 11 percent.

Spinach also has 28 percent of the magnesium you need to maintain a healthy blood pressure. It also contains calcium, but the benefits are actually neutralized by oxalates, which are substances in spinach that contribute to the formation of kidney stones in people with a predisposition toward them. Obviously, people who have had kidney stones should be eating spinach in moderation.

SPINACH
BEST FOR HELPING YOU:
Repair DNA
Maintain a healthy heart
Prevent stroke
Keep your blood pressure steady
Prevent cancer
Prevent macular degeneration

Tomatoes: The Power
to Prevent Prostate Cancer

Who would've thought that those giant summer sandwiches stuffed with vine-ripened tomatoes could protect men from prostate cancer?

Who would've thought that the giant pizzas our children scarfed down in high school could do the same?

"They can," says Steven K. Clinton, M.D., Ph.D., director of the Dana-Farber Cancer Institute and a professor at Harvard Medical School in Boston. While prostate cancer accounts for nearly half of all new cancers in American men, a study recently conducted at Harvard Medical School found that men who eat five to seven servings of tomatoes concentrated in sauces,

---

SPINACH BASICS

HOW TO BUY: Fresh. Look for crisp leaves with a deep green color.
HOW TO STORE: Unwashed. Put it in a plastic bag, then toss the whole thing in the crisper of your refrigerator.
HOW TO USE: Wash well, remove any thick stems, then cook, covered, in your microwave with a teaspoon of olive or canola oil to help your body absorb the lutein. Stir-frying equally releases the power of spinach.

pizzas, or salsas every week reduced their risk of prostate cancer by a whopping 40 percent. What's more, laboratory studies indicate that concentrated tomato products delayed tumor growth in mice that already had the cancer.

Addressing a group of scientists from around the country who had gathered at a lakefront retreat near Chicago to share their work, Dr. Clinton explained that simply incorporating a single serving of concentrated tomato-based products in the diet every day might be enough to prevent the onset of prostate cancer. And if it doesn't and cancer does get started, tomato-based products might be able to delay tumor growth until we're too old to care.

"We don't mind if we die at 120 with prostate cancer," says Dr. Clinton—as long as it doesn't bother us until then.

Prostate cancer is a disease that takes decades to develop, he explains. Studies have found that it exists in 20 to 60 percent of men in their 30s, although, typically, the disease isn't generally symptomatic until somewhere in the 60s.

That may mean that it's possible to prevent or delay prostate cancer, particularly if tomato-based products are incorporated into the diet during those periods critical to the prostate's development—in the mother's diet while a male child's prostate is developing in utero, during adolescence when a boy's prostate increases fivefold, and during the early 30s when a man's prostate once again begins to grow.

The protective constituent, researchers suspect, is a potent antioxidant called lycopene which gives tomatoes their bright red color—and which is known to accumulate in the prostate itself. Scientists figure that it's got to be in there for a reason, although, as Dr. Clinton points out, it might just be a marker for something else. Supporting the notion that lycopenes are involved, however, is

TOMATOES

BEST FOR HELPING YOU:

Prevent prostate cancer

TOMATO BASICS

HOW TO BUY: Fresh. Look for smooth, heavy tomatoes that are bright red. Leave the green-topped lightweights on the shelf.

HOW TO STORE: Ripe tomatoes should be stored in the crisper and used within three days. Unripe tomatoes can be left in a cool area out of the light until they ripen, then popped in the crisper.

HOW TO USE: Cooked, with a monounsaturated oil like olive oil. Heat actually breaks down cell walls and releases lycopene from a web of substances that keep it locked inside the tissues of a raw tomato. And the small amount of olive oil you should add—to a sauce, for example—enables your body to absorb the lycopenes that have been released.

If you don't have time to make your own sauce, feel free to use a canned paste or bottled sauce. Both will supply just as many lycopenes as a homemade product.

One caveat: Studies indicate that tomato juice apparently does not protect against prostate cancer. The jury's still out on why that might be—although some researchers suspect that the reason is that it's consumed without any fat to aid absorption.

a new study at Harvard which indicates that, no matter what your age, the more lycopenes you consume, the lower your risk of prostate cancer. As amazing as the effect of the tomato is on prostate cancer, there's still one more accomplishment we need to lay at its feet: in a study of 1,379 European men, researchers found that those who ate the most lycopene were half as likely to have a heart attack as those who consumed the least.

Clearly, for men who intend to live long and prosper, any dish that contains a tomato is a step in the right direction.

Watermelon: Summertime Nutrition

Slurping down the icy-cold fruit of a watermelon and spitting seeds off the front porch is as much a part of an American summer as Huckleberry Finn and the Fourth of July. Every year we manage to scarf down almost 3 billion pounds—and give ourselves a nice shot of five potent nutrients that help us stay young and healthy.

One of those nutrients is glutathione, a powerful antioxidant that neutralizes deadly molecules created by cigarette smoke, stress, air pollution, sunlight and other substances. Since these molecules would otherwise have gone on to damage our bodies' cellular blueprints and trigger many of the diseases we associate with aging, it's a good bet that watermelon is one of the foods that helps keep us young.

How effective is glutathione? No one knows for sure. But a study at the University of Michigan indicates that it may be pretty powerful. The Michigan researchers checked blood levels of glutathione in 33 people over the age of 60, then compared those levels to the number of health problems reported by study participants. They found that the more glutathione people had, the lower their blood pressure, cholesterol, and weight, and the fewer health problems they reported. On the other hand, the less glutathione people had, the more likely they were to report arthritis, diabetes, and heart disease.

WATERMELON

BEST FOR HELPING YOU:

Get rid of excess fluid

Fight cancer

Maintain healthy levels of cholesterol, blood pressure, and weight

---

WATERMELON BASICS

HOW TO BUY: Look for a round, smooth-skinned melon with no nicks or cuts. A glossy green top and yellow bottom indicate it's ripe. Despite all the melon thumpers in the market, thumping a melon really doesn't help you figure out whether or not it's ripe. Avoid buying sliced watermelon unless it's just been cut in front of you. Cut watermelon rapidly begins to lose some of its nutrients.

HOW TO STORE: No matter where you need to shove everything else, store watermelon in the refrigerator. Once cut, watermelon slices can be wrapped and stored in the crisper for no more than a day.

HOW TO USE: Rinse, slice, and slurp. You can get complicated with cutlery if you want to, but that kind of defeats a watermelon's purpose: to keep your life as simple as it is healthful.

But watermelon isn't just a one-nutrient band. A single serving also contains 20 percent of the vitamin A you need to protect cell walls from invading viruses, plus a big bite of vitamin C to help keep cholesterol down. It also contains cucurbitacin, a substance that fights cancer, and citrulline, a naturally occurring diuretic that helps get rid of excess fluid that accumulates in your hands and feet during hot weather.

Yogurt: Armor-Plating Your Gut and Vagina

Glancing down at his Mickey Mouse watch, Bruce Chassey, Ph.D., head of nutrition and food science at the University of Illinois, checks the time, then looks back at his colleague across the table. It's been a long day. Scientists from all over the country have gathered at a conference center near Chicago to talk about their research, and in a very few minutes coffee will be served and the conference coordinator will wind things up. In the meantime, however, yet another colleague has taken advantage of

SPIT IT OUT!

Wanna get kids to eat more watermelon? Sponsor a seed-spitting contest. Set out markers and see whose seed goes the farthest. The world record for seed-spitting is 66 feet 11 inches.

Dr. Chassey's presence to quiz him about "probiotics"—a scientific buzz word that literally means "for life."

I try to follow the conversation, but the two men are slicing through a world of chemical reactions and biological relationships that need more than a year of college biology to understand. What I gather, however, and what Dr. Chassey later confirms, is that the microbes contained in yogurt actually set up housekeeping in the lining of the intestine—and that several strains of bacteria found in yogurt may actually help create and maintain a healthy gut and vagina.

Streptococcus thermophilus and *Lactobacillus bulgaricus*, for instance, are the two bacteria that give yogurt its smooth texture

YOGURT

BEST FOR HELPING YOU:

Jump-start a sluggish bowel

Prevent osteoporosis

Avoid vaginal infections

Zip up the immune system

ARE LYCOPENE SUPPLEMENTS BETTER?

Probably not. Anyone interested in preventing prostate cancer and heart disease should probably stick to cooked, whole tomato products like stewed tomatoes or tomato paste. Researchers don't know for sure whether the tomato's therapeutic effects are from the lycopene in the tomato, the lycopene interacting with another tomato compound, or an as-yet undiscovered compound that simply rides along with the lycopene. So until researchers figure it out, you're probably better off reaching for a bottle of spaghetti sauce, not a bottle of pills.

Besides, let's get real: A bottle of 30 pills can cost up to $21. A can of tomato paste costs around 21 cents.

and sour taste. But they also produce lactase, an enzyme that breaks down milk sugars so dairy products can be digested. Most of us make our own lactase as infants, but we seem to lose much of that ability as we age. In fact, except for northern Europeans and their descendants, most of us develop a downright deficiency of lactase as we age. And that means we're likely to get cramps and bloating whenever we eat dairy products—a real problem not only because it's uncomfortable, but because it stops us from eating the calcium-rich dairy products we need to help maintain bone mass and avoid osteoporosis.

Enzyme replacements such as Lact-Aid are available to counteract a lactase deficiency, of course, but yogurt already contains its own natural lactase replacement—and it doesn't cost an extra dime.

As helpful as *Streptococcus thermophilus* and *Lactobacillus bulgaricus* are, however, there are two other bacteria that frequently occur in yogurt that are sending ripples of excitement through the scientific community: *Lactobacillus acidophilus* and *Bifidobacterium*.

Yogurt that contains acidophilus has been touted as a folk remedy for vaginal yeast infections for years. But many doc-

---

HOW TO MAKE AUNT ELLEN'S WATERMELON BASKET

Down at my Aunt Ellen's in South Carolina, a pretty way of presenting fruit on a hot summer day is to pile it into a deep, cool watermelon basket.

To make the basket, rinse and pat dry one whole watermelon. Slice a small, thin piece off the bottom of the melon (the yellow side) so that it will lie flat. Place a thick tea towel on the counter for traction, then place the melon on the towel, flat side down. Using the point of a small, sharply pointed knife, lightly trace a line lengthwise around the entire circumference of the melon. Begin at the stem and just go right around the whole thing. To make the handle, trace two parallel lines about 1½ to 2 inches apart across the width of the melon, stopping on either side of the melon at the line you've already traced.

Now, using a long serrated knife, cut into the melon along the edges of the handle you just drew (along each of the parallel lines). Cut about halfway into the melon, stopping at the first line of circumference you drew. Now, cut along the line that marks the circumference stopping on each side when you reach the handle. When you've finished, you should be able to lift out one-quarter of the melon as a single section.

To finish, scoop all the ripe, pink flesh out of the melon—including the arch that forms the handle (though be careful not to make the handle too thin or it will break). If desired, make alternating cuts left and right along the rim to create a saw-toothed edge. Remove seeds from the scooped-out melon, shape it into bite-sized balls with a melon baller, and return the balls to the basket. Mix in other melon balls, such as cantaloupe or honeydew, and bite-sized pieces of fruit, such as peaches or grapes, until the basket overflows. Then toss in a handful of blueberries for color.

The entire project takes about 20 minutes and makes a fabulous centerpiece for any summer picnic or barbecue. You can slice the leftover sections into chunks and serve along with the basket—or you can sneak them back into the fridge and save them for tomorrow morning's breakfast.

tors openly dismissed the notion until 1996, when an Israeli study found that five ounces of acidophilus-rich yogurt a day reduced the incidence of chronic vaginal infections by 35 percent. That study, which compared 23 women with recurrent vaginal infections who ate acidophilus-rich yogurt with an equal number of infection-prone women who simply ate regular pasteurized yogurt, found that the acidophilus bacteria actually took up residence in cells lining the rectum and vagina of those who ingested it. No one's really sure how the acidophilus interacts with the yeast, although some researchers suspect that it produces a chemical compound which prevents *Candida albicans*—the itchy little yeast with which most women are intimately familiar—from surviving.

Solving this particular health problem would be more than enough to justify its existence on the planet. But acidophilus may have one or two other gifts as well. A study at the University of Nebraska at Lincoln found that at least one strain of acidophilus stimulates the production of several immune system cells, while laboratory studies at the National Institute for

---

YOGURT BASICS

HOW TO BUY: As promising as these studies are, it is sometimes difficult to get all of the health benefits they suggest from commercially processed yogurt. The longer acidophilus is stored, the fewer health-giving bacteria it contains, says Dr. Chassey. The same occurs in bifido-containing yogurts. The bacterium simply doesn't like being exposed to oxygen, nor does it like acid—not the kind that naturally occurs in your stomach or the kind that naturally occurs as milk evolves into yogurt.

So how do you get the yogurt you need?

Commercially, any yogurt labeled "live, active cultures" or "LAC" will contain a minimum of 100 million live bacteria per gram. Most of those bacteria are likely to be the kind that makes lactase. So if you're eating yogurt as a rich source of calcium to help prevent osteoporosis, buying containers marked "LAC" will get you what you want.

If you're eating yogurt to gain the health benefits of acidophilus or bifido, however, you'll want to buy containers which are labeled "LAC" and which list acidophilus or bifido. Acidophilus is common; bifido is not. Look for it in appropriately marked containers of Stonyfield Farms yogurt, which is also organic.

TWO CAVEATS: Since many of the healthful bacteria start dying the moment milk turns into yogurt, check the expiration date on any yogurt you buy—and buy the ones with the dates farthest away. And avoid any yogurt that's been heat-treated. Heat kills bacteria.

HOW TO STORE: In the refrigerator.

HOW TO USE: Promptly. The longer you let yogurt sit in the refrigerator, the fewer healthful bacteria you get. Use it not only "as is," but as a delightful topping for cereal and fruit, or as a fabulous replacement for sour cream—both on potatoes and in baked goods. Just keep in mind that a single serving of yogurt's bacteria can only survive in your gut for a few days. To maintain its healthful benefits, you'll need to eat it on a regular basis.

the Study of Cancer Treatment in Milan, Italy, have found that the growth of breast cancer cells is inhibited by 85 percent when they're exposed to acidophilus.

But as therapeutic as acidophilus may be, *Bifidobacterium*—or bifido as its researchers usually call it—seems to have equal potential. One study indicates that women who ate 250 grams—about seven ounces—of bifido-containing yogurt every day were able to significantly speed up the amount of time it takes for food to pass through the gut. For older folks who frequently suffer from painful constipa-tion or a "sluggish" bowel that makes them feel nauseated a couple of hours after every meal, bifido may be a godsend.

There is also a preliminary study from the American Health Foundation in Valhalla, New York, which indicates that eating a particular strain of bifido may actually prevent the formation of tumors in the colon. And a survey of research over a 30-year period by researchers at the University of Washington in Seattle indicates that both bifido and acidophilus will prevent the nasty diarrhea that frequently accompanies the use of antibiotics.

Stir-Fried Artichoke and Scallops with Angel Hair Pasta

*H*eat wok on medium-high heat and add oil. Add garlic, onion and red pepper and stir-fry about 4 to 5 minutes or until the onion is softened. Remove the vegetables from the wok.

In a large pot, bring three quarts of water to a boil to cook the pasta.

To the hot wok, add the scallops and cook about 3 minutes. Add the saved vegetables, artichoke hearts, chopped tomatoes, and basil to the wok. Cover and cook about 2 minutes.

Boil the angel hair pasta for 2 minutes. Drain. Add to the wok and combine well with the scallops. Garnish with basil.

INGREDIENTS

YIELD: 4 SERVINGS

1 tablespoon olive oil
2 cloves garlic, minced
1 medium onion, thinly sliced
½ sweet red pepper, chopped
1 pound sea scallops
1 can (14 ounces) or 1 package (9 ounces) frozen artichoke hearts, quartered
1 cup chopped, peeled tomato with juice, canned or fresh
1 teaspoon sweet basil
8 ounces angel hair pasta
Basil for garnish

PER SERVING

Calories	363
Carbohydrates	56 g
Fat	6.6 g
Saturated fat	1 g
Dietary fiber	8 g
Cholesterol	18 mg
Sodium	374 mg

Mediterranean Pita Pizza

*T*hese pita pizzas can be quickly made to order—great for eating on the run.

Preheat the oven to 400 F.

Place the pitas on an ungreased baking sheet. Brush each pita with ½ teaspoon olive oil. Spread the garlic over the olive oil, dividing it evenly among the 6 pitas. Then top each pita with about 2 tablespoons chopped broccoli, 1 quartered artichoke heart, a tablespoon of chopped pimiento, a tablespoon of crumbled Feta cheese, and about ½ teaspoon of Parmesan cheese. Finally sprinkle some oregano over the top.

Bake for 10 minutes or until the Feta is melted. Serve immediately.

INGREDIENTS

YIELD: 6 SERVINGS

6 pitas
3 teaspoons olive oil
3 cloves garlic, minced
¾ cup chopped frozen broccoli, thawed
6 artichoke hearts, quartered (canned or frozen)
1 jar (4 ounces) chopped pimiento
6 tablespoons crumbled Feta cheese
3 teaspoons grated Parmesan cheese
1 teaspoon oregano

PER SERVING

Calories	232
Carbohydrates	39 g
Fat	5 g
Saturated fat	3 g
Dietary fiber	4 g
Cholesterol	9 mg
Sodium	467 mg

Toasted Cheese and Veggie Sandwich

*C*ut this sandwich in half to reveal the attractive row of cut asparagus.

Wash the asparagus and break off and discard the mature ends. Bring an inch of water to a boil in a skillet. Add asparagus, cover, lower heat, and steam for 10 to 13 minutes or until tender. Drain.

To make sandwich, place one of the slices of bread on a plate. Make a layer of asparagus by placing the asparagus side by side on the bread. Then cover with the tomato, onion, and then cheese. Finally top with the slice of bread.

In the skillet, heat the oil and add the garlic. Heat for a few seconds and stir to combine with the oil. Add the sandwich with the asparagus side down. When the bread is golden brown on one side, turn and heat until the cheese is melted and the bread is golden brown on the other side.

Cut in half and serve immediately.

INGREDIENTS

YIELD: 1 SERVING

¼ pound asparagus (about 6 stalks)
2 slices homemade bread (flaxseed bread would be excellent)
2 slices tomato
1 thin slice mild onion
¾ ounces reduced-fat cheddar cheese
1 teaspoon canola oil
½ clove minced garlic

PER SERVING

Calories	442
Carbohydrates	70 g
Fat	11 g
Saturated fat	2 g
Dietary fiber	7 g
Cholesterol	5 mg
Sodium	736 mg
Folate	160 mcg

Bow Ties with Asparagus

*I*n a large saucepan, cook the bow-tie noodles according to package directions. However, after the noodles have cooked for 8 minutes, add the asparagus and continue cooking for 4 more minutes or until both noodles and asparagus are tender. Drain.

Meanwhile, heat the olive oil in a small skillet. Add the onion, red pepper, and garlic and sauté for 5 minutes or until the onions have softened. Add the chicken broth, Parmesan, and sweet basil. Heat through.

Spoon the cooked noodles and asparagus into a serving bowl. Pour the hot stock with vegetables over the noodles and coat the noodles. Garnish with basil and pass the Parmesan.

INGREDIENTS

YIELD: 4 SERVINGS

6 ounces bow-tie noodles
1½ cups asparagus cut into 1-inch diagonal lengths
2 teaspoons olive oil
¼ cup chopped onion
½ cup chopped red pepper
1 clove garlic, minced
½ cup fat-free chicken broth
2 tablespoons grated Parmesan cheese
¼ teaspoon dried sweet basil
Basil for garnish

PER SERVING

Calories	228
Carbohydrates	39 g
Fat	4 g
Saturated fat	1 g
Dietary fiber	3 g
Cholesterol	3 mg
Sodium	131 mg

South of the Border Pizza

You can reduce the fat in this delicious pizza by substituting low-fat cheese, or mixing low-fat and nonfat cheeses. You can also use less avocado.

Preheat the oven to 400 F.

Place the pizza shell on a baking sheet, cover the shell with the cheese, and bake for 10 minutes or until the cheese is melted. Remove from oven.

Meanwhile combine the tomatoes, garlic, cilantro, scallion, and chile pepper. Spread over the melted Monterey Jack cheese. Cover with avocado slices and serve.

INGREDIENTS

YIELD: 8 SERVINGS

1 pizza shell (10 inches)
1 cup shredded Monterey Jack cheese
3 plum tomatoes, seeded and chopped
1 teaspoon minced garlic
2 tablespoons chopped fresh cilantro
1 scallion, thinly sliced
1 tablespoon chopped chile pepper
½ avocado, thinly sliced

PER SERVING

Calories	154
Carbohydrates	19 g
Fat	6 g
Saturated fat	2 g
Protein	8 g
Dietary fiber	10 g
Cholesterol	10 mg
Sodium	311 mg

Apple-Cranberry Date Crisp

Preheat oven to 375 F. Spray an 8-inch x 8-inch square pan with nonstick spray.

Combine apples, dates, and craisins in the prepared pan. In a bowl combine the flour, brown sugar, and margarine. Add the oats and almonds to the flour mixture. Cover the fruit mixture with this topping.

Bake for 40 to 45 minutes or until the apples are soft and the topping is browned.

INGREDIENTS

YIELD: 9 SERVINGS

8 apples, cored, peeled, and sliced
½ cup chopped dates
¼ cup craisins
½ cup unbleached or whole wheat flour
2 tablespoons brown sugar
2 tablespoons canola oil
¼ cup oats
2 tablespoons sliced almonds

PER SERVING

Calories	176
Carbohydrates	37 g
Fat	4 g
Saturated fat	0 g
Dietary fiber	4 g
Cholesterol	0 mg
Sodium	16 mg

Bull's Avocado Chicken Soup

This recipe comes to me by way of my daughter's friend, who is nicknamed Bull. It is a simple soup with lots of flavor, most of which comes from the avocado slices and crushed tortilla chips in the bottom of the bowl. You don't need salt: It's already in the tortilla chips. This is a main-dish soup; just add bread and a salad.

Heat the olive oil in a large soup pot. Add the chicken and sauté until golden brown on both sides. Remove chicken from the pot and set aside.

Add the garlic, onion, cumin, and turmeric to the hot pot and cook until the onions are softened.

Add the chicken broth and tomato sauce or tomatoes and bring to a simmer. Cut the chicken into bite-size pieces and add back into the pot. Simmer for 30 minutes or up to one hour. The longer the soup cooks, the more the flavors will blend together.

To serve, place the avocado and some broken tortilla chips into the bottom of a soup bowl and then ladle a cup of soup over them. The tortilla chips and avocado can be passed at the table as another option.

INGREDIENTS

YIELD: 6 SERVINGS

1 tablespoon olive oil
1 pound boneless, skinless chicken breasts
2 cloves garlic, minced
1 large onion, chopped
1 teaspoon ground cumin
¼ teaspoon turmeric
4 cups chicken broth
1 can (16 ounces) tomato sauce or diced tomatoes
1 avocado, peeled and thinly sliced
2 cups low-fat tortilla chips

PER SERVING

Calories	319
Carbohydrates	27 g
Fat	11 g
Saturated fat	2 g
Monounsaturated Fat	5 g
Dietary fiber	5 g
Cholesterol	58 mg
Sodium	270 mg

Cantaloupe with Blueberry-Mint Sauce

Rinse blueberries and remove stems. Combine cleaned blueberries with water, sugar, and mint leaves in a small saucepan. Cook on medium heat about 10 minutes or until the berries begin to release their juices and break down. Stir occasionally. The berries will be simmering the last 5 minutes.

Allow to cool. Cut the cantaloupe into chunks or balls. Serve the cantaloupe topped with the blueberry-mint sauce.

NOTE: The sauce can be puréed if a smooth texture is preferred.

INGREDIENTS

YIELD: 6 SERVINGS

1 pint fresh blueberries (about 2½ cups)
2 tablespoons water
¼ cup sugar
1 spring mint (about 10 leaves)
1 cantaloupe

PER SERVING

Calories	98
Carbohydrates	25 g
Fat	0.5 g
Saturated fat	0 g
Dietary fiber	2 g
Cholesterol	0 mg
Sodium	12 mg

Cantaloupe and Strawberry Salsa

*T*hese two fruits make a delightful and beautiful combination with the added chopped chives. The salsa is very simple but gives a gourmet (and healthy) touch to poached fish.

Combine the cantaloupe, strawberries, and chives. Allow to stand and combine flavors for about 15 minutes.

This salsa goes well with poached fish. It can also be served on a bed of lettuce as a small salad.

INGREDIENTS

YIELD: 4 SERVINGS

1 cup finely chopped cantaloupe
1 cup finely chopped strawberries
1 tablespoon snipped chives

PER SERVING

Calories	27
Carbohydrates	6 g
Fat	0.3 g
Saturated fat	0 g
Dietary fiber	1 g
Cholesterol	0 mg
Sodium	4 mg

Crispy Haddock on a Bed of Sautéed Julienne Vegetables

*H*eat a large nonstick skillet sprayed with nonstick spray. Add the carrots, celery, leeks and garlic and sauté for 5 minutes or until the vegetables are tender crisp. Add some of the chicken stock if the vegetables are sticking to the pan. When the vegetables are tender, remove them to a serving platter. Cover the platter with a sheet of aluminum foil and put in the oven on warm to retain heat while the haddock cooks.

Dip the haddock fillets into the egg substitute and then into the bread crumbs. Heat the olive oil in the same nonstick skillet and brown the fish on one side, turn, and brown the fish on the other side. Add some chicken stock if necessary to keep the fish from sticking to the pan. If the fish is not cooked throughout by the time it is browned on the second side, cover the pan and steam the fish for a few minutes.

Place the cooked fish on the bed of julienne vegetables. Serve.

INGREDIENTS

YIELD: 4 SERVINGS

2 carrots, cut into julienne strips
2 celery ribs, cut into julienne strips
2 leeks, cut into julienne strips
2 cloves garlic, minced
½ cup fat-free chicken stock
1 pound haddock fillets
¼ cup egg substitute
½ cup dry bread crumbs
1 tablespoon olive oil

PER SERVING

Calories	239
Carbohydrates	21 g
Fat	5 g
Saturated fat	0.9 g
Omega-3 Fatty Acids	0.4 g
Omega-6 Fatty Acids	0.6 g
Dietary fiber	3 g
Cholesterol	0 mg
Sodium	268 mg

Celery Slaw

With only 3 grams of fat per serving, this slaw is a dieter's delight!

Combine the celery, carrots, raisins, and walnuts in a bowl. In a separate bowl, combine the yogurt, mayonnaise, and pepper. Add the dressing to the vegetables and mix well.

Serve on a bed of romaine.

INGREDIENTS

YIELD: 6 SERVINGS (1 CUP EA.)

2 thinly sliced celery stalks
1 coarsely shredded carrot
¼ cup raisins
2 tablespoons coarsely chopped walnuts
3 tablespoons plain nonfat yogurt
2 tablespoons light mayonnaise
¼ teaspoon white pepper
Romaine

PER SERVING

Calories 69
Carbohydrates .... 10 g
Fat .... 3 g
Saturated fat .... 0.5 g
Dietary fiber .... 1 g
Cholesterol .... 0 mg
Sodium .... 83 mg

Spinach and Grapefruit Salad with Broccoli Sprouts

Here's another salad that's low in calories—only 109—but high in fat (6 grams). The fat is in the olive oil, though—one of the good fats. So don't be afraid to enjoy!

Peel and section the grapefruit, halve each section, and place them in a salad bowl. Add the washed spinach leaves and finally the oil and roasted soybeans. Toss. Serve topped with the broccoli sprouts.

INGREDIENTS

YIELD: 4 SERVINGS

2 red grapefruit
5 ounces washed spinach leaves
4 teaspoons olive oil
2 tablespoons roasted unsalted soybeans
½ cup broccoli sprouts

PER SERVING

Calories 112
Carbohydrates .... 13 g
Fat .... 6 g
Saturated fat .... 0.9 g
Monounsaturated Fat .... 4 g
Dietary fiber .... 3 g
Cholesterol .... 0 mg
Sodium .... 29 mg

Tomato and Chile Cornbread

This cornbread is made the old-fashioned way—by pouring the batter into a heated iron skillet and then baking it in the oven. So get out your iron skillet...and prepare this traditional Southwestern-style cornbread.

Preheat the oven to 425 F.

Pour 1 tablespoon of the canola oil into a 10-inch iron skillet and put the skillet in the oven.

Combine the cornmeal, flour, sugar, baking powder, and salt in a large bowl. In a smaller bowl, beat the egg substitute. Add the remaining 2 tablespoons of oil. Beat in the remaining 2 tablespoons of oil, then stir in the tomatoes and chiles. Add this liquid mixture to the cornmeal mixture.

Remove the heated pan from the oven and pour in the batter. Smooth over the entire surface with a spatula and place the pan back into the oven for 20 to 25 minutes or until the bread is lightly browned and a toothpick inserted in the center comes out clean.

Spread the shredded cheese on top of the cornbread, cut into eight slices, and serve immediately.

INGREDIENTS

YIELD: 8 SERVINGS

3 tablespoons canola oil
1¼ cups fine yellow cornmeal
½ cup unbleached flour
1 tablespoon sugar
1 teaspoon baking powder
½ teaspoon salt
¼ cup egg substitute
1 can (10 ounces) diced tomatoes and green chiles*
½ cup shredded low-fat Monterey Jack or cheddar cheese

PER SERVING

Calories	187
Carbohydrates	24 g
Fat	8 g
Saturated fat	2 g
Dietary fiber	2 g
Cholesterol	5 mg
Sodium	426 mg

*NOTE: Canned diced tomatoes and chiles are available in most supermarkets. I used the Ro-Tel brand, which is distributed by International Home Foods. If you can't find a commercial brand, substitute 1 cup of chopped tomatoes and 2 ounces (¼ cup) of canned mild or hot chiles, or add 1 to 2 tablespoons chopped fresh jalapeños.

Refreshing Fruit Salad

Peel and section the oranges and add to a medium bowl. Halve the mango and cut into ½-inch cubes and add to the bowl. Peel and cut the pineapple half into small triangles and combine with the fruit. Add the lemon zest and the yogurt. Mix well. Finally top the salad with slivered almonds.

INGREDIENTS

YIELD: 12 SERVINGS

2 oranges
1 mango
½ fresh pineapple
2 teaspoons lemon zest
1 container (8 ounces) fat-free vanilla yogurt
2 tablespoons slivered almonds (garnish)

PER SERVING

Calories	61
Carbohydrates	13 g
Fat	1 g
Saturated fat	0 g
Dietary fiber	1.5 g
Cholesterol	0 mg
Sodium	14 mg

Hearty Soy-Corn Soup

This is a thick soup filled with vegetables and brown rice. You can substitute canned tomatoes and chiles for the salsa.

Heat the oil in a 3- to 4-quart pot. Add the garlic, chopped onions, celery, and carrots. Sauté for 10 minutes on low until the vegetables begin to soften. Add the broth and cook for 10 minutes or until vegetables are tender. Add the soybeans, corn, salsa, parsley, quick brown rice, tarragon, and oregano. Cover and simmer for 10 minutes to blend the flavors. Garnish with parsley and serve with extra salsa.

INGREDIENTS

YIELD: 10 SERVINGS

2 teaspoons canola oil
1 clove garlic, minced
1 cup chopped onions
1 cup chopped celery
1 cup chopped carrots
4 cups low-fat, low-sodium chicken broth
1 can (15 ounces) cooked soybeans
1 package (10 ounces) frozen corn
½ cup medium hot salsa
½ cup chopped parsley
½ cup quick brown rice
1 tablespoon fresh tarragon or 1 teaspoon dried
2 teaspoons fresh oregano or ½ teaspoon dried
Chopped parsley for garnish

PER SERVING

Calories	155
Carbohydrates	19 g
Fat	6 g
Saturated fat	1 g
Dietary fiber	5 g
Cholesterol	2 mg
Sodium	112 mg

Barley-Corn Pancakes

These pancakes can be used as a main dish for supper. Just add a tossed green salad.

In a medium bowl, beat the egg substitute until foamy. Add the milk, oil, flours, honey, baking powder, and salt. Mix until the flour disappears. Add the corn and the chile powder (if desired).

Heat a nonstick pan. Pour the batter into the pan, using about ¼ cup per pancake. Brown on both sides.

Serve with salsa instead of syrup.

INGREDIENTS

YIELD: 12 SERVINGS

¼ cup egg substitute
1¼ cups nonfat milk
2 tablespoons canola oil
1 cup barley flour
¼ cup whole wheat flour
2 teaspoons honey
1½ teaspoons baking powder
½ teaspoon salt
1 cup frozen, canned or cooked corn kernels
1 teaspoon chile powder (optional)

PER SERVING

Calories	81
Carbohydrates	13 g
Fat	3 g
Saturated fat	0.2 g
Dietary fiber	2 g
Cholesterol	0.5 mg
Sodium	211 mg

Shrimp and Broccoli with Sesame Seeds

The flavor of the sesame seeds is enhanced by the use of sesame oil as well. The Kame brand of sesame oil I used is a combination of toasted sesame oil and canola oil.

Heat a large skillet. Add the sesame seeds to the dry skillet and toast until they are golden or change color. Shake the skillet so the seeds do not stick and burn. Remove the seeds from the skillet and set them aside.

Heat the sesame oil in the skillet. Add the broccoli, onion, red pepper, and shrimp and cook and stir until the vegetables are tender and the shrimp are pink.

Add the toasted sesame seeds and the soy sauce and stir. Serve.

INGREDIENTS

YIELD: 4 SERVINGS

1 tablespoon sesame seeds
1 tablespoon sesame oil
6 cups broccoli, cut into 1-inch lengths
1 large onion, sliced
½ red pepper, chopped
1 pound shrimp, washed, shelled, and deveined
1 tablespoon low-sodium soy sauce

PER SERVING

Calories	178
Carbohydrates	13 g
Fat	6 g
Saturated fat	1 g
Dietary fiber	6 g
Cholesterol	135 mg
Sodium	346 mg

Brussels Sprouts in Garlic Butter

"When you get to the brussels sprouts recipes, don't let them smell up the kitchen!" Ellen requested. "Can you make them so they won't have any odor?" To tell the truth, I love brussels sprouts, and I don't notice a bad smell. There are people who can't stand garlic, and we know how good that is for us!

I think the secret to odor prevention in brussels sprouts is to not cook them too long, and especially don't overcook them. Use a metal steamer insert for your saucepan, add water, bring the water to a boil, add the brussels sprouts, cover, and cook them on high for seven minutes. Then taste one! It should be tender, crisp, green, and sweet.

INGREDIENTS

YIELD: 4 SERVINGS

10 ounces raw brussels sprouts
2 teaspoons butter or olive oil
2 teaspoons minced garlic

PER SERVING

Calories	50
Fat	2 g
Saturated fat	1 g
Dietary fiber	3 g
Cholesterol	5 mg
Sodium	38 mg

You don't have to use the butter I did in this recipe. You can use olive oil. I just like the butter flavor with brussels sprouts. The recipe uses only two teaspoons of butter or oil for four servings—and the garlic butter might tempt the many who think they don't like or want to try brussels sprouts.

Wash the brussels sprouts, slice off a bit of the bottoms and remove yellowed leaves. They can be halved, an X can be cut into the bottom, or they can be left alone.

Bring 2 cups of water to a boil in a saucepan. Insert a metal steamer. Add the brussels sprouts, cover, and let steam on high for 7 minutes. Test for doneness by inserting a knife into the sprout. If it goes in easily, the sprouts are finished. Remove the sprouts from the pan so they do not cook any further. Drain.

Meanwhile, melt the butter or heat the oil in another pan. Add the garlic and sauté until slightly browned. Remove from the heat.

When the brussels sprouts are cooked and drained, add them to the garlic butter and toss to coat. Serve.

Oriental-Style Chicken Soup with Cabbage

This is a light chicken soup, low in fat and calories (only 105 in a cup).

In a 6-quart to 8-quart pot, heat a tablespoon of oil. Add the onions, carrot, and celery and cook for 5 minutes or until softened. Add the chicken broth and chicken, cover the pot and cook for 10 minutes or until chicken is cooked through. Remove the chicken from the pot and cut into bite-size pieces.

Add the chicken back into the pot with the cabbage and soy sauce. Cover and continue cooking for 10 to 15 minutes or until the cabbage is tender.

INGREDIENTS

YIELD: 8 SERVINGS

1 tablespoon olive oil or canola oil
½ cup chopped onions
1 carrot, chopped
1 celery rib, chopped
6 cups chicken broth
½ pound raw skinless, boneless chicken breast
1 pound savoy cabbage, thinly sliced (about 6 cups)
1 tablespoon low-sodium soy sauce

PER SERVING

Calories	105
Carbohydrates	6 g
Fat	3 g
Saturated fat	0.5 g
Dietary fiber	2 g
Cholesterol	22 mg
Sodium	236 mg

Cauliflower with Ham, Onion, Garlic, and Turmeric

This is a very delicious way to eat cauliflower. You'll want more than one serving.

Bring 2 cups of water to a boil in a saucepan fitted with a steamer insert. Add the cauliflower. Cover and steam for 7 to 10 minutes or until just tender. Remove the lid from the pan so that the cauliflower will not cook further and remove from the heat.

Meanwhile, heat the olive oil in a saucepan. Add the onion, ham, garlic, and turmeric and sauté until the onion is tender. Add the cooked and drained cauliflower and toss to coat. Cover and reheat if necessary. Serve.

INGREDIENTS

YIELD: 4 SERVINGS

2 to 3 cups raw cauliflower florets (about 10 ounces)
2 teaspoons olive oil
¼ cup chopped onion
2 tablespoons chopped low-fat ham
1 teaspoon minced garlic
¼ teaspoon turmeric

PER SERVING

Calories	50
Carbohydrates	5 g
Fat	3 g
Saturated fat	0.4 g
Dietary fiber	2 g
Cholesterol	2 mg
Sodium	80 mg

Garlic and Zucchini Fettuccini

I used two teaspoons of garlic in this recipe, but garlic lovers can use more. This recipe is a good way to use up the zucchini that most gardeners grow in abundance every summer. Zucchini doesn't have a lot of nutrients, but is great for its dietary fiber. Plus, it doesn't have sodium, fat, cholesterol, or calories! There are only about fourteen calories in a half-cup of sliced zucchini.

Bring a pot of water to a boil and cook the fettuccini according to the package directions. Drain and set aside.

Cut the zucchini into 2-inch matchstick or julienne cuts. Set aside.

Heat the oil in a large skillet. Add the garlic and the cut zucchini and sauté on medium-low until the zucchini is softened, about 10 minutes. Add the drained fettuccini and toss with the zucchini. Add the sour cream and the Parmesan cheese and mix well. Serve. Top with some fresh basil.

INGREDIENTS

YIELD: 4 SERVINGS (¾ CUP EA.)

8 ounces fettuccini
8 ounces zucchini (about 1 medium)
1 tablespoon olive oil
2 teaspoons minced fresh garlic
1 tablespoon fresh basil or 1 teaspoon dried
¼ cup low-fat or fat-free sour cream
2 tablespoons grated Parmesan cheese
Fresh basil for garnish

PER SERVING

Calories	287
Carbohydrates	48 g
Fat	7 g
Saturated fat	2 g
Dietary fiber	5 g
Cholesterol	7 mg
Sodium	72 mg

Zippy Tomato-Broccoli Salad

P eel the broccoli stalk and cut it and the florets into ½-inch pieces. Pour about an inch of water into a pot, add the broccoli and cover. Steam for 5 minutes or until just tender. Drain and cool.

Put the cooled, cooked broccoli in a small bowl. Add the tomato and onion.

In a small bowl, combine the yogurt, mayonnaise, and horseradish. Add to the vegetables. Combine well and serve. This salad can be served on romaine or as an individual salad.

INGREDIENTS

YIELD: 6 SERVINGS (½ CUP EA.)

1 broccoli stalk (about 8 ounces)
1 large tomato, chopped
2 tablespoons chopped mild onion
¼ cup plain yogurt
2 teaspoons light mayonnaise
2 teaspoons horseradish

PER SERVING

Calories	28
Carbohydrates	4 g
Fat	1 g
Saturated fat	0.2 g
Dietary fiber	2 g
Cholesterol	0 mg
Sodium	34 mg

Key Lime Pie

*L*ate one winter night in January, my husband and I were driving through Quakertown, Pennsylvania, and stopped at a Clemens Market because we'd heard of their reputation for having great produce and unusual stock. I found Key limes, which I had never actually seen before. They are small, firm, and dark green. I bought nine limes and used them in this recipe.

I decided to use silken tofu in this recipe because I wanted to have at least one tofu dessert that would be acceptable to confirmed tofu haters. I tested this recipe on a few of those and it passed—no one knew it was there.

Prepare crust according to recipe for Barley Crust in Bottom Cupboard chapter and bake according to directions above.

For filling, beat together the nonfat sweetened condensed milk, silken tofu, lime zest and lime juice. Pour 2 tablespoons of cold water into a glass measuring cup and add the gelatin. Allow to soften for 2 minutes and then microwave on high for 30 seconds; stir thoroughly and let stand 2 minutes or until gelatin is completely dissolved. The gelatin can also be dissolved in a small saucepan on top of the stove.

Add the dissolved gelatin into the milk mixture and whip thoroughly, using a wire whisk. Pour the mixture into the cooled pie shell and allow to set about 5 minutes.

For meringue: Preheat oven to 375 F. Beat the egg whites until frothy. Add the cream of tartar and whip until stiff. Gradually beat in the sugar one tablespoon at a time. Beat in the vanilla. Spread the meringue on the pie filling. Place in oven and bake 10 minutes or until the top is lightly browned.

INGREDIENTS

YIELD: 8 SERVINGS

PASTRY:
Use a one-crust pastry or the recipe for Barley Pastry found in The Bottom Cupboard chapter in this book. Bake the crust in a nonstick sprayed 9-inch pie plate for 7 minutes at 375 F.

FILLING:
1 can (14 ounces) nonfat sweetened condensed milk
⅔ cup firm silken tofu
2 teaspoons grated lime zest
⅓ cup fresh key lime or regular lime juice
1 envelope plain gelatin (¼ ounce)

MERINGUE:
3 egg whites
¼ teaspoon cream of tartar
⅓ cup granulated sugar
1 teaspoon vanilla

PER SERVING

Calories	316
Carbohydrates	55 g
Fat	8 g
Saturated fat	0 g
Monounsaturated Fat	3 g
Dietary fiber	3 g
Cholesterol	3.4 mg
Sodium	82 mg

Smooth and Creamy Vegetable and Lentil Soup

This easy, nutritious soup is made creamy by the puréed vegetables and skim milk.

Heat the olive oil in a 3-quart to 4-quart pot. Add the garlic, onions, carrots, celery, and turmeric and sauté until the onions are tender.

Add the water, chicken broth, tomato sauce, lentils, rice, cumin, and black pepper. Bring to a boil, lower heat, cover and simmer for 40 to 50 minutes or until the lentils are tender.

Purée the soup in batches in a food processor or blender. Pour the puréed soup back into the pot and add the skim milk. Heat just to boiling. Serve. Pass the plain fat-free yogurt.

INGREDIENTS

YIELD: 6 SERVINGS (1½ CUP EA.)

1 tablespoon olive oil
2 cloves garlic, minced
1 cup chopped onions
1 cup chopped carrots
½ cup chopped celery
½ teaspoon turmeric
2 cups water
4 cups fat-free chicken broth
1 can (8 ounces) tomato sauce
1 cup dried lentils
⅓ cup uncooked rice
1 teaspoon cumin
¼ teaspoon black pepper
2 cups skim milk
Plain yogurt for garnish (optional)

PER SERVING

Calories	239
Carbohydrates	38 g
Fat	3 g
Saturated fat	0.5 g
Dietary fiber	12 g
Cholesterol	2 mg
Sodium	627 mg

Quick and Easy Mushroom-Spinach Lasagna

Lasagna is a fabulous one-dish meal that not only tastes great and makes a great leftover, but can also be used as a vehicle for adding vegetables to the diet. Here is a quick and delicious version of a veggie lasagna. Use a variety of mushrooms and save cooking time by using quick noodles. Just layer the noodles as they come from the box.

Preheat oven to 350 F. Spray two 8-inch x 8-inch baking pans with nonstick spray.

In a large skillet, heat the tablespoon of olive oil. Add the onion, garlic, and mushrooms and sauté until softened, about 10 minutes. Add the wine and simmer about 10 minutes more on medium-low heat until they are well softened.

Beat together the ricotta cheese, the eggs, and the lemon rind in a large bowl.

Pour ½ cup of the pasta sauce in each of the pans. In each pan, lay two lasagna noodles side by side on top of the sauce. Divide the ricotta mixture between the pans and add another layer of 2 lasagna noodles. Cover each one with 1 package of spinach. Cover the spinach with the remaining sauce, using 1½ cups in each pan. Add another 2 noodles to each pan. Finally, divide the mushroom mixture between each of the pans and top with 2 tablespoons of grated Parmesan.

Cover each pan with a sheet of aluminum foil and bake for 15 minutes. Uncover and bake for 15 minutes more. Cool slightly and cut each pan into 6 servings.

NOTE: Per serving is approximate, depending upon the calories, fat and sodium content of the commercial sauce used.

INGREDIENTS

YIELD: 12 SERVINGS

1 tablespoon olive oil
1 large onion, chopped
2 cloves garlic, minced
16 ounces mushrooms, sliced (use a combination of buttons, portobellos, shiitakes)
⅓ cup dry red wine
2 pounds reduced-fat ricotta
½ cup egg substitute or 2 eggs
1 tablespoon grated lemon rind
4 cups jarred pasta sauce
12 quick lasagna noodles
2 packages (10 ounces) frozen chopped spinach, thawed, drained, and squeezed almost dry
¼ cup grated Parmesan

PER SERVING

Calories	276
Carbohydrates	32 g
Fat	8 g
Saturated fat	4 g
Dietary fiber	5 g
Cholesterol	25 mg
Sodium	459 mg

Shiitake Mushrooms and Rice

Both dried and fresh shiitake mushrooms are wonderful in this grain dish. The dried mushrooms need to be soaked before using. To soak dried mushrooms, cover them with lukewarm water and soak for thirty minutes or cover them with boiling water and soak for two to five minutes. The resulting soaking broth is very flavorful and should be saved.

The stems of the shiitakes can be tough, especially from the dried mushrooms, so you may want to remove them. Test before discarding; some stems will be tender. Tough stems may be chopped and used. Because these mushrooms are expensive, I would try to save as much as possible.

INGREDIENTS
YIELD: 4 SERVINGS

4 ounces fresh shiitakes or 1 ounce dried and soaked
2 teaspoons olive oil
2 cloves garlic, minced
⅓ cup water or (⅔ cup water if using dried and soaked shiitakes)
1 teaspoon low-sodium soy sauce or tamari soy sauce
1 large basil leaf, chopped
1 cup uncooked quick brown rice

PER SERVING	
Calories	215
Carbohydrates	42 g
Fat	4 g
Saturated fat	0.6 g
Dietary fiber	2.5 g
Cholesterol	0 mg
Sodium	49 mg

DRIED/FRESH EQUIVALENTS:

½ ounce dried shiitakes = 10 small mushrooms
1 ounce dried and soaked = 4 ounces fresh shiitakes

SELECTION AND CARE:

Most fresh shiitakes in the supermarkets are prepackaged in 3½-ounce containers. If sold loose and by the pound, select those that have firm, smooth, dark tops. There should be no mold on them and they should not be dried out. A white powdery look to some of the tops is normal and can be wiped off. The mushrooms should keep several days at home if wrapped loosely in plastic. Mushrooms are best wiped clean or lightly rinsed.

Slice the mushrooms. If using the dried shiitakes instead of fresh, first drain and retain the liquid, and then slice. Heat the olive oil in a saucepan. Add the garlic and the mushrooms and sauté for 10 minutes, or until mushrooms are softened. Add the water, soy sauce and basil and bring to a boil. Lower heat and simmer for 3 minutes.

Add 1¼ cups water to the saucepan and bring to a boil. If soaking liquid was retained, use this plus enough water to make 1¼ cups. Add the rice, lower the heat, cover and cook for 10 minutes. Allow to stand for several minutes off the heat with the lid on. Then fluff with a fork before serving.

Charleston Gumbo

Tomato, Okra and Black-Eyed Pea Soup

In a saucepan, add the black-eyed peas and enough water to cover. Bring the water to a boil, turn off the heat, cover, and allow to soak for 1 hour. Pour off the water, add 4 cups of fresh water, the bay leaves, coriander and turmeric. Bring the water to a boil, lower heat, and allow to cook for 1 hour or until the peas are tender.

In a small saucepan, heat the olive oil. Add the celery, onion, and peppers. Sauté on medium-low until softened.

When the black-eyed peas are tender, add the sautéed vegetables and the sliced okra. Slice the tomatoes and add them and their juice to the pot. Bring the soup to a boil, turn down the heat and simmer for 15 minutes or until the okra is tender.

*NOTE: Canned black-eyed peas can be substituted for the dried. Use 2 cans (15 ounces) and add them to the pot with 2 cups of water and the dried herbs. Proceed with the sautéing of the vegetables.

INGREDIENTS

YIELD: 8 SERVINGS (1 CUP EA.)

1½ cups dried black-eyed peas*
2 bay leaves
1 teaspoon ground coriander
½ teaspoon turmeric
1 tablespoon olive oil
1 cup chopped celery
1 cup chopped onion
1 sweet red pepper, chopped
1 hot red pepper, chopped
½ pound fresh okra, sliced or 1 package (10 ounces), frozen
1 can (28 ounces) tomatoes

PER SERVING

Calories	89
Carbohydrates	16 g
Fat	2 g
Saturated fat	0.3 g
Dietary fiber	5 g
Cholesterol	0 mg
Sodium	27 mg

Radish and Cucumber Yogurt

My grandmother loved to eat radishes with sour cream; this is a modification of that tasty lunch. And it is much lower in fat!

Wash and sliced the cucumber. Place in a bowl with the radishes and chopped onion. Combine the yogurt, cider vinegar, and water. Add to the vegetables and mix well. Top with the chopped chives. Serve.

INGREDIENTS

YIELD: 4–6 SERVINGS

1 small pickling cucumber (5 to 6 inches)
1 cup sliced radishes
¼ cup finely chopped onion
¼ cup nonfat plain yogurt
1 tablespoon apple cider vinegar
1 tablespoon water
1 teaspoon chopped chives

PER SERVING

Calories	25
Carbohydrates	5 g
Fat	0.3 g
Saturated fat	0 g
Dietary fiber	1 g
Cholesterol	0 mg
Sodium	21 mg

Tortilla Roll-Ups

*T*hese tortilla roll-ups are great for a family meal fortified with a bowl of soup or chili. Just set out a buffet of ingredients and let everyone be creative. This is a good way to add vegetables, including spinach, to the diet. The rolls can also be prepared and wrapped for picnics and lunches.

Place a tortilla on a plate. Cover with ½ teaspoon light mayonnaise. Then layer with a slice of turkey roll, and then spinach leaves. Place a line of shredded carrots down the center, top it with the parsley and red pepper and then roll the tortilla. Repeat with the second tortilla.

The roll can be served this way or it can be cut into 8 slices. These slices can be turned to the side so that the cut side is up and the vegetables and the colorful side show.

INGREDIENTS

YIELD: 1 SERVING (2 ROLLS)

2 (8-in) flour tortillas
1 teaspoon light mayonnaise
2 thin slices low-fat, low-sodium deli turkey
8 spinach leaves
⅓ cup shredded carrots
1 tablespoon fresh chopped parsley
4 julienne strips roasted red pepper

PER SERVING

Calories	321
Carbohydrates	41 g
Fat	96 g
Saturated fat	3 g
Dietary fiber	4 g
Cholesterol	0 mg
Sodium	341 mg

Cauliflower with Marinara Sauce and Linguini

*W*ash and cut cauliflower into florets.

Cook cauliflower by adding about 1 cup of water to a large pot. Bring the water to a boil, add the cauliflower, cover, and cook for 5 minutes or until tender.

Cook linguini according to package directions. Drain.

When the cauliflower is just tender, without draining, add the marinara sauce, combine with the cauliflower and continue cooking on medium until the sauce is hot.

Serve the sauce over the linguini. Top with minced fresh parsley. Pass the grated Parmesan if desired.

INGREDIENTS

YIELD: 6–8 SERVINGS

1 head cauliflower
1 jar (28 ounces) marinara or spaghetti sauce
    or 3 cups homemade marinara sauce
1 pound linguini or spaghetti
⅓ cup minced fresh parsley
Grated Parmesan cheese (optional)

PER SERVING

Calories	398
Carbohydrates	7.5 g
Fat	5 g
Saturated fat	7 g
Dietary fiber	11 g
Cholesterol	0 mg
Sodium	566 mg

Chunky Vegetable Marinara Sauce

Some of the new commercial vegetable primavera sauces are very good and contain chunks of vegetables. This is my interpretation of one of these sauces full of healing ingredients. Keep the vegetables chunky when chopping them.

To peel the tomatoes, dip them into boiling water for 1 minute. Remove them from the boiling water with a spoon and transfer them quickly to a bowl of ice water. As soon as they are cool enough to handle, simply peel off the skins. Cut the tomatoes into chunks.

Heat the olive oil in a large, heavy pot (6-quart), and sauté the onion and garlic for 5 minutes. Stir in the peppers, carrots, celery, zucchini, parsley, mushrooms, tomatoes, oregano, and basil. Simmer, uncovered, about 1 hour or until thickened. Can be frozen to store.

INGREDIENTS

YIELD: 4 CUPS

2½ pounds plum tomatoes or fresh, in-season high-flavor tomatoes (about 16)
1 tablespoon olive oil
1 large onion, chopped (1½ cups)
3 cloves garlic, chopped
1 chopped red pepper
2 chopped carrots
1 stalk chopped celery
1 zucchini or yellow squash, chopped
4 tablespoons finely chopped parsley
4 to 5 large mushrooms, chopped
1 tablespoon fresh oregano or 1 teaspoon dried oregano
1 tablespoon fresh basil or 2 teaspoons dried basil
Salt and pepper (optional and to taste)

PER ½-CUP SERVING

Calories	82
Carbohydrates	15 g
Fat	2 g
Saturated fat	0 g
Dietary fiber	4 g
Cholesterol	0 mg
Sodium	28 mg

Pineapple-Cranberry Dessert

My cousin Cindy told me about this easy frozen dessert. She likes this combination of fruits with yogurt. It can be served from the refrigerator or it can be frozen and served as a sherbet.

Combine the ingredients in a bowl or freezer container. Refrigerate or freeze. Garnish with mint leaves and serve.

INGREDIENTS

YIELD: 6–8 SERVINGS

1 cup fat-free vanilla yogurt
1 can (16 ounces) whole cranberry sauce
1 can (10 ounces) crushed pineapple, drained
Mint leaves for garnish

PER SERVING

Calories	170
Carbohydrates	41 g
Fat	0 g
Saturated fat	0.9 g
Dietary fiber	2 g
Cholesterol	1 mg
Sodium	38 mg

Easy Morning Breakfast

*P*our the yogurt into a cereal bowl. Top with the granola, then the sliced apricots and the berries. Serve.

Walnut-Coated Baked Apples with Blackberry Sauce

*T*he inspiration for this recipe comes from Devorah Leah Mangel of Dayton, Ohio, who likes to use Cortland apples for baking.

Preheat the oven to 350 F. Spray a baking pan large enough to hold the apples.

Beat the egg whites in a medium bowl until soft peaks form. Combine the walnuts and sugar in a small bowl.

Dip the whole apples in the egg whites and then in the nut-sugar mixture to coat completely. Place the coated apples in the baking pan and bake for 50 minutes or until the apples are lightly browned and tender on the inside. The outside of the apple will toughen and dry slightly.

Prepare the sauce: Heat the berries in a saucepan over low heat until warmed and thawed. Combine the cornstarch with the cold water in a small measuring cup and pour over the berries. Combine and cook over low heat until the sauce has thickened slightly.

To serve, place baked apple in a dessert dish and pour sauce over it.

*NOTE: If you are using unsweetened berries, you may have to add a little honey or sugar to taste.

Curried Chicken with Apricots, Onions, and Rice

*U*se fresh ripe apricots in this recipe; the sweetness of the apricots is needed to complement the tartness of the yogurt.

Heat the oil in a large nonstick skillet.

Combine the flour, cornmeal, curry, turmeric, cardamom, cayenne, salt, and pepper in a small bowl. Remove a tablespoon of the mixture and reserve.

Place the chicken tenders in another bowl. Pour the lemon juice over the chicken and stir to coat the chicken.

Dip and coat each chicken tender in the flour mixture and add to the hot skillet. When all the fingers are coated and in the skillet, brown them on all sides. When browned, remove them to a clean plate and set aside.

Sauté the fenugreek seeds, garlic, and onions in the same pan for 5 to 10 minutes or until softened. If necessary, add some of the chicken stock to keep the onions from sticking.

Add the remaining chicken stock and bring to a simmer. Add the chicken back into the pan and heat until the chicken is done. This may only take 5 to 10 minutes, depending on the size of the fingers. Cut into one of the tenders to make sure it is cooked completely.

Combine the reserved tablespoon of seasoned flour with the yogurt and add to the chicken mixture with the sliced apricots. Continue cooking until the apricots and yogurt are heated through. Serve over rice.

INGREDIENTS

YIELD: 6–8 SERVINGS

2 tablespoons olive oil
3 tablespoons unbleached flour
3 tablespoons cornmeal
1¼ teaspoons curry powder
¼ teaspoon turmeric
¼ teaspoon cardamom
Dash cayenne, salt, and black pepper
1 pound chicken tenders
1 lemon, juiced (about 3 to 4 tablespoons)
½ teaspoon fenugreek seeds
2 cloves garlic, minced
2 onions, thinly sliced
1 cup chicken stock, defatted
1 cup nonfat plain yogurt
2 fresh apricots, pitted and sliced or 4 canned apricot halves, sliced
6 to 8 cups cooked long grain brown rice

PER SERVING

Calories	424
Carbohydrates	61 g
Fat	8 g
Saturated fat	0 g
Monounsaturated Fat	4 g
Dietary fiber	5 g
Cholesterol	45 mg
Sodium	121 mg

Honey-Chile Garlic Sauce

When any food that I eat tastes bland to me, I spark up the dish with heat from a commercial sweet chile sauce from Thailand. So I've developed a recipe for this spectacular sauce. You'll find it hot and sweet, and it will add to your enjoyment of an entrée or side dish that you feel needs a little upgrade.

This recipe makes ¼ cup; the recipe can be doubled.

Combine the ingredients and allow to set about an hour to blend flavors. Store in a glass jar in the refrigerator.

INGREDIENTS

YIELD: ¼ SERVING

¼ cup honey
1 teaspoon cider vinegar
½ teaspoon dried hot chile pepper
½ teaspoon minced garlic
⅛ teaspoon salt

PER 2-TEASPOON SERVING

Calories	45
Carbohydrates	12 g
Fat	0 g
Saturated fat	0 g
Dietary fiber	0 g
Cholesterol	0 mg
Sodium	49 mg

Green-and-White Party Dip

I don't like to serve dips. It seems most people want to dip chips in them, which are just extra calories—and not necessarily healthy ones. But this dip, which is made with chopped kale, is a healthy one. So don't spoil it: use fresh vegetables as a dipper. If you don't have kale, chopped collards or even spinach will be great. The other reason I like this dip is that people don't know they're eating kale—and discover they like it.

To cook the package of frozen chopped kale, bring 1 cup of water to a boil, add the kale, lower heat, cover, and cook for 20 minutes. When tender, drain well, squeezing out the water.

Place the kale in a bowl and add the remaining ingredients. Combine. Chill.

INGREDIENTS

YIELD: 2 CUPS

1 package (10 ounces) frozen chopped kale
    or collards
2 cups nonfat plain yogurt
2 cloves garlic, minced
1 green onion, finely sliced
2 tablespoons fresh chopped parsley
½ teaspoon sugar
¼ teaspoon salt
Dash black pepper

PER TABLESPOON SERVING (15G)

Calories	12
Carbohydrates	2 g
Fat	0 g
Saturated fat	0 g
Dietary fiber	0.1 g
Cholesterol	0 mg
Sodium	31 mg

Southern-Style Clam Chowder

Adding okra to a clam chowder is what makes this soup Southern style—and delicious too.

Heat the oil in a soup pot. Add the garlic, onion, celery, and carrots and sauté for 10 minutes or until the onions are softened. Add the potatoes, chicken broth, and drained juice from the clams. Bring to a boil. Lower the heat and add the thyme, sage, bay leaf, and tomatoes. Cover and allow to simmer for 10 minutes. Add the okra and cook for 10 minutes. Add the clams and heat just until they are hot.

Serve. Garnish with chopped parsley if desired.

INGREDIENTS

YIELD: 10 TO 12 SERVINGS

1 tablespoon olive oil
1 clove garlic, minced
1 cup chopped onion
1 cup chopped celery
1 cup chopped carrots
1½ cups cubed potato
2 cups defatted chicken broth
2 cans (6½ ounces each) chopped clams in juice
1 cup saved clam juice
1 teaspoon thyme
½ teaspoon sage
1 bay leaf
1 can (14½ ounces) diced tomatoes
1 package (10 ounces) frozen okra
Chopped parsley for garnish

PER SERVING

Calories 77
Carbohydrates .... 12 g
Fat .... 2 g
Saturated fat .... 0 g
Dietary fiber .... 3 g
Cholesterol .... 1 mg
Sodium .... 232 mg

Honey-Roasted Onions with Garlic

Preheat the oven to 425 F. Spray an 8-inch square baking ban with non-stick spray.

Peel and cut onions in half so rings are revealed. Place the cut side down in pan.

Bake for 15 minutes. Meanwhile, combine the honey and garlic, and after the 15 minutes are up, turn the onions over to reveal the ring side. Drizzle the honey mixture over the tops of the onions and bake another 10 minutes or until the onions are tender.

If a browned top of the onion is preferred, broil the onions for two minutes after they've cooked.

Serve as a side dish or as a healthy garnish to a main dish.

INGREDIENTS

YIELD: 4 SERVINGS (½ ONION)

2 medium onions
4 teaspoons honey
4 cloves garlic, minced

PER SERVING

Calories 47
Carbohydrates .... 12 g
Fat .... 0.1 g
Saturated fat .... 1 g
Dietary fiber .... 1 g
Cholesterol .... 0 mg
Sodium .... 2 mg

French Onion Soup

What makes it "French" onion soup is the long, slow cooking of the onions, which caramelizes them and makes them sweet. I've eliminated the heavy coating of Gruyère cheese as well as the butter. This soup is very flavorful and light.

Heat 1 tablespoon of the olive oil in a heavy soup pot. Add the onions and garlic and cook slowly on medium heat for about 30 minutes until the onions are lightly browned and softened. Add the stock, parsley, and sherry and bring to a boil. Turn to low, cover, and cook for 20 minutes or until the onions are tender. Season with salt and pepper to taste.

Meanwhile, toast the Italian bread. Before toasting, brush the tops with the remaining 2 tablespoons of olive oil and sprinkle some garlic powder and grated Parmesan on them.

To serve, spoon about 1 cup of soup into a bowl, add a slice of toast in the center of the bowl, and serve. If you have crocks, you can add a slice of cheese on top and melt the cheese in the oven.

INGREDIENTS

YIELD: 8 CUPS OR 2 QUARTS

3 tablespoons virgin olive oil, aromatic and flavorful
1 pound onions (about 4 large), thinly sliced
4 cloves garlic, minced
2 quarts chicken stock, skimmed of fat
⅓ cup chopped fresh parsley
¼ cup sherry
Salt and pepper to taste
8 slices Italian bread
½ teaspoon garlic powder
2 teaspoons grated Parmesan cheese
8 slices low-fat Jarlsburg cheese (optional)

PER SERVING

Calories	184
Carbohydrates	16 g
Fat	6 g
Saturated fat	0 g
Monounsaturated Fat	4 g
Dietary fiber	2 g
Cholesterol	0 mg
Sodium	399 mg

Fresh Tomato and Onion Pizza

Preheat the oven to 375 F.
Place the pizza crust on a baking pan. Brush the crust with the oil. Spread the garlic over the crust. Then top with the mozzarella cheese. Cover the cheese with the sliced tomatoes and onions. Then shake the oregano, basil, and grated Parmesan over all.

Bake for 10 to 12 minutes or until the mozzarella is melted and the top is lightly browned.

INGREDIENTS

YIELD: 8 SERVINGS

1 prebaked 10-inch to 12-inch pizza crust
1 teaspoon olive oil
2 cloves garlic, minced
1 cup (4 ounces) shredded part-skim
   mozzarella cheese
2 tomatoes, thinly sliced
1 onion, thinly sliced
½ teaspoon oregano
½ teaspoon basil
1 tablespoon grated Parmesan

PER SERVING

Calories	184
Carbohydrates	23 g
Fat	6 g
Saturated fat	3 g
Dietary fiber	2 g
Cholesterol	15 mg
Sodium	370 mg

Radish and Greens Salad with Orange Vinaigrette

Combine the lettuce, orange slices, and radish slices in a bowl. With a fork, mix the orange juice and olive oil and pour over the salad. Toss. Divide between two salad plates. Garnish with the thinly sliced green onion.

INGREDIENTS

YIELD: 2 SERVINGS

2 cups washed leaf lettuce
1 orange, peeled and sliced
8 thinly sliced radishes
2 tablespoons orange juice
1 teaspoon olive oil
1 thinly sliced green onion

PER SERVING

Calories	69
Carbohydrates	12 g
Fat	3 g
Saturated fat	0 g
Monounsaturated Fat	2 g
Dietary fiber	3 g
Cholesterol	0 mg
Sodium	7 mg

Soft-Shell Crabs with a Cajun Rub

*B*efore sautéing your favorite soft-shell crab, try rubbing into it a Cajun or "jerk" rub. Rubs are a mixture of seasoning that are smoothed onto a food before cooking and can be used on ribs, chops, chicken, and seafood.

A Cajun rub, or jerk rub, is usually very spicy. The hottest peppers, such as ground Jamaican hot or Scotch bonnet, are usually used. Other spices that can be added are onion powder, garlic powder, coriander, ginger, black pepper, thyme, allspice, cinnamon, cloves, and nutmeg.

After combining the spices, rub them over the outside of the food. If you have a spice grinder, mix your own combinations. Choose the heat of your mixture by varying the amount of pepper.

Combine the dried herbs and spices. Rub over the crabs.

Heat a nonstick skillet that will be large enough for the crabs. When hot, add the oil. Add the crabs and sauté until cooked on one side and then turn and cook on the other side. It should take about 3 to 4 minutes per side.

INGREDIENTS

YIELD: 2 SERVINGS

(2 SOFT-SHELL CRABS PER PERSON AND 2 TO 3 TEASPOONS SEASONING PER CRAB)

5 teaspoons paprika
2 teaspoons garlic powder
2 teaspoons onion powder
2½ teaspoons dried thyme
½ teaspoon black pepper
½ teaspoon allspice
½ to ¾ teaspoon crushed red pepper or hot pepper
4 cleaned soft-shell crabs
1 to 2 tablespoons peanut oil

PER SERVING

Calories	140
Carbohydrates	9 g
Fat	8 g
Saturated fat	2 g
Monounsaturated Fat	3 g
Oewmga-6 fatty acids	2.7 g
Dietary fiber	3 g
Cholesterol	33 mg
Sodium	129 mg

Creamy Chilled Mango Soup

A quick and easy and delicious soup made in the food processor or blender. Use one mango per person and top the soup with a dash of ground allspice.

Peel and cut the mango from the pit. Add the pulp to a food processor or blender. Purée. Add the yogurt and combine. Pour into a soup bowl. Garnish with allspice.

INGREDIENTS

YIELD: 1 SERVING

1 ripe mango
½ cup plain nonfat yogurt
Dash allspice

PER SERVING

Calories	204
Carbohydrates	45 g
Fat	1 g
Saturated fat	0 g
Dietary fiber	4 g
Cholesterol	2 mg
Sodium	98 mg

Anita's Fat Substitute for Baking

*C*hances are you've used applesauce or nonfat yogurt as a substitute for fat in baking. Cutting back on the amount of fat and then substituting applesauce results in an appealing product. But this product does dry out faster than one made with fat. Fat keeps food moist.

You can now buy prune purée for the same purpose, but I thought apricot purée would be a good substitute. So I experimented with an apricot purée and, like applesauce and prune purée, it left some baked goods a little dry. But I did combine ground flaxseed with an apricot puree, which I found to work very well. I tested it on chocolate chip cookies and all my tasters liked the result.

INGREDIENTS

YIELD: 2 CUPS

½ pound fresh apricots*
2 tablespoons water
2 cups freshly ground flaxseed

PER TABLESPOON SERVING	
Calories	51
Carbohydrates	4 g
Fat	3 g
Saturated fat	0 g
Monounsaturated Fat	1 g
Polyunsaturated Fat	1 g
Dietary fiber	3 g
Cholesterol	0 mg
Sodium	3 mg
Folate	28 mcg

This substitute, which has a third of the fat and half the calories of butter or margarine, worked very well substituted in equal parts for the usual fats in chocolate chip cookies.

Flax does have oil in it too, so this really isn't a fat-free fat substitute. But flax is one of the good fats—polyunsaturated—and its seeds are high in healthy isoflavones. It's also high in fiber and contains no trans fatty acids or cholesterol.

Wash and slice the apricots. Discard the pits. Add the sliced apricots to a small saucepan with the water. Bring to a slow boil, lower the heat, and simmer for about 10 minutes. Drain, saving the liquid. Purée the apricots in a blender or a processor. Add the flaxseed and combine well. If necessary, add some of the saved liquid.

Keep this mixture refrigerated and use as a substitute in quick breads or cookies instead of the fat. It can be substituted in equal parts for the fat that is omitted from the original recipe.

If you will not be using the mixture within a few days, the apricot substitute can be frozen in quarter- or half-cup quantities and thawed as needed.

*NOTE: Canned apricots can be substituted for the fresh. A 15-ounce can of apricots in extra light syrup or juice can be drained and then puréed. Combine with the ground flaxseed.

Hearty Kale Soup
with Vegetables and Soybeans

*C*anned black soybeans are used in this recipe, but white canned soybeans can be substituted.

In a soup pot, heat the oil. Add the garlic, onion, celery and carrots. Cook on medium-low for 10 minutes or until the onions are softened.

Add the chicken stock, kale and zucchini and bring to a boil. Lower the heat and simmer for 20 minutes, covered.

Finally add the drained soybeans and continue cooking for 5 minutes or until the beans are heated through.

Serve garnished with chopped parsley. Add salt and pepper if desired.

INGREDIENTS

YIELD: 6 SERVINGS

2 teaspoons olive oil
1 clove garlic, minced
1 large onion, chopped
1 stalk of celery with leaves, chopped
2 carrots, chopped
4 cups defatted chicken stock
10 ounces chopped frozen kale
1 small zucchini, coarsely chopped
1 can (15 ounces) black soybeans
Parsley (for garnish)
Salt and pepper to taste

PER SERVING

Calories 129
Carbohydrates .... 13 g
Fat.. 3 g
Monounsaturated Fat .... 1 g
Dietary fiber.. 6 g
Cholesterol .... 0 mg
Sodium... 136 mg

Clam Cakes

*T*hese clam cakes can be served on a roll or with a salad for a light lunch or dinner.

Preheat the oven to 400 F. and spray a nonstick baking sheet.

Combine the clams, chopped tomato, red pepper, onion, thyme, sage, and dill in a medium bowl. Add the egg substitute and mix well. Add the bread crumbs.

Use your hands to form 4 patties or cakes and place them on the baking sheet. Bake for 20 minutes. Turn the cakes after 10 minutes and bake on the other side for the remaining minutes or until golden brown.

INGREDIENTS

YIELD: 4 PATTIES OR CAKES

2 cans (6½ ounces) cans chopped clams, drained
½ cup chopped tomato
¼ cup chopped red pepper
¼ cup chopped onion
1 teaspoon thyme
½ teaspoon sage
½ teaspoon dill leaves
¼ cup egg substitute or 1 egg
¼ cup bread crumbs

PER SERVING

Calories 131
Carbohydrates .... 11 g
Fat.. 2 g
Saturated fat .... 0 g
Dietary fiber.. 1 g
Cholesterol .... 38 mg
Sodium... 151 mg

Grilled Chicken with Watermelon and Sweet-and-Sour Ginger Dressing

This recipe makes a lovely platter for a summer afternoon. The watermelon is a cool touch. Pass the dressing for heightened flavor.

Place chicken fingers in a glass pan. Combine the rice vinegar, soy sauce, honey, ginger, peanut oil, and sesame oil in a measuring cup and combine well. Pour two tablespoons of the sauce over the chicken fingers, turning to coat. Reserve the remaining sauce to pass at the table.

Heat a nonstick grill pan or pan with grill marks in it. Add the chicken to the heated pan. Brown on both sides. Remove from pan.

Set up a serving platter or four individual plates. Line the platter or plates with the romaine. On one side place the grilled chicken fingers.

Cut the watermelon from the rind and then cut the watermelon into sticks or fingers. They can be about 4 inches in length. Place the watermelon on the romaine next to the chicken.

Spread the cut green onion over the platter. Add chopped cilantro or parsley, if desired. Top with some of the rice noodles.

Pass the reserved sweet-and-sour sauce.

INGREDIENTS

YIELD: 4 SERVINGS

¾ pound chicken fingers (skinless, boneless chicken breast)
¼ cup rice vinegar
1½ tablespoons soy sauce
2 teaspoons honey
1 teaspoon grated ginger root
1 tablespoon peanut oil
1 teaspoon sesame oil
4 romaine leaves
2½-pound watermelon section
1 green onion, thinly sliced
Chopped cilantro or parsley for garnish
3 ounces rice noodles

PER SERVING

Calories	276
Carbohydrates	32 g
Fat	6 g
Saturated Fat	0 g
Monounsaturated Fat	2 g
Dietary fiber	1 g
Cholesterol	49 mg
Sodium	449 mg

The Vegetable Bin

The Roots of Good Nutrition

The garden was warm as I carefully picked my way around the lettuce, stepped over the young corn, and headed toward the beets. I had never grown root vegetables before. But encouraged by studies showing that many of them could protect my heart, lower cholesterol, reduce blood pressure, and prevent diabetes and stroke, I decided to give them a try. Not only would fresh-picked vegetables assure me of maximum nutrition, I thought, but the added flavor of a vegetable yanked from the ground at peak ripeness might encourage me to work more of these nutritious foods into my family's diet.

Now, looking down at the dark, blue-green leaves of the baby beets, I was glad I'd given in to the impulse. I could harvest the first leafy thinnings for a salad, then return in a few weeks to pull up the warm, purple globes that had been nurtured by the earth. By mid-summer, the carrots would be ready, and by late summer, the potatoes could be dug.

The effort would be minimal. And in return I'd be assured of a vegetable bin full of nutrients to ensure my family's health.

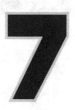

7

VEGETABLE BIN

BEST FOR HELPING YOU:

Lower cholesterol

Prevent diabetes

Reduce high blood pressure

Prevent stroke

Unfortunately, few of us are eating anywhere near the numbers or varieties of the roots and gourds we need to keep us healthy. A survey by the United States Department of Agriculture found, for example, that fewer than 10 percent of Americans eat even a single serving per day of the dark yellow vegetables like carrots, sweet potatoes, and squash that have been found to protect against everything from heart attack and stroke to lung cancer and high blood pressure.

How effective are these veggies? In some studies a single serving every other day prevented lung cancer—even among those who smoked. In a decade in which lung cancer now kills more women and men than any other disease, roots and gourds should regularly appear on our plates and those of our families.

Here's the lowdown on which veggie does what—and how you can benefit.

Beets: The Healthy Roots of Purple Passion

Beets, the most colorful of my earthy seedlings, are loaded with folate, a vitamin that protects your heart, prevents

133

spinal birth defects, and helps your body repair damaged cells that can lead to cervical cancer. They also contain a dash of fiber, iron, manganese, and potassium to help maintain basic body health.

And that's just what's in the roots. In the leaves, which rarely even make it to the table, there's a hidden store of lutein, a carotenoid that guards against macular degeneration, the leading cause of blindness among older adults. It's a disease that affects one in three people over the age of 75. Yet, if you eat enough foods rich in antioxidants, it's an entirely preventable problem.

In one study, for example, researchers evaluated the amount of carotenoids eaten by 356 people between the ages of 55 and 80 who had macular degeneration. Then they looked at the diets of 520 similar folks who did not. The result?

Those who ate the most carotenoids had reduced their risk of macular degeneration by 43 percent.

Carrots: A Natural Source of Carotenoids

Carrots have been a symbol of health for decades. Their bright yellow-orange color indicates that they're packed with carotenoids, a group of plant chemicals that lower cholesterol and prevent cancer. What's more, they actually prevent heart attacks by increasing tPA—a natural clot-busting substance that roams your blood look-

---

BEETS

BEST FOR HELPING YOU:

Prevent age-related blindness

Avoid birth defects

Protect your heart

BEET BASICS

HOW TO BUY: Canned beets lose a serious percentage of nutrients during processing, and they don't have those nutritious beet greens attached. So forget the canned stuff and pick up a bunch of fresh beets from the produce section of your market whenever you see them. Look for small, hard beets with a deep red color and smooth skin. The leaves should be small, perky, and a deep, dark green; the taproot should be slender.

HOW TO STORE: Whack off the leaves about an inch from the root, rinse, shake dry, and store in a plastic bag in your refrigerator's vegetable bin—or crisper, as its sometimes called. Store the purple part of the beets whole and unwashed in a plastic bag next to them. If you don't have a vegetable bin in the refrigerator, toss the leaves in the bottom of your refrigerator and store the beets themselves in a vegetable bin kept in a dark corner of a cool cellar. Use within a couple of days.

HOW TO USE: Because of their rich, earthy color, beets can easily take center stage at almost any meal—baked as a side dish, boiled and puréed as a cold soup, or steamed, then sliced and grated into a salad.

Prepare beets by washing gently before cooking. Do not peel or use a vegetable brush—the beet will lose both color and nutrients. Cook until a knife easily pierces the skin, then peel and serve.

Beet greens should not be cooked—they'll lose much of the lutein stored inside their leaves. Instead, mix them with other greens and drizzle with a little balsamic vinegar and olive oil. The oil will actually help your body absorb the lutein.

ing for clots that might jam up your coronary arteries.

Study after study has demonstrated a strong relationship between eating carrots and a healthy heart:

- In Scotland, researchers found that those who ate seven ounces of raw carrots a day reduced their cholesterol levels by 11 percent.
- In Sweden, researchers found that the more carrots a group of men between the ages of 30 and 60 ate, the more natural tPA they had in their blood.
- And in Italy, researchers found that women between the ages of 22 and 69 who had a diet rich in carrots were one-third less likely to have a heart attack than those who preferred other foods.

Carrots may also help prevent some forms of cancer. Researchers in Belgium found that those who ate carrots reduced their risk of colon cancer by as much as 24 percent, while researchers at the National Institute of Environmental Health Sciences in North Carolina found that women who ate carrots more than twice a week reduced their risk of breast cancer by 44 percent.

Unfortunately, the relationship between carrots and cancer is not quite as clear as the one between carrots and heart disease. The problem is that although carrots are loaded

CARROTS

BEST FOR HELPING YOU:

Prevent heart attacks

Lower cholesterol

Prevent colon cancer

Reduce your risk
of breast cancer

CARROT BASICS

HOW TO BUY: Look for small, cylindrically shaped carrots with dark green foliage still attached and crisp. Avoid any carrots that are cracked, dark at the top, or sprouting rootlets. Generally, the smaller the carrot, the sweeter the taste. My favorites are the tiny ready-to-eat ones wrapped with a tiny container of low-fat ranch dressing. Lots of crunch and a no-brainer for calorie control.

HOW TO STORE: Wrapped in perforated plastic and tucked in your refrigerator's vegetable bin or in a cool, dark part of your cellar. Keep them far away from fruits such as apples and pears. Both give off ethylene gas, a substance that may cause your carrots to go bad.

HOW TO USE: Carrot skin tends to absorb pesticides. So unless your bunch is certified organic, peel off every inch of the outer layer. Then serve the carrots either raw or cooked.

Carrots are one of the few vegetables for which cooking actually increases the available nutrients. A 3.5-ounce serving of raw carrots has 10,650 units of alphacarotene and 18,250 units of beta carotene. A 3.5-ounce serving of cooked carrots has 15,000 units of alphacarotene and 25,650 units of beta carotene. Unfortunately, our bodies have trouble absorbing carotenoids in general. Eating a little fat along with your carrots—even just a drop of olive oil in the cooking water—helps your body use the carotenoids they provide.

with alphacarotene, a carotenoid that inhibits the spread of cancer cells, they also contain beta carotene, a carotenoid that scientists are uneasy about because several studies have shown that taking beta carotene supplements increases the risk of lung cancer in some smokers.

The bottom line? Common sense seems to dictate that all of us should eat a balanced diet that includes carrots. But we might want to avoid the concentrated sources of beta carotene found in whole pitchers of carrot juice or beta carotene supplements.

Potatoes:
An Anti-Aging Torpedo

Baked, whipped, roasted, or boiled, potatoes are packed with an arsenal of nutrients to block the diseases that can make old age miserable. They cut your risk of stroke, knock down your blood pressure, inhibit the spread of cancer cells, reduce the pain-causing inflammation of arthritis and bursitis, help steady your heartbeat, and perhaps even play a role in protecting you from the onset of Parkinson's disease as you age.

Not bad for a little guy who spends most of his life underground, is it?

Scientists began to realize the potato's tremendous therapeutic potential when a group of researchers at the University of California in San Diego found that those who ate even a single extra serving a day of a potassium-rich food like the potato were cutting their risk of stroke death by a full 40 percent.

But that was only the beginning. Since then, researchers at Temple University in Philadelphia have found that a diet rich in the potato's potassium can counteract the blood pressure spikes triggered by the typical salty American diet. Other researchers have found that potatoes also contain powerful protease inhibitors—substances that interrupt the spread of cancer cells and discourage the reproduction of various viral invaders, even the virus that causes AIDS. And they've found that potatoes also contain quercetin, a naturally occurring substance that encourages your immune system to stay on an even keel and not go into the kind of inflammatory hyperdrive that produces arthritis, allergies, and bursitis.

What's more, potatoes also contain alpha lipoic acid. This powerful antioxi-

POTATOES

BEST FOR HELPING YOU:

Cut your risk
of Parkinson's disease

Protect your brain
from a stroke

Reduce blood pressure

Stop the spread of cancer

Maintain a steady heartbeat

Reduce arthritic pain

KEEP YOUR HEART ON A STEADY BEAT

In a stunning study from Harvard University Medical School, researchers have found that the more alpha-linolenic acid in your diet from foods like potatoes, the less likely you are to drop dead from a fatal cardiac rhythm disturbance. The study, which questioned 76,763 women about their food habits over a 16-year period, found that women who consumed a diet of foods rich in alpha-linolenic acid reduced their risk of sudden death by 46 percent.

If you have difficulty finding organically grown potatoes at your local supermarket, here are two outfits that will ship potatoes to your door:

Willow Wind Farms
HCR Box 381
Ford, WA 99013

New Penny Farm
P.O. Box 448
Presque Isle, ME 04769

dant neutralizes many of the free radicals that damage cells and trigger the diseases of old age. It also preserves and protects other nutrients such as vitamins C and E that also disarm these molecules. There's even some thought among scientists that it lowers the risk of death from heart disease—possibly by helping the heart maintain a strong, steady beat.

Potatoes are also a wonderful friend to those of us who constantly struggle with extra pounds. A study at the University of Leeds in Great Britain found, for example, that those who ate a meal that includ-

POTATO BASICS

HOW TO BUY: Buy organically grown potatoes if you intend to eat the peel. Look for firm potatoes with no signs of sprouting and not the slightest tinge of green. The green is a toxic substance called solanine that forms just under the skin when a potato is exposed to light. Small amounts can cause diarrhea, stomachaches and headaches; large amounts can affect your nervous system.

HOW TO STORE: For a week in your refrigerator's vegetable bin, or for 4-15 weeks in a very dark, very cool vegetable bin in your cellar. Do not store in plastic. Store loose or in a paper bag. A study at Aristotle University in Greece suggests that tucking English lavender and rosemary among potatoes when they're stored will inhibit sprouting.

HOW TO USE: Americans love potatoes. They account for roughly one-third of each person's intake of vegetables every day. Unfortunately, 20 percent of us eat them fried—the best way possible to generate the cell-trashing free radicals that destroy the body and lead to many of the diseases that wrinkle our skins and turn our arteries into lead pipes.

Instead of frying, use potatoes baked, boiled, or steamed. The method you use is determined pretty much by the starch content of the potato you choose. Potatoes with lots of starch—the russets most of us use as bakers, for example—have a cellular structure which gives them a mealy texture that easily absorbs moisture. That means they will make terrific mashed potatoes because they'll soak up lots of milk and air when whipped. Unfortunately, they make a lousy potato for potato salad—they simply fall apart into a soggy mass when boiled.

Potatoes with a medium starch content—yellow fins, Yukon golds, and red potatoes, for instance—are moist with a solid texture that holds its shape. They make great roasters—especially when they're cut into chunks, lightly sprayed with olive oil, covered with minced onion, salted, then tucked in a 350°F oven for 40 minutes.

Potatoes with a low starch content—butterfingers, for example—have a solid cellular structure that makes them hold their shape under duress. They're great for boiling, so toss them in stews or potato salad.

If you're headed for elective surgery, make sure you don't load up on mashed potatoes the week before. A study at the University of California Medical Center has found that even tiny amounts of chemicals frequently found in potatoes—solanaceous glycoalkaloids—can block your body's ability to process many of the anesthetics and muscle relaxants commonly used to keep you comfortable.

ed potato ate a total of 21 percent fewer calories than those who did not.

Some studies also indicate that potato skins contain an anticancer substance called chlorogenic acid. But whether or not it will do you any good is a controversial question. Some scientists feel that you shouldn't eat the peel because it absorbs pesticides commonly applied by commercial growers. Eat the peel, these scientists say, and the potential health threat from pesticides cancels out any benefit. Other scientists feel that the amount of pesticides in food is so negligible that you should feel free to scarf it down.

Whether or not you eat the peel, make sure you regularly include the insides of potatoes on your menu. Parkinson's disease is a degenerative disease that causes limbs to tremble. Researchers at the University of Magdeburg in Germany have found that a key difference between the diets of those who develop Parkinson's and those who don't is potatoes; those who eat a lot of potatoes seem to be protected from the disease. Other dietary factors are involved—those who get Parkinson's tend to eat more sweets and raw meat, for example—so researchers are by no means ready to say that potatoes prevent Parkinson's.

THE NEW POTATOES

That big old white Katahdin is still the sweetest baker on the face of the earth. But a daily diet of even your favorite baked potato is bound to get boring. So try alternating that beautiful Katahdin with the rainbow of potatoes from around the world that are gradually turning up in our markets today. Red, blue, purple, yellow, or striped all contain the same healthy dose of nutrients that make the potato a key weapon in the fight against disease. Here's a guide to the ones you're most likely to find in your market—and the best way to prepare them.

VARIETY	COLOR	BEST PREPARATION & USE
All Blue	blue inside & out	mashed
All Red	red inside & out	mashed
Butterfinger	yellow flesh	boiled for potato salad
Caribe	blue skin; white flesh	mashed
Purple Peruvian	purple inside & out	steamed
Red potatoes	red skin; white flesh	boiled for potato salad
Ruby Crescent	red-brown skin; white flesh	boiled for potato salad
Yellow Fins	pale yellow flesh	roasted
Yukon Gold	bright yellow flesh	roasted

There is an association, however. So do yourself and the potato industry a favor—put 'em on your plate as often as you can.

Sweet Potatoes: A Gift from the South

Unless you come from the South, chances are that your relationship to the sweet potato has been limited to an occasional meeting at Thanksgiving or Christmas. And then the sweet potato is wearing a brown sugar overcoat. But given the amazing number of nutrients packed into the fruit of this native American vine, it's a relationship you should nurture.

That's because a single sweet potato contains a whopping dose of potassium that keeps your blood pressure normal and your heart tripping along with a healthy rhythm. It also contains a nice amount of fiber—3.3 grams, or as much as a whole bowl of many cereals—and a good chunk of three antioxidants: vitamin A, vitamin C, and vitamin E. All three antioxidants play an important role in neutralizing the free radicals that damage blood vessels and set the stage for heart disease, stroke, macular degeneration, and cataracts.

Studies have found that those who eat a single serving of yellow-orange vegetables like sweet potatoes every other day have half the risk of lung cancer as those who don't. Even among those who smoke, the protection is significant.

> **SWEET POTATOES**
>
> BEST FOR HELPING YOU:
>
> Fight off cataracts
>
> Prevent a heart attack
>
> Avoid a stroke
>
> Reduce your risk of lung cancer

SWEET POTATO BASICS

HOW TO BUY: Look for dense, blemish-free tubers sold individually in the produce section of your supermarket, particularly during the fall, which is when they're harvested. Avoid canned and frozen varieties. They have significantly less vitamin A and vitamin C. And be aware that sweet potatoes are sometimes called yams in your local market. Real yams are tubers indigenous to Africa that can weigh up to 120 pounds each. They rarely show up in the fresh produce section of foreign supermarkets—and only in chunks.

HOW TO STORE: Sweets will keep for a week in your kitchen vegetable bin at room temperature. To keep them for a month, put them in a vegetable bin that's kept in a cool, dark area of your home.

HOW TO USE: Whipped with a splash of orange juice and a pinch of cinnamon, baked with a spoonful of light sour cream, or smooshed into a casserole with maple syrup, a smidgen of canola oil, and ¼ teaspoon each of cinnamon, nutmeg, and ginger. You can also make sweet potato chips for an after-school snack. Just slice up a raw sweet, sauté it in a tablespoon of canola oil, and drain it on a paper towel with a sprinkling of salt. When the chips reach room temperature, serve them to your little people with a tall glass of milk. One caveat: Don't bother trying to peel a sweet. Just scrub before cooking. The skin is so thin that most of it comes off as you scrub.

We may love potatoes today, but when Spanish explorers first brought them to Europe from South America in the 16th century, nobody knew how to cook them. So instead of just baking or boiling the tuber itself as we do today, many cooks tossed the whole plant—leaves, stem, and tuber—into the pot. Unfortunately, the leaves and stems are toxic. Large numbers of people became ill, doctors came to believe it caused leprosy, and the government of at least one French province labeled potatoes a poisonous and mischievous root and then banned them from the area!

Eventually, folks figured out what the problem was. They started cooking just the tuber and the potato's reputation as a tasty, nutritious vegetable was launched.

The Gourds

More than just something to use as table decorations after the fall harvest, gourds are versatile foods loaded with carotenoids and other disease-fighting antioxidants.

Winter squashes, such as acorn, butternut, hubbard, and pumpkin, are

SWEET GOURDS

BEST FOR HELPING YOU:

Watch your weight

Prevent cervical cancer

Side-step heart disease

Avoid stroke

Prevent age-related blindness

usually packed with beta carotene, plus vitamins A, C, and E to help prevent heart disease, stroke, macular degeneration and cancer. They also have a good shot of magnesium and potassium to maintain a sound heartbeat and ensure smoothly functioning muscles. In a study at the University of Wash-

GOURD BASICS

HOW TO BUY: Look for the deepest-colored squash you can find. It indicates the highest possible nutritional content for that particular squash. Winter squash, which is available mostly in the fall, can be as big as you like—the longer a winter squash, the sweeter it is. In all squash, look for firm, unmarked skin.

HOW TO STORE: Winter squash is a great keeper. Stored whole in your vegetable bin in a dark, cool place, it will stay fresh for up to three months. On the other hand, summer squash is more delicate. Slip it into a plastic bag, store in your refrigerator's vegetable bin, and it will stay fresh for two or three weeks.

HOW TO USE: Scrub the outer skin. If it's tough, you may want to peel it. Otherwise, plan on using the whole squash—yes, including the skin and seeds—in whatever it is you make. Winter squash is best when it's baked because baking preserves its beta carotene content. It also caramelizes some of the sugars, making this one of the sweetest vegetables ever grown. Because of its high water content, summer squash is best sliced and sautéed over a high heat with other vegetables. A pinch of salt sprinkled over the vegetable before cooking will help it retain as much water during cooking as possible.

ington, for example, women who regularly ate winter squash cut their risk of cervical cancer by 40 percent.

If you must use gourds for decoration, choose summer squashes—what you generally find in the market labeled yellow straightneck, patty pan, or zucchini. Though they contain fiber, they have so few nutrients that their chief value is their looks.

A PASSION FOR PUMPKIN

When the leaves fall, the acorns drop, and deer come down off the ridge to nibble corn spilled in the empty fields, I know its only a matter of days until I get my first taste of fresh pumpkin.

Hopefully, I cruise by the pumpkin patch just down the road and scout the local farm stands. And when the first PUMPKIN FOR SALE sign goes up, my wallet comes out. I buy little ones for pumpkin pie, medium ones for pumpkin butter, and large ones for pumpkin seeds. And when that supply runs out in late November, I turn to canned pumpkin. It's not quite as good as fresh, but in my kitchen, not-as-good pumpkin is still better than the best of anything else.

For those of you who share my obsession with this incredible vegetable, here's my favorite mid-winter pumpkin fix. With only a little fat and a lot of taste, it's a great way to satisfy pumpkin passion without adding any more winter padding to my hips.

1 box phyllo mini shells (in the frozen pastry section of your supermarket)
½ cup canned pumpkin
½ cup light (not nonfat) sour cream
½ teaspoon cinnamon
Pinch of nutmeg
Sugar and cinnamon for garnish

Place shells on cookie sheet. Mix the other ingredients and heap into the shells. Bake according to directions on the phyllo box. Chill and serve with a dusting of cinnamon and sugar. Rich in both bone-building calcium and heart-healthy beta carotene, these little pastries also make a great snack for kids.

Baked Apples and Sweet Potatoes

*P*reheat the oven to 350° F.

Peel and thinly slice the sweet potatoes. Layer half of them into a 3-quart casserole.

Core, peel, and slice the apples about ½ inch thick. Layer half over the sweet potatoes. Then add the remaining sweet potatoes, and finally the remaining apples.

Combine the apple cider and cornstarch in a saucepan. Mix well. Heat until slightly thickened. Add the honey. When well combined, pour over the apples and sweet potatoes. Combine the sugar and cinnamon and sprinkle over the top.

Bake for 45 minutes or until sweet potatoes are tender and apples on top are golden brown.

INGREDIENTS

YIELD: 6–8 SERVINGS

2 large sweet potatoes (1¼ pounds)
3 apples (1 pound)
1 cup apple cider or juice
2 tablespoons cornstarch
½ cup honey
1 teaspoon sugar
¼ teaspoon cinnamon

PER SERVING

Calories	260
Carbohydrates	65 g
Saturated fat	0.1 g
Dietary fiber	5 g
Cholesterol	0 mg
Sodium	15 mg

Garlic Mashed Potatoes

*S*ounds heavenly… and they are. These potatoes are cooked in milk with a clove of garlic. You'll be surprised at the creaminess that comes from the added fat-free cream cheese. A traditional Irish dish is Colcannon, which is a combination of mashed potatoes and cabbage. To give the Garlic Mashed Potatoes that Irish flavor, serve them in a large dish surrounded by chopped cooked cabbage and top with sliced and sautéed turkey sausage.

Wash, peel, and cut the potatoes into 1-inch cubes. Add to a heavy-bottomed saucepan. Add the garlic and milk and bring to a simmer over medium heat. Then lower heat slightly, cover, and cook for about 15 minutes or until the potatoes are tender when a sharp knife is inserted into the center of the potatoes. (Check the potatoes occasionally, making sure the temperature is hot enough to cook them but low enough not to scorch them.)

Remove the pan from the heat and add the cream cheese. Mash the potatoes and garlic, using a potato masher or a fork, until all the milk has been incorporated and the potatoes are fluffy.

INGREDIENTS

YIELD: 4 SERVINGS (2 CUPS)

1½ pounds russet potatoes
2 cloves garlic, peeled
1 cup low-fat milk (1%)
2 tablespoons fat-free cream cheese

PER SERVING

Calories	164
Carbohydrates	34 g
Fat	1 g
Saturated fat	0.5 g
Dietary fiber	3 g
Cholesterol	3 mg
Sodium	78 mg

Barley Borscht

Vegetarian

Borscht is the Polish name for a soup made with beets. You can also make this rich red soup with beef and other vegetables.

In a 4-quart soup pot, add the barley and water and bring to a boil. Turn the heat off, cover the pot, and allow the barley to soak for 1 hour.

Meanwhile wash, peel, and cut the beets into chunks. Chop the onion, carrots, celery, and garlic. Set aside. When the barley is finished soaking, pour off the water. Add the beets, onion, carrots, celery, garlic, and bay leaves. Add 6 cups of water. Bring to a boil, lower heat, cover, and simmer for 45 to 50 minutes or until the beets and barley are tender.

Add the tomatoes, chopped beet or turnip greens, and lemon juice. Cook another 15 minutes or until all the vegetables are tender and hot.

Serve hot with a dollop of yogurt for garnish.

INGREDIENTS

YIELD: 12 CUPS

½ cup hulled barley
1½ cups water
2 pounds raw beets
1 medium onion
2 carrots
2 stalks celery
2 cloves garlic
2 bay leaves
6 cups water
2 cups chopped tomatoes
10 ounces fresh or frozen chopped beet or
　　turnip greens
1 lemon, juiced
Plain nonfat yogurt for garnish

PER SERVING

Calories	83
Carbohydrates	18 g
Fat	0.5 g
Saturated fat	0.1 g
Dietary fiber	4 g
Cholesterol	0 mg
Sodium	125 mg

Acorn Squash
Stuffed with Mushrooms and Wild Rice

One acorn squash will make two servings. The acorn squash can be cooked in the microwave and then stuffed and finished in a standard oven.

Preheat the oven to 350 F.

Cut the acorn squash in half. Place the cut side down on a microwavable dish or waxed paper. Microwave on high for 7 to 8 minutes or until tender. Allow to stand for 5 minutes.

Heat the oil and sauté the mushrooms for 10 minutes or until softened.

Combine the mushrooms with the wild rice in a bowl and add the scallions, apples, almonds, parsley, and half the cheddar cheese.

Place about ½ cup of the filling in the center of each acorn squash. Place the squash in a baking dish that can be used in a standard oven. Bake for 15 minutes, covered. Remove the cover and top with the remaining shredded cheese. Return to the oven and allow the cheese to melt, about 5 more minutes.

INGREDIENTS

YIELD: 4 SERVINGS

2 acorn squash
1 tablespoon olive oil
4 ounces raw mushrooms, chopped
1½ cups cooked wild rice
2 scallions, thinly sliced, including the green tops
½ apple, chopped
2 tablespoons slivered almond
2 tablespoons chopped parsley
2 ounces shredded low-fat cheddar cheese

PER SERVING

Calories	248
Carbohydrates	41 g
Fat	7 g
Saturated fat	1 g
Dietary fiber	6 g
Cholesterol	3 mg
Sodium	99 mg

Oven-Roasted Pumpkin Chips

It is easier to peel a pumpkin if the pumpkin is first heated in the microwave to soften the skin. To do this, first wash the skin. Then pierce the skin all over with a sharp knife and place the pumpkin in the microwave on a double layer of paper towels.

Microwave on high for 3 minutes, then turn the pumpkin over and microwave the other side on high for 3 more minutes.

These baked chips are great hot or cold.

Preheat the oven to 450 F.

When the pumpkin has cooled after softening the skin in the microwave, cut it in half. Remove the seeds and center fibers. Peel it. Slice the pumpkin into ¾-inch chips.

Spray a cookie sheet with a nonstick spray. Spread the pumpkin chips over the pan. Combine the sugar and cinnamon and sprinkle on the chips.

Roast the chips for about 10 minutes. When they are browned on the bottom, turn them over with a pancake turner and sprinkle with the sugar/cinnamon mixture and roast for another 10 minutes or until browned on the other side.

INGREDIENTS

YIELD: 4 CUPS

1 pumpkin (2 pounds) or crookneck squash
1 tablespoon sugar
1 teaspoon cinnamon

PER SERVING

Calories	27
Carbohydrates	6 g
Fat	0.3 g
Saturated fat	0 g
Dietary fiber	2 g
Cholesterol	0 mg
Sodium	1 mg

Red Cabbage and Beets

The combination of red cabbage and red beets makes a beautiful side dish.

Heat the olive oil in a large soup pot. Add the sliced onion and cook on medium-low for 10 minutes or until the onion is softened.

Meanwhile, wash, peel, and cube the beets; wash and chop the beet greens and wash and slice the cabbage. Add the beets, beet greens, and cabbage to the pot with the water and vinegar.

Bring to a boil, lower the heat, and cook on low for about 30 minutes or until the beets and cabbage are tender.

INGREDIENTS

YIELD: 8–10 SERVINGS

1 tablespoon olive oil
1 large whole onion, sliced
3 raw red beets
6 beet green leaves
½ head red cabbage
1 cup water
2 tablespoons red-wine vinegar

PER SERVING

Calories	57
Carbohydrates	9 g
Fat	2 g
Saturated fat	0.3 g
Dietary fiber	3 g
Cholesterol	0 mg
Sodium	78 mg

Stewed Carrots and Tomatoes

$\mathcal{I}$n a large saucepan, bring the carrots and water to a boil. Cover and steam until tender. More water can be added if necessary.

When the carrots are tender, add the remaining ingredients to the pot. Bring to a boil. Cover and take the pot off the heat. Allow the combination to cool and marinate.

This can be served hot, cold, or at room temperature.

INGREDIENTS

YIELD: 6–8 SERVINGS OR 2½ CUPS

6 carrots, peeled and sliced
½ cup water
2 cloves garlic, minced
1 can (14½ ounces) no-salt stewed tomatoes
2 tablespoons lemon juice
1 tablespoon fruity olive oil
2 teaspoons sugar
¼ teaspoon dry mustard
⅛ teaspoon ground turmeric

PER SERVING

Calories	79
Carbohydrates	13 g
Fat	2 g
Saturated fat	0 g
Monounsaturated Fat	2 g
Dietary fiber	3 g
Cholesterol	0 mg
Sodium	34 mg

Carrot and Barley Salad

$\mathcal{T}$his vegetable and grain salad can be prepared and served immediately or stored in the refrigerator and served cold. Cooked barley can be kept frozen and used as needed in recipes.

In a microwave-safe container with a lid, place two tablespoons water and the carrots. Microwave on high for 3 minutes and then allow to stand for 2 minutes.

Add the cooked carrots and any of the liquid to a serving bowl. Add the remaining ingredients and toss. Serve over greens.

INGREDIENTS

YIELD: 4 SERVINGS (½ CUP EA.)

2 carrots, peeled and chopped (about 2 cups)
1 cup cooked hulled barley
1 scallion, thinly sliced (optional)
2 teaspoons balsamic vinegar
2 teaspoons olive oil
1 teaspoon minced fresh tarragon or 2
    teaspoon dried tarragon
½ teaspoon minced garlic

PER SERVING

Calories	107
Carbohydrates	19 g
Fat	3 g
Saturated fat	0.4 g
Dietary fiber	5 g
Cholesterol	0 mg
Sodium	14 mg

The Freezer

Open my freezer door on any given day and you'll likely find a range of fat, cold-water fish like salmon or mackerel, plus chicken and turkey neatly stacked inside. Occasionally, when my son is home from college, you'll also find a pound of lamb—a high-fat meat that makes no pretensions of being healthful, but one without which it's impossible to make an authentic Irish Stew.

What you won't find is beef. Or pork. Or veal. And that's because fish, chicken, and turkey contain everything my family needs from a source of protein without any negative side effects. They're widely available without additives, and fish even has some extra benefits—heart-healthy fats that have been proven to increase my family's chances of having strong, healthy hearts that will beat well into the next century.

On the other hand, beef, pork, and veal don't have any extra benefits that would allow them into my freezer—and they do have plenty of negatives: studies show that beef has a clear relationship to heart disease, and a re-

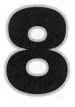

8

FREEZER

BEST FOR HELPING YOU:

Control irregular heartbeat

Prevent heart attacks

Avoid Alzheimer's disease

Lower blood pressure

Lower cholesterol

Prevent gallstones

Reduce rheumatoid arthritis pain

Soothe ulcerative colitis

Relieve itchiness

Maintain a healthy weight

cent study at Wayne State University in Detroit has linked it to DNA damage in women. Pork, which usually contains antibiotics, contributes to the life-threatening growth of antibiotic-resistant bacteria throughout the world and has also been linked to DNA damage. And veal has all the drawbacks of beef—plus it's produced by keeping a baby calf upright and immobile in a pen every moment of every day of its short, miserable life.

Obviously, not including these three products in my freezer is a deeply personal choice. But it's a choice that increasing numbers of people are making every day. Twenty years ago, surveys showed that each of us ate 89 pounds of beef a year; today we eat 64. Pork consumption has also declined 11 percent over the past two decades. What's more, surveys now show we eat as much poultry as beef, and more fish than ever before.

These new eating styles may be one very good reason heart disease rates have dropped roughly 25 percent over the past 20 years. It's also why this chapter of *The Healing Kitchen* validates those choices and encourages you to ignore food industry hype as you maintain the common-sense approach that is leading you and your family to a healthier life. Beef is NOT what's for dinner in the Healing Kitchen!

Fish: A Net Full of Health

Standing in an ice-cold stream in the Pacific Northwest may not be your idea of healthy living. But if you manage to catch and then eat the salmon swimming past your waders, you've probably done more for your heart than a whole school of cardiologists can.

Salmon—and other cold-water fish such as herring, mackerel, and sardines—all contain a rich oil made up of substances that scientists call "omega-3 fatty acids." In fish, these omega-3s keep the little swimmer warm as it dives through ice-cold waters. In humans, omega-3s seem to be responsible for a whole host of health-giving benefits: studies show they reduce your risk of high blood pressure, high cholesterol, heart disease, irregular heart rhythms, heart attack, Alzheimer's disease, and even gallstones. What's more, scientists have found that a diet rich in fish reduces pain in those with rheumatoid arthritis, soothes a grouchy bowel if you have ulcerative colitis, and relieves the itchiness of the skin diseases psoriasis and dermatitis.

University of Washington researchers, for example, studied the diets of 334 peo-

FISH

BEST FOR HELPING YOU:

Control irregular heartbeat

Prevent heart attacks

Avoid Alzheimer's disease

Lower blood pressure

Lower cholesterol

Prevent gallstones

Reduce rheumatoid arthritis pain

Soothe ulcerative colitis

Relieve itchiness

Maintain a healthy weight

ple who had died of cardiac arrest, then compared them to the diets of 493 similar people who had not. They found that those who ate just one serving of fatty fish a week had cut their risk of premature death by 50 percent. Even better was a study in which researchers at Northwestern University followed the diets of more than 2,000 men between the ages of 40 and 55 for over 30 years. This study found that those who ate just over an ounce of fish every day cut their risk of death from a heart attack by 67 percent.

Just how fish does all this remains to be seen. Scientists suspect it has something to do with the ability of the fish's omega-3s to alter the body's chemical balance by blocking its production of a variety of leukotrienes, prostaglandins, and thromboxane— some or all of which seem responsible for sending pain messages to the brain, triggering inflammation, causing blood vessels to constrict, and encouraging platelets to form clots that can get stuck in your arteries.

But don't get stuck in a trough with only fatty fish. Freshwater species—trout and white bass, for example—also seem to have the ability to guarantee good health. When researchers at the University of Washington in Seattle compared a group of African tribespeople who lived on freshwater fish from a local lake with a group that lived on vegetables and grains grown in the surrounding hills, they found that those who lived on fish had 40 percent less of a particularly nasty type of cholesterol—Lp(a)—roaming their arteries. What's more, a team of Italian researchers who studied the same two groups found that 16 percent of the grain and vegetables eaters had high blood pressure, while only 3 percent of the fish eaters did.

How much fish did it take to get these life-giving benefits? A lot. The Africans who lived on fish ate three or four fish meals a day, totaling about 23 percent of their total intake.

But you don't have to eat that much to reap the many benefits of fish. Two or three fish meals a week will pay off big. Most fish is a low-fat alternative to meat. It's loaded with muscle-building protein—a single serving of halibut has about 27 grams or half a day's supply—plus a whopping dose of vitamin B12. And canned salmon, which generally contains a bunch of small, edible bones, is also a fabulous source of calcium.

Two caveats: First, since some fish can contain trace amounts of mercury, a highly toxic metal, or pollutants known

---

FISH BASICS

HOW TO BUY: Shop with your nose. Fish should not smell "fishy." Eyes should be clear; flesh should be firm. There should be no slime anywhere on it. Your best bet is to shop at a fish market rather than a store that sells fish as one of many foods. Ask the owner where the fish came from and how it was handled on the ship. If he or she doesn't know, find another place to shop. For fish taken from the ocean, fish that is flash-frozen on the ship that takes it from the sea should be your first choice. You can't get it any fresher. And avoid fish that's on sale. It won't be a bargain—just an old fish with fishy nutrition.

Canned fish is also a good choice, as long as it's packed in water and not oil. The vegetable oil in which it's packed simply adds calories, not nutrients. Draining the oil is an option, of course, but it drains away much of the heart-healthy omega-3s as well.

HOW TO STORE: Fresh fish should be rinsed, wrapped in plastic, and immediately stored in the freezer. Fish already frozen should be transported from store to home in a bag of ice—just ask the clerk to double-bag the fish with some ice in the outer bag—and placed in your freezer as soon as you get home.

HOW TO USE: Fish fresh from the freezer is always fast and convenient. That's why I always keep a stack of individually wrapped fillets on hand. Just rinse the fish under cold running water, remove any tiny bones, brush it with a touch of garlic-infused oil, and toss in the pan or on the grill. The Canadian Fisheries and Marine Service suggests you cook fish 10 minutes per inch of thickness—more if it's still frozen. Turn the fish so it's cooked evenly on both sides. Steaming it in the microwave is also a good option—particularly since this method preserves the most omega-3s.

Canned fish is an even quicker way to get the health benefits of fish. Add a few drops of garlic-infused oil and some celery to canned salmon and you've got a first-class Neptune salad for lunch.

However you serve fish, always try to prepare it with a rich source of vitamin E, such as almonds, sunflower seeds, or sunflower oil. The vitamin E in these sources prevents the fish oils from oxidizing and turning a healthful fat into a harmful one.

All fish are not created equal. Only those with the most omega-3 fatty acids are likely to stabilize heart rhythm, cut your risk of a heart attack, reduce the pain of rheumatoid arthritis, soothe a grouchy bowel, or prevent Alzheimer's when you reach old age. So based on their omega-3 content here, in rank order, are the top eight healthiest fish. Fish high in omega-3s but likely to contain pollutants like mercury are not included.

1 Atlantic herring
2. Anchovies
3. Pink salmon
4. Bluefin tuna
5. Atlantic sardines
6. Sockeye salmon
7. Oysters
8. Rainbow smelts

as PCBs, pregnant and nursing women should check with their state department of fisheries about which fish are safe to eat for themselves and for young children. Second, since one of the ways ome-ga-3s prevent heart attacks is to "thin" the blood, common sense suggests that those who are taking "blood-thinning" medication to prevent heart attacks or stroke, or those who have a history of stroke in their family, should check with their doctor before increasing their intake of fish.

Poultry: The New American Standard

In the race to reduce fat, build muscle, and avoid the negative health effects of meat, many of us build our meals around turkey and chicken.

It's not a bad idea. A three-ounce serving of roasted turkey breast has a whopping 25 grams of muscle-building protein, less than three grams of fat, plus more than a quarter of the amount of niacin and vitamin B6 you need every day to convert body fat to energy and build the antibodies of your immune system. A 3-ounce serving of roasted chicken breast has an incredible 26 grams of protein—and just a whisker more than three grams of fat. But it also has a whopping dose of B vitamins: more than 60 percent of the amount of niacin you need every day,

A few warm-water fish that thrive in the shallows of the Caribbean and the Pacific Ocean have been found to contain a nasty toxin called ciguatera. Found mostly in grouper, snapper, barracuda, amberjack, and moray eel, the toxin cannot be detected by touch, taste, or smell, nor is it killed in cooking or processing.

Three to six hours after you eat an infected fish, ciguatera announces its presence with nausea, cramps, vomiting, and diarrhea. A day or two later, the toxin attacks your nervous system and causes dizziness, fatigue, numbness in arms and/or legs, muscle pain, joint pain, and extreme weakness. It also screws up your body's thermostat: hot objects feel cold, cold objects feel hot. Sometimes your feet, hands, or mouth become itchy.

If any of these symptoms appear, contact your doctor immediately. There's no known antidote, but once the toxin is identified, your doctor can make you more comfortable.

plus more than 25 percent of the B6 and 15 percent of the B12 you need to build strong nerves and a healthy brain.

If your goal is to build a strong body, poultry's not a bad way to start. Like so many things, however, poultry has its good and bad sides. Its good side is the lean, white breasts that are naturally low in fat. Its bad side is the darker meats— the leg or drumstick— that can have double the fat of the lighter meat.

But even the dark meat's not all bad. It usually boasts a nice chunk of zinc—anywhere from 20 to 25 percent of your daily requirement—to boost your immune system to up to maximum strength.

Meat: Oprah Was Right

I love meat. The thicker the steak, the juicier the roast, the fatter the ribs, the happier I am. But I love myself and my family, as well. And a steady diet of thick, juicy steaks, corpulent pot roast, or thick country bacon is one of the fastest ways I can think of to kill us all off.

Now, having said that, I'm going to live in mortal terror that rabid representatives of the meat industry are going to come after me the way they did Oprah Winfrey and try to take my family home. But the truth is the truth. And unless a whole passel of scientists over the past decade have been wrong—always possible, I admit— then none of us should be eating meat.

POULTRY

BEST FOR HELPING YOU:

Build muscles, organs, and enzymes

Maintain strong nerves

Build a healthy brain

Provide energy

Make immune system antibodies

MEAT

BEST FOR HELPING YOU:

Build muscle

Prevent anemia

Build a sound immune system

Maintain strong nerves

Keep up with cellular repair

Let's look at the pros and cons. First, here's what's good about meat:

- It's a great source of iron for premenopausal women. Not only does a single serving frequently contain anywhere from 5 to 30 percent of the iron we need on a daily basis, it contains heme iron, a form that is more readily absorbed by the body than the non-heme iron found in plants.

- It's a good source of easily absorbed zinc. A single serving of most beef will provide somewhere around one-third of the amount you need every day to keep your immune system on its toes.

- It's a good source of B vitamins, which are necessary for strong nerves, healthy skin, cellular repair, and an active metabolism.

- It's a terrific source of protein, with a single serving containing nearly all the protein a child under 10 needs to build muscle for an entire day.

Now the bad:

- Meat is generally loaded with fat, particularly saturated fat—the kind that causes blocked arteries and heart attacks.

- A single serving of meat generally contains nearly one-third the total cholesterol you should eat for an entire day.

- Meat is calorically dense—three bites of just about anything runs around 175 calories.

And the ugly:

- A study of 1,000 women at the University of Milan found that women who ate a lot of beef and other red meat increased their risk of endometriosis between 80 and 100 percent.
- A study of 70,000 women at the Harvard School of Public health found that eating a single serving of meat a day increased the risk of Type 2 diabetes by 26 percent. Eating two servings a day increased the risk by 40 percent.
- Your body turns two chemicals in meat into homocysteine, a compound that scars blood vessel walls and sets the stage for heart disease.

If it was simply a case of the good outweighing the bad or the good and bad being even, I'd probably feel free to eat at least one serving of meat a day. But study after study seems to indicate that every

---

POULTRY BASICS

HOW TO BUY: Frozen. If you buy chicken or turkey in a market, pick either the whole chicken or turkey or its selected parts from below the freezer line in your grocer's freezer. Then check the "sell-by" date on the label. That date is 7 to10 days from the day a chicken or turkey was slaughtered so it's pretty easy to see which chicken is the freshest. Avoid capons, which are bred to be full of fat.

To be honest, I try to buy only free-range "organic" chicken and turkey that have been raised on a farm—preferably one that I've visited. Dietitians will tell you that there's no difference in nutrition between an organically raised chicken or turkey and one that was raised in an overcrowded pen and stuffed with antibiotics and hormones. Supposedly, they all have relatively the same protein, the same vitamins, and the same minerals.

But having spent the last decade watching food scientists discover literally hundreds of substances in foods that have a direct impact on our health, I can't help wondering if there's something good for me in organic chickens that they're about to discover as well. So I've decided to err on the side of caution. And since, with one or two exceptions, the more processed, handled, and abused foods are, the less natural, protective substances they contain, I've decided to buy poultry the way I buy produce: with as few sprays, shots, chemicals, and hormones added as possible.

I may be wrong. But I have a friend who used to always say, "What goes around, comes around." If that's true in poultry, all of us had better start looking harder at the way chickens and turkeys are handled before they get to our plates.

HOW TO STORE: Frozen. Slip the already-frozen poultry you've purchased into a lock-top plastic bag and burrow it in the coldest part of your freezer.

HOW TO USE: Thaw the bird in your refrigerator, then wash it within an inch of its life, keeping in mind that life-threatening bacteria lurk in every nook and cranny. Roast, broil, or microwave it, then remove the skin and serve. Once you've removed the skin, you've removed most of the fat and cholesterol on any piece of chicken.

bite of meat puts me a step closer to a funeral home. In a study at Haukeland University Hospital in Norway, for example, scientists monitored the diets and blood levels of homocysteine for nearly five years in 587 people who already had heart disease. They found that 3.8 percent of those with homocysteine levels below nine micromoles per liter had died, while 24.7 percent of those with homocysteine levels of 15 micromoles per liter were dead.

Breaking it down even more minutely, the researchers found that those with 9 to 14.9 micromoles per liter of homocysteine nearly doubled their risk of death. Those with 15 to 19 micromoles of homocysteine almost tripled their risk. And those with more than 20 micromoles of homocysteine increased their risk almost fivefold. Clearly, the more homocysteine people had, the more likely they were to die from heart disease.

Another study, this one a joint effort among Tufts University in Boston, the Framingham Heart Study in Framingham, Massachusetts, Boston University, and several other American institutions, looked at the relationship between homocysteine levels and the clogged neck arteries that set the stage for stroke. After checking the homocysteine levels and arteries of more than 1,000 elderly folks in Massachusetts, the researchers found that higher homocysteine levels actually doubled the risk of a blocked neck artery and, hence, the risk of stroke.

Your gut doesn't fare any better than your neck. A study of more than 88,000 women between the ages of 34 and 50 found that women who ate beef, pork, or lamb every day had more than twice the risk of colon cancer than women who ate meat less than once a month.

What's more, a South American study that compared the diets of 169 women with breast cancer and 253 women without the disease found that eating any kind of meat tripled the women's risk of breast cancer—and red meat had quadrupled it.

I don't know about you, but that's enough for me. If you still choose to eat meat after all that, here's how to mitigate some of its effects:

Eat less than three ounces a day. This recommendation comes from the American Institute for Cancer Research, a non-profit organization that drew together a panel of international experts on meat. The experts subsequently issued a 600-page report that said, in part: "If eat-

---

MEAT BASICS

HOW TO BUY: Rarely. Check "The Real 'Choice' Meats" on page 155 and let it be your guide. Look for a bright, cherry-red color indicating that it's still well oxygenated and avoid any hint of marbling and external fat.

HOW TO STORE: Frozen. Drop store-wrapped meat into a plastic freezer bag and store in the back of your freezer.

HOW TO USE: Defrost in the refrigerator, wash within an inch of its life, then use as a condiment. A few strips of meat in a stir fry, a couple of bones thrown into a soup, a medallion or two flanked by a geometric arrangement of veggies. Those who have high blood pressure shouldn't even eat that much. A study at the University of Bergen in Norway indicates that high levels of homocysteine interact with high blood pressure to put you at even greater risk of a heart attack.

en at all, limit intake of red meat to less than three ounces daily. It is preferable to choose fish, poultry, and meat from non-domesticated—'wild'—animals in place of red meat."

Avoid ground meat, whether it's beef, pork, or lamb. Serving for serving, ground meat generally has two to three times the saturated fat of other types of meat. The same goes for processed meat products like hot dogs and hamburgers, which frequently use ground meat. And don't let the "lean" label on some packages of ground beef fool you. It means that the package on which it appears contains meat that is "no more than 22.5 percent fat by weight." By anybody's count but the meat industry's, that's not lean. Unfortunately, ground beef accounts for close to half of all beef sold in the United States.

Eat leafy greens. For every bite of meat, take 10 bites of leafy green vegetables. And talk to your doctor about using a B-complex supplement as a chaser.

Folic acid plus vitamins B6 and B12 lower homocysteine levels in the blood, says Jacob Selhub, Ph.D., a researcher at Tufts University's USDA Human Nutrition Research Center on Aging.

Finish your meal with a vitamin C supplement. Studies indicate that eating a meal loaded with fat causes your heart's arteries to constrict, thus setting up anyone with clogged arteries for an immediate heart attack. Conversely, taking a vitamin C supplement seems to counteract this effect. Check with your doctor for the dose that's right for you.

Clear the air of smoke. A study at the University of Bergen in Norway found that high homocysteine levels apparently interact with tobacco smoke to increase the risk of a heart attack—particularly in women. Now, chances are you don't smoke. But since you inhale just as many chemicals from smoke when you're standing or sitting next to someone who does, common sense says you should stay

---

THE NEW PORK: IS IT REALLY THE "OTHER WHITE MEAT"? OR A WOLF IN SHEEP'S CLOTHING?

The pork industry has been bragging about the leanness of a new generation of pork for some time. But call one of the industry's consumer hot lines and ask for the amount of saturated fat in a particular company's products and the folks on the other end of the phone turn coy: "I don't know how much fat it has," one perky pork person said happily when I called. "All I know is it has 60 percent less fat than it did."

"So I'd have to read the label on your product in order to find out how much that is?"

"Guess so," came the cheerful reply.

Made suspicious by the fact that she wouldn't quote the fat content, that's exactly what I did. And to my surprise, she was right. Or pretty close to it. New techniques in breeding, feeding, raising, and packaging pork have reduced the fat content of pork by nearly a third over the past 15 years. That doesn't mean you can go hog wild, of course, and fatten yourself for market. Tenderloins and top loins aren't too bad, but there are still some cuts you may want to avoid. A few strips of bacon still equals over 500 calories and 49 grams of fat—17 of them saturated.

away from places that permit smoking. Or move to Vermont. It's actually against the law here to smoke in public places.

Wild Creatures: A Healthy Alternative to Beef

The snow started before dawn.

By 9 A.M., the early morning hunters were hunkered down at the Hungry Bear on Route 5, just inside the eastern Vermont border. Still wearing their thick plaid hunting shirts and heavy boots, they slumped over the counter and eyed the snow squall outside from behind cups of dark, steaming coffee.

By 10 A.M., the hunters had gone home, the squall had given way to a steady snowfall, and several inches of fresh powder covered the white-framed houses and

THE REAL "CHOICE" MEATS

When you get that primitive urge to swing from the trees and eat a hunk of meat, some choices are better than others. If you remember to trim the fat and keep your portions under four ounces, here's the best of the lot:

PORTION	CALORIES	SATURATED FAT	TOTAL FAT
Ham, canned, ex. lean	136	2 grams	5 grams
Pork tenderloin	164	2 grams	5 grams
Beef eye round	180	2 grams	5 grams
Lamb foreshank	187	2 grams	6 grams
Beef top round	230	2 grams	6 grams
Lamb shank	180	2 grams	7 grams
Beef bottom round	200	2 grams	7 grams
Pork top loin	194	3 grams	7 grams

MAY THEY REST IN PEACE

Several cuts you're not likely to find in a Healing Kitchen:

PORTION	CALORIES	SATURATED FAT	TOTAL FAT
Prime rib	420	14 grams	35 grams
Pork spareribs	450	13 grams	34 grams
Lamb rib roast	390	13 grams	31 grams
Beef chuck blade	390	12 grams	29 grams
Beef brisket	380	11 grams	28 grams
Beef arm pot roast	370	10 grams	25 grams
Porterhouse steak	340	10 grams	25 grams
Rib eye steak	340	10 grams	24 grams

churches along the main street of Bradford, a small Vermont village just up the road.

By noon, Connie Chipman was in the Bradford United Church of Christ Congregational kitchen checking on 175 pounds of field-dressed venison roasting in the ovens, while Bobby Mosenthal, a senior member of the church, was calmly counting out paper placemats in the dining room.

It was the Saturday before Thanksgiving. And snow or no snow, every member of the church who was not dead or in the hospital was at or on the way to his or her post for the 42nd Annual Bradford Wild Game Supper.

Outside the back door, Gary Tomlinson was firing up the grill to cook boar. Across the road at the Methodist church, Anita Perry and her daughter were preparing platoon-sized pans of pheasant and rice. Up the road, Craig White had opened up the high school kitchen, put on his running shoes, and started cooking the 700 pounds of potatoes he and his crew had peeled, halved, and soaked the night before. The salad makers arrived— mother, daughter, and son-in-law—soon after, closely followed by the vegetable crew and the gingerbread squad.

Within two hours, church members and assorted friends had completed final preparations for the supper. One hundred and twenty rabbits, 24 pheasant, 16 beaver, 10 deer, 4 boar, 3 bear, and half a moose—most of it donated by state game wardens, game preserves, game farms, and local hunters—had been roasted, baked, stewed, or stuffed in one church kitchen or another.

More than 1,200 pounds of salad, potatoes, and squash were ready at the high school. And all 1,150 chunks of gingerbread— freshly baked at the high school the night before—were on their way to the UCC church.

Once there, the gingerbread and the rest of this wild banquet would meet up with more than 1,000 visitors from 48 states. It was going to be a feast. No one would go away hungry. And most would have satisfied their craving for meat—without inciting their cholesterol levels to riot.

WILD CREATURES

BEST FOR HELPING YOU:

Prevent anemia

Prevent fatigue

Maintain a healthy weight

Cut Saturated Fat in Half

Wild game has always been a healthful alternative to beef. In fact, according to the USDA's Nutrient Database, wild game generally has about half the saturated fat of those high-fat steaks, roasts, and patties we buy in the supermarket.

The average amount of fat in cooked beef trimmed of its extra fat is a whopping 21.54 grams of fat per 3½-ounce serving. Yet rabbit has only 6.31 grams of fat, roasted pheasant has 3.25, cooked deer has 3.19, bison has 2.42, elk has 1.9, and moose comes in at an amazing .97.

Clearly, it's also a better choice to keep the lid on your cholesterol levels. Although both beef and game have about the same amounts of dietary cholesterol in each serving—ranging from 50 to 90 milligrams per three ounces of meat— the higher amounts of saturated fat in beef can send the cholesterol levels in your body soaring, while the low levels in game won't.

What's more, game can provide your body with the fat it needs to absorb valuable antioxidants like vitamin E without putting you at risk for high cholesterol, heart disease, breast cancer, and obesity.

Game is also a rich source of the B vitamins necessary to turn your food into cellular fuel and counteract the amino acids in meat that contribute to heart disease. And a single serving contains about one-third the amount of iron nutritionists recommend to help premenopausal women replace red blood cells lost during their periods—thus helping to prevent the fatigue and low-level anemia that plague many women just before they menstruate.

Wild Cuisine

Fortunately, nobody has to take out a hunting license or fire a gun to get good game any more. The number of game farms across the country is increasing at a rapid rate and many forms of game—particularly deer, pheasant, boar, and bison—are being domestically raised and shipped from one end of the continent to the other.

At the Bradford Game Supper, for example, Supper cochairperson Connie Chipman wanted to give folks a taste of something they weren't likely to find in her neck of the woods. So in addition to making friends with every game warden in the area, she also called up an ostrich farm in the Midwest and ordered enough meat to make ostrich burgers for all 1,000 Game Supper diners.

How Did It Taste?

That's what I went to the 42nd Annual Game Supper to find out.

As we entered the hall and headed toward the buffet table, Cecil took our tickets and Bill handed each of us a plate. Then we slowly shuffled past pan after pan of game. Peep plopped a steaming spoonful of venison chili on my plate, while Jim added a few slices of venison steak and roast. Jane tossed a couple of moose patties and ostrich burgers on the side, and Carol added a slice of rabbit pie.

My plate began to get heavy, but I was only halfway down the line. Rob somehow found room for rabbit roast, Bonnie added boar roast, and Juanita snuck in a tiny boar sausage. Fran added some game stuffing, while Darlene smooshed everything to one side so she could give me at least a few slivers of roast beaver and buffalo.

Arriving at the end of the buffet—potatoes, squash, and salad were already on

---

GAME BASICS

HOW TO BUY: Buy frozen game from a local specialty shop, or check with your local state game commission for the names of local suppliers. Avoid field-dressed game that's been allowed to "age," unless you personally can vouch for the handling of the game. Improperly dressed game can result in the production of life-threatening toxins like salmonella.

HOW TO STORE: In a zero-degree freezer for three to six months. Defrost in the refrigerator before cooking—allow four hours per pound.

HOW TO USE: Since the fat on wild game can frequently have an "off" taste, trim any visible fat. Then braise the meat in liquid. Or roast it, basting frequently. (See "Cooking Wild: Vermont Venison" on page 158.)

the tables—Bobby handed me a printed sheet with "The Toothpick Code." Since nobody could ever remember which piece of meat was which, they began sticking a color-coded toothpick into each serving. And Bobby's handout told me—a wild game neophyte—how to tell beaver from pheasant.

Penny Randall, Connie's cochair, handed us over to a couple of young apprentices with sweet smiles and helping hands who seated us along one side of a long banquet table. Families on either side of us were fork-deep in their game suppers and across the table a father and his two adult sons debated the merits of beaver.

"It tastes like rotten skunk, Dad," warned the eldest as his parent took a forkful.

"Naw," disagreed his stalwart sibling. "Just a little gamy. The way beaver should."

Cautiously I looked down at my plate and tried to remember which colored toothpick signaled beaver. I couldn't tell, but, checking Bobby's chart, I found it was marked with a blue toothpick. I ID'd its location and decided to save it for last. I had never eaten wild game. I was not going to start with anything that was under debate.

My 19-year-old son Matthew had no such hesitation. After studying Bobby's handout for a moment, he started right in. A bite here, a munch there, and with a nod of satisfaction, my own personally bred carnivore was content to sample the wild side of the table.

COOKING WILD: VERMONT VENISON

"People who cook game like it's beef will be disappointed with the result," says 55-year-old Connie Chipman, cochair of the 42nd Annual Bradford Wild Game Supper in Bradford, Vermont, and an experienced game cook.

Why? "Because most game is so low in fat, it needs to be braised in liquid rather than baked or roasted," she explains. That's why all roasts at the game supper are cooked in bags with liquid added. It's also, she adds, why the supper's meat is moist and full of flavor.

Here's Connie's recipe for one of the supper's favorite offerings—roast venison (which usually refers to deer meat):

Soak a 12-pound roast overnight in cider vinegar. Don't add any seasoning. The point is to let the cider take the edge off the gamy taste, but not kill the wild flavor—which is what will happen if you let the seasoning hang around overnight. When you're ready to cook the roast the next day, set the oven to 300 degrees. Then make a marinade of the listed ingredients.

INGREDIENTS

2 parts cassis, a cordial
2 parts port wine
2 parts maple syrup
6 parts red wine
a fistful of cranberries
4 raw chestnuts, sliced
2 cloves
1 tablespoon fresh thyme
1 tablespoon fresh rosemary
1 tablespoon sage
¼ teaspoon freshly ground pepper

Put 2 cups of marinade in a roasting bag with the 12-pound roast, seal it, and cook for 25 minutes to the pound.

The result is unmistakably Vermont.

On the other side of me, however, was my husband Wayne, a 40-something fitness nut who lives on fruit, vegetables, yogurt, and whole grains, supplemented by a serving of chicken or fish once a day. There is the occasional orgy of Ben & Jerry's to keep him human, but otherwise his eating patterns are obnoxiously pure. And meat is not his thing. So while the rest of us sniffed, picked, and rolled new flavors over our taste buds, Wayne contented himself with a few forkfuls of pheasant and rice.

"Good," he conceded. "Tastes like chicken."

And, surprisingly, it did. In fact, the difference between the beef, chicken, and pork that most of us eat every day and the wild game we ate that night was subtle—like the addition or deletion of a particular spice or vinegar (see "Cooking Wild" on previous page).

The strongest difference was, as my table neighbor had cautioned, the beaver. But with its rich, full-bodied flavor reminding me of the very best pot roast I'd ever eaten, I wasn't about to complain.

In fact, an hour later, as I walked out into the snowy night with my son and husband, each of us replete with the warmth of good food and good company, I was reminded of the simple but poignant prayer printed at the bottom of Bobby's handout:

We thank Thee for these gifts of Thy bounty:

For the sacred way of sacrifice of food and life.
Lead us toward responsible dominion
Over Thy wild creatures.

(And) Help us to be faithful to The gifts of nature . . .

Open-Face Turkey Reuben

Turkey tenders take the place of fatty corned beef in this healthy, hearty sandwich.

Heat a nonstick skillet over medium-high heat. Add the turkey tenders and brown on both sides. When browned, cover them with the rinsed sauerkraut, then the shredded cheese. Cover the pan and allow the cheese to melt.

Toast the rye bread and spread with the Russian dressing. When the cheese has melted, divide the turkey and toppings and place on the rye bread. Serve.

INGREDIENTS

YIELD: 4 SERVINGS

4 turkey tenders (12–16 ounces total weight)
8 ounces canned sauerkraut, rinsed and drained
3 ounces low-fat Swiss or sharp cheddar cheese, shredded
4 ounces fat-free Russian dressing
4 slices rye bread

PER SERVING (ESTIMATED)

Calories	251
Carbohydrates	23 g
Fat	4 g
Saturated fat	1 g
Dietary fiber	3 g
Cholesterol	69 mg
Sodium	811 mg

Curried Vegetables with Turkey

The turkey in the recipe is ground turkey formed into meatballs and browned in a little olive oil. A combination of Indian spices is added to onion, pepper, potatoes, peas, and cabbage. This braised mixture can be served with rice.

Combine the ground turkey and chopped onions and form into 16 meatballs. Heat the olive oil in a large, heavy pot. Add the meatballs and brown on all sides. Remove the browned turkey balls from the pot and reserve.

Add the sliced onions, garlic, and red pepper to the pot. Cook for 5 minutes or until softened.

Add the chicken stock and the coriander, cumin, ginger, cardamom, turmeric, and allspice. Bring to a boil. Lower heat and add the potatoes and cabbage. Cover and cook for 10 minutes.

Add the reserved meatballs and the peas and cook for another 5 minutes or until the peas and meatballs are hot.

Serve over rice.

INGREDIENTS

YIELD: 8 SERVINGS

1 pound ground turkey breast
½ cup chopped onions
1 tablespoon olive oil
1 onion, thinly sliced
1 clove garlic, minced
½ red pepper, chopped
1 cup fat-free chicken stock or water
2 teaspoons ground coriander
1 teaspoon cumin
½ teaspoon powdered ginger
¼ teaspoon cardamom
½ teaspoon turmeric
¼ teaspoon allspice
2 potatoes, cubed
½ head cabbage, coarsely chopped
1 package (10 ounces) frozen peas
Salt and pepper to taste

PER SERVING

Calories	169
Carbohydrates	18 g
Fat	3 g
Saturated fat	5 g
Dietary fiber	5 g
Cholesterol	39 mg
Sodium	90 mg

Low-fat Buffalo Burgers

Buffalo meat can be purchased in some local markets in the freezer section. If you can purchase ground buffalo meat by the pound, divide it into five patties after it is defrosted. Buffalo meat is very low in fat; in one of these patties, there are only 99 calories and two grams of fat.

These patties can be served on the Flaxseed Rolls in The Breadbox chapter (p. 65). Serve the burgers with lettuce, sliced tomato and sliced onion and pass the condiments.

INGREDIENTS
YIELD: 5 BURGERS

1 pound ground buffalo
Barbecue Sauce (optional)
5 Flaxseed Rolls

PER BURGER WITH ROLL	
Calories	264
Carbohydrates	29 g
Fat	6 g
Saturated fat	0.9 g
Dietary fiber	4 g
Cholesterol	56 mg
Sodium	245 mg

Form the ground buffalo into 5 burgers.

Heat a nonstick skillet on medium-high heat. If desired, the burgers can be brushed with a commercial barbecue sauce or the Barbecue Sauce in The Snack Cupboard chapter (p. 226). Place the burgers in the skillet and brown on one side, turn, and brown the other side.

Cook quickly. The burgers will shrink somewhat and since they are so low in fat, they will be dry if they are overcooked.

Serve on warmed Flaxseed Rolls with lettuce, sliced onion, and sliced tomato.

Broiled Flounder with Honey-Mustard Garlic Sauce

Delicious and fast, this recipe can be made with Orange Roughy, tilapia, or sole, says my friend Arlene. The fish can be baked or microwaved. Arlene serves the fish with orzo and peas.

Place the rinsed fillets on a nonstick spray-coated pan.

In a small dish or custard cup, combine the honey, mustard, and garlic. Spread over the top of the fillets.

Broil the fish about 8 inches from the heat for 10 to 15 minutes or until the top is browned and the fish is cooked through.

INGREDIENTS
YIELD: 4 SERVINGS

1 pound fresh flounder fillets
5 teaspoons honey
4 teaspoons Dijon mustard
4 cloves garlic, minced

PER SERVING	
Calories	141
Carbohydrates	9 g
Fat	2 g
Saturated fat	0.4 g
Monounstaurated Fat	0.5 g
Dietary fiber	0.1 g
Cholesterol	54 mg
Sodium	219 mg

Oven-Poached Salmon

Whole poached salmon or a side of salmon makes a sophisticated presentation for a buffet meal. This recipe is an easy way to make salmon for a family meal as well. Serve with a grain, such as rice.

Your fishmonger can bone and skin a side or the whole salmon for you. A whole salmon weighs about four to five pounds minimum, so half or a side should not be less than two pounds. For a buffet presentation, you can buy a larger fish (but make sure you have a big enough pan). For a two- to three-pound side, a nine-inch by nine-inch pan would work.

Preheat the oven to 325°F.

In a saucepan, add the water, wine, dill, peppercorns, and bay leaves. Bring to a boil. Remove from heat and save this poaching liquid.

INGREDIENTS

YIELD: 8–12 MAIN DISH PORTIONS
(12–16 BUFFET PORTIONS)

2 quarts water
1 cup white wine
1 tablespoon dill leaves or fresh dill
1 teaspoon black peppercorns
2 bay leaves
2- to 3-pound fillet or 4-pound whole salmon
Fresh dill, washed greens, lemon slices for
    garnish

PER 4-OUNCE PORTION

Calories	209
Carbohydrates	0 mg
Fat	9 g
Saturated fat	2 g
Omega-3 Fatty Acids	1.78 g
Dietary fiber	0 g
Cholesterol	65 mg
Sodium	60 mg

Place the salmon in a 9-inch x 13-inch pan. If you have a rack that fits into the pan, the fish can be placed on it for easier removal when cooked. Place the pan with the fish in it in the oven and then add the prepared poaching liquid. The fish should be covered with liquid, but add only enough to just cover the fish. It is important to put the pan in the oven first and then add the liquid so that the liquid does not splash as the pan is being transferred to the oven

Bake for 24 to 30 minutes. Make a slice at the thickest part to check if it is cooked through. The fish will be pink throughout; not red in the middle.

Remove the pan from the oven and gently remove the fish onto a platter. The fish will be tender and needs to be treated carefully so that it remains whole for the buffet or presentation. The fish can be served immediately or chilled and served cold. Serve with a horseradish sauce and garnish with fresh dill, washed greens, and lemon slices.

Super Sardine Sub

Sardines are a great food, high in omega-6 fatty acids, good tasting, and quick to prepare and serve. The best-looking of the canned varieties are the skinless and boneless varieties that are packed in soy oil. I find the King Oscar brand, a product of Morocco, the most attractive. Brisling Sardines are small, black-skinned, and packed closely together in the can. This type is good for antipasto or for mashing into a spread.

Sardines are also sold packed in tomato sauce and in mustard sauce. Sardines packed in mustard sauce usually contain turmeric, a definite plus because of the spice's healing powers. And because they're not packed in oil, they contain less fat.

A friend from Singapore told me her mother sautés onions and hot pepper, adds a can of sardines in tomato sauce, and serves it over rice. Sounds good and easy to me.

Other varieties available in cans are low-sodium and water-packed. You can also find some packed in olive oil. Check out several markets and you're sure to find the type that suits you.

Most varieties claim a 4-ounce can as a serving. If you don't drain it, this could be as much as 19 grams of fat per serving. When the sardines are the larger size, a serving is considered about three sardines, which could contain six to seven grams of fat.

Spread a thin layer of mayonnaise over the cut roll. Top with lettuce leaves, then 2 to 3 sardines, tomato slices, onion slices, and finally radish slices.

INGREDIENTS

YIELD: 4 SANDWICHES

4 sub rolls or steak rolls (8 in)
4 teaspoons light mayonnaise or horseradish sauce
8 lettuce leaves
2 cans (4⅜ ounces) lightly smoked sardines
2 plum tomatoes, thinly sliced
4 to 8 slices mild onion
2 radishes, thinly sliced

PER SERVING

Calories	335
Carbohydrates	37 g
Fat	11 g
Saturated fat	2 g
Monounsaturated Fat	4 g
Polyunsaturated Fat	4 g
Omega-6 fatty Acids	2.42 g
Dietary fiber	0 g
Cholesterol	88 mg
Sodium	685 mg

Orange-Poached Sole

I could have used several kinds of ocean-dwelling fin fish for this recipe—halibut, flounder, hake, pollack, or cod. Even tuna, mahi-mahi, and wahoo. Though I love their taste, I avoid tropical ocean fish such as snapper, grouper, and Spanish mackerel because of the risk that they carry a food-borne illness called ciguatera, which can cause nervous system damage.

Rinse fish and set aside.

Heat the olive oil in a large skillet on medium-high. Add sliced scallions. Sauté for 3 minutes. Add the chopped tomato, orange juice, orange rind, and sliced green olives. Bring to a boil.

Place the fish over the tomato mixture, turn the heat to medium-high, cover, and poach for 5 minutes or until the fish is cooked through.

Serve immediately with the poaching liquid, topped with white pepper and parsley.

INGREDIENTS

YIELD: 4 SERVINGS

1 pound sole fillets, about 4 thin slices or portions
1 tablespoon virgin olive oil
8 scallions, thinly sliced
1 tomato, cubed, or 1 cup chopped tomato
½ cup orange juice
2 teaspoons finely chopped orange rind
8 stuffed green olives, sliced
White pepper to taste
Parsley for garnish

PER SERVING

Calories	196
Carbohydrates	10 g
Fat	6 g
Saturated fat	0.9 g
Monounsaturated Fat	3 g
Dietary fiber	2.9 g
Cholesterol	42 mg
Sodium	252 mg

Broiled Atlantic Mackerel with Ginger and Garlic

There are several kinds of mackerel, all coming from the Atlantic Ocean. In the area of northeastern U.S. there is the Atlantic mackerel, which has a strong flavor. In the area around Florida there are wahoo, cero, and Spanish mackerel. These are white when cooked and have a milder flavor. (Shy away from Spanish mackerel, however, because of the possibility of ciguatera poisoning.) The Atlantic and Spanish varieties are usually found in local markets. Wahoo is a larger fish, like the tuna, and found in the Florida area. In Hawaii Wahoo is known as ono.

Mackerel contains the most fat in the fall. Over the winter they lose their fat, so by spring they're lean. That means to get the most omega fatty acids, you're best using mackerel in the fall.

Rinse the mackerel fillets, remove the skin, and cut into 4 portions. Place on broiler pan.

Combine the lemon juice, soy sauce, garlic, and ginger. Spoon over the fish.

Broil the fish for 4 minutes about 4 to 5 inches from the heat. Then turn carefully. Spoon any remaining marinade over the fish and broil for 4 to 5 more minutes or until the fish is cooked through.

Serve garnished with thinly sliced lemon.

INGREDIENTS

YIELD: 4 SERVINGS

1 pound Atlantic mackerel fillets
2 tablespoons lemon juice
2 teaspoons light soy sauce
2 cloves garlic, minced
2 teaspoons grated fresh ginger
Lemon wheels for garnish

PER SERVING

Calories	164
Carbohydrates	2 g
Fat	7 g
Saturated fat	2 g
Monounstayrated Fat	3 g
Polyunsaturated Fat	3 g
Omdega-3 fatty Acids	2 g
Dietary fiber	0 g
Cholesterol	86 mg
Sodium	156 mg

Caramelized Sweet Peppers and Onions with Chicken over Rice

Bring the water to a boil, add the rice, cover, and cook on low for 45 minutes.

Heat the olive oil in a large skillet. Add the peppers and onion and sauté for 10 minutes on medium heat. Turn the heat to medium-low, cover, and continue cooking for 20 more minutes. Stir occasionally and add water or a few tablespoons of chicken stock if moisture is needed.

Remove the peppers and onions to a bowl and set aside. Add the chicken and basil to the hot skillet and sauté the chicken until cooked through. Add the pepper and onion mixture to the chicken and combine well. Heat through. Serve over cooked rice and top with the slivered almonds.

INGREDIENTS

YIELD: 6 SERVINGS

2½ cups water
1 cup long grain brown rice
1 tablespoon olive oil
3 cups julienne sliced red, green, and yellow peppers or a 12-ounce bag frozen sliced peppers
1 large onion, thinly sliced
12 ounces raw chicken breast, cut into cubes
1 teaspoon dried basil or 1 tablespoon minced fresh basil
2 tablespoons slivered almonds

PER SERVING

Calories	240
Carbohydrates	30 g
Fat	5.5 g
Saturated fat	0.8 g
Monounsaturated Fat	3 g
Polyunsaturated fat	1 g
Omega-6 Fatty Acids	1 g
Dietary fiber	3.5 g
Cholesterol	33 mg
Sodium	44 mg

Chicken Stir-Fry with Broccoli and Cashews

This stir-fry has the characteristics of a Thai dish, with ginger, black sweet soy sauce, and tamarind paste. Serve it with Honey-Chile Garlic Sauce (p. 125) for a spicy-sweet flavor.

Heat a wok. Add the oil. Add the minced garlic and cook on high for 1 minute. Add the chicken and stir-fry until the chicken is almost cooked through. Add the onion and pepper and stir-fry for 1 minute. Add the ginger, chicken stock, tamarind paste, and sweet black soy sauce and stir fry for 1 minute to combine ingredients. Add the broccoli and cashews, cover the wok, and allow to steam for 5 to 6 minutes or until the broccoli is tender.

Serve over rice.

INGREDIENTS

YIELD: 6 SERVINGS

2 tablespoons peanut oil
3 to 4 cloves garlic, minced
¾ pound skinless, boneless chicken breast, thinly sliced
5 green onions, thinly sliced into diagonals
1 sweet red pepper, slivered
1 teaspoon minced ginger
½ cup water or chicken stock
4 teaspoons tamarind paste
2 tablespoons sweet black soy sauce
3 broccoli stalks, or 4 cups florets only
¾ cup unsalted roasted cashews
3 cups cooked Jasmine rice

PER SERVING

Calories	283
Carbohydrates	33 g
Fat	9 g
Saturated fat	2 g
Monounsaturated Fat	4
Dietary fiber	3.3 g
Cholesterol	33 mg
Sodium	358 mg

The Spice Rack

Spices may bring an intense splash of color and flavor to food, but they also bring an equally intense dose of potent, naturally occurring chemicals that can pep up your immune system, protect your heart, soothe your digestive tract, relieve pain, and help you sleep.

Some of these spices are old friends. Onion, garlic, cinnamon, rosemary, and parsley are found in just about every kitchen spice rack. But turmeric, a powerful antioxidant that provides the intense yellow color that characterizes Indian curry, is a new friend you're probably still getting to know when you dine out. Same with cilantro, coriander, and fenugreek.

Yet all of these spices are equally deserving of a place in your kitchen. Because, with just these four powerhouses alone, you can prevent cancer, stave off hot flashes, stabilize diabetes, halt infections, and soothe colic.

If that sounds amazing, wait until you read through the following pages. You'll see how these and other spices are turning our kitchens into the most powerful centers of natural healing in the world. You'll also come to understand why our use of spices has increased 45 percent over the last decade. When every shake of the spice bottle adds a burst of flavor and a shot of health, you can bet your oven mitts that every cook in the world is trying to spice up every dish on the table.

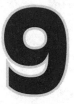

SPICE RACK

BEST FOR HELPING YOU:

Prevent cancer

Stave off hot flashes

Stabilize blood sugar

Protect your heart

Sooth your digestive tract

Relieve pain

Prevent insomnia

Slow infections

Soothe colic

ALLSPICE

BEST FOR HELPING YOU:

Relieve muscle aches & pains

Soothe an upset stomach

Fight yeast infections

Allspice: Boost Your Allspice, Boost Your Digestive Enzymes

Allspice, which smells like a whisper of cloves, cinnamon, and nutmeg all rolled into one, comes from the berry-sized fruits of a 40-foot tall tree that grows primarily in Jamaica. The fruits are hand-picked and dried just before they ripen when their fragrance—and the therapeutic oils that create it—are at their peak.

You may take a pinch of the dried fruit, crush it between your fingers, and drop it into a variety of soups and stews just as the Jamaicans do—or into a chocolate cookie

RX FOR ACHING MUSCLES

Mix one ounce of ground allspice with enough warm water to make a paste, then spoon the mixture onto half of a clean cloth. Fold the cloth over so that the paste is completely encased in fabric.

Make sure you're not hypersensitive to the allspice by touching the poultice to a small area of skin. If there's even a hint of redness, toss the poultice in the compost. If your skin remains clear, however, place the poultice on your over-taxed aching muscle and relax as it cools—and as your pain melts away.

---

batter as my friend Anita does in her "Chocolate Allspice Cookies" on page 193. Yet crushing the spice will do far more than release the intoxicating scent of allspice. It will also unleash eugenol, a naturally occurring chemical that boosts the activity of a powerful digestive enzyme called trypsin in your body. This means that when you eat a dish flavored with allspice, you're less likely to experience digestive upset. Take a bowl of a stomach-eating Jamaican stew, add a pinch of allspice, and you'll be able to enjoy the Caribbean's exotic flavors without fear of post-stew discomfort.

When used topically, minute amounts of the eugenol in allspice also seems to relieve minor aches and pains. It also fights fungal infections on the skin better than many pharmaceutical agents do. In one laboratory study, for example, eugenol killed roughly twice as many yeast cells as did equivalent amounts of the antifungal drug nystatin.

ANISE

BEST FOR HELPING YOU:

Beat premenstrual fatigue

Sweeten your breath

Digest food

Reduce gas

Prevent anemia

Anise: A Tummy-Soothing Breath Freshener

Anise seed provides that big, bold flavor you associate with licorice candy. But

ALLSPICE BASICS

HOW TO BUY: Both whole and ground (powdered) allspice is readily available in supermarket spice shelves.

HOW TO STORE: Tightly covered, away from light.

HOW TO USE: To prevent indigestion, simply sprinkle a pinch of powdered allspice on your food during cooking. It tastes best on fruit compotes, root vegetables, and meats.

To soothe an upset tummy, simmer one teaspoon of whole dried allspice in a pot of mulled cider for 10 minutes, then strain and serve as an after-dinner drink.

You can also try tapping allspice's ability to relieve muscle aches by making a poultice. (See "Rx for Aching Muscles" above.)

Unfortunately, the use of allspice to cure yeast infections is tricky because of eugenol's irritating effect on what are frequently delicate skin cells. Do not use it for this purpose without your doctor's advice.

it's also a first-class breath freshener and tummy soother that dates back to Greek and Roman times.

In the first century, for example, its crushed seeds were frequently sprinkled into a kind of cake that was served at the end of the meal. Not only did it help guests digest their hostess' cooking, it also kept them from airing, shall we say, any internal disturbances her more original dishes may have caused.

Aside from that, anise is a good spice for premenstrual women to keep on hand. A single tablespoon of anise provides roughly 16 percent of the amount of iron you need every day to counteract blood loss during your period. Keeping iron stores up will produce healthy red blood cells that transport oxygen to every cell in your body. And that will help you prevent anemia and keep premenstrual fatigue at bay.

Cayenne Pepper: The Hot Spice that Chills Sinus Pain

Adding a pulsating note of heat to the healthy dishes we've been preparing in our kitchens over the past couple of years, cayenne pepper has become so popular that its consumption has increased 125 percent in the past two decades.

And why not? Cayenne not only adds zip to your chili and spice to your rice, it also relieves sinus headaches, aids digestion, cuts cholesterol, and helps prevent heart attacks and strokes. And if preliminary studies in India pan out, it may also reduce a substance involved in triggering arthritic pain by 88 percent.

Ground from the dried red fruit of a capsicum (pepper) plant, cayenne contains capsaicin, a naturally occurring plant chemical that tingles your taste buds while it liquefies sinus-clogging mucus produced by your immune system. It also reduces the tendency of your blood to form artery-clogging clots.

How capsaicin affects your blood chemistry is still something of a mystery. But scientists have found that it turns on cellular spigots throughout your body to wash out nasal passages, sinus cavities, and airways that are clogged with thick mucus during a cold or allergy. And since most sinus headaches start when mucus blocks the holes through which the sinuses normally drain, unclogging those same sinuses will frequently relieve a sinus headache.

CAYENNE PEPPER

BEST FOR HELPING YOU:

Relieve sinus headaches

Reduce arthritic inflammation

Protect your stomach

Cut cholesterol

Prevent heart attacks and strokes

ANISE BASICS

HOW TO BUY: Anise is readily available in your supermarket as whole or crushed seeds or as an extract.

HOW TO STORE: In a tightly closed container, out of sunlight.

HOW TO USE: Drop the crushed seeds into breads, cakes, cobblers, cookies, and pies. Or chew a handful of the whole seeds to freshen your breath. Try the extract in candy where a heavy burst of licorice won't overshadow subtler flavors.

What's more, the fluids released by capsaicin will also clear your airway when you have a cold.

Capsaicin will also protect your stomach lining from the irritating effects of alcohol and acidic foods—a particular benefit if you accidentally overindulge in one or the other.

Mixed into a cream that's sold under the trade name Zostrix, capsaicin is also a topical pain reliever. Spread over an arthritic joint, on shingles, across a psoriatic plaque, or on a nerve-damaged diabetic foot, the cream forces nerves in the affected area to use up all their substance P, a neurochemical that transmits pain messages to the brain. Fortunately, once nerves have cleared out their supply of substance P, they can't seem to make any more—at least not as long as you continue to rub the area with capsaicin.

Unfortunately, the capsaicin in cayenne is likely to take your skin off if you try smearing a homemade paste directly on your skin. So if you'd like to try it as a topical pain reliever, check with your doctor first. He or she can help you figure out the appropriate strength and dosage of Zostrix.

Celery Seed: A One-Two Punch against High Blood Pressure

Celery seeds not only add a muted bitter note to your favorite salad dressings and slaws; they may also help lower blood pressure, reduce cholesterol, and prevent cancer.

Studies show that, among other things, celery seeds contain butyl phthalide, a naturally occurring chemical that seems to have a powerful effect on blood vessels. In the lab, it reduces the amounts of hormones in the body that constrict arteries.

It also causes arteries to dilate (open up).

This one-two punch on blood vessels can have an amazing effect on blood pressure. In a study at the University of Chicago, the blood pressure of lab animals given butyl phthalide dropped an astonishing 12 points. In a human being, that could mean the difference between having to take high blood pressure medication and being able to control the condition with just exercise and diet.

Other studies indicate that butyl phthalide may have a similar lowering effect on cholesterol, while still others show that it may reduce the numbers of tumors in those who are exposed to cancer-causing agents.

One caveat: Celery seed also contains a chemical constituent that makes you more susceptible to sunlight. So if you notice that you're more likely to get a sunburn after eating a food liberally sprinkled with celery seed, cut back on the amount you use.

CELERY SEED

BEST FOR HELPING YOU:

Lower blood pressure

Reduce cholesterol

Prevent cancer

CILANTRO/CORIANDER

BEST FOR HELPING YOU:

Quell a queasy stomach

Heal minor cuts and scrapes

Cilantro and Coriander: Double Health

A single plant that originated around the Mediterranean over 3,500 years ago produces both cilantro and coriander. Cilantro comes from its leaves; coriander from the seeds. Both taste great when used to zip up nouvelle cuisines—and both can give a hefty boost to digestion. Laboratory scientists have found that coriander in particular contains an essential oil that kills bacteria and fungi, relaxes muscles, and aids digestion—all of which makes it an excellent remedy

CELERY SEED BASICS

HOW TO BUY: Celery seed is available in your local supermarket.

HOW TO STORE: In tightly closed glass bottles, out of the light.

HOW TO USE: Sprinkle celery seeds anywhere you like the taste of celery. Mix it into tomato sauces and soups, chicken salad, and salad dressing. Or sprinkle it over potatoes, potato salad, even meat.

for upset stomachs. It's also a good aid to healing minor cuts and scrapes.

You can also use the powdered seed to help heal minor cuts and scrapes. Wash the affected area thoroughly with soap and water, then sprinkle a pinch of coriander over the area. Do not cover. The coriander will attack stray germs on contact.

Cinnamon: An Aromatic Infection Fighter

If you've ever succumbed to the tantalizing aromas of a sticky bun store at your local mall, chances are it's the smell of cinnamon that did you in.

But so what if you ended up eating what looked like 3,000 calories of gooey glory? So what if melting icing smeared across your cheeks and dripped down your chin? So what if your husband took one look, handed you a napkin, and excused himself to look at shoes?

With the amount of cinnamon in that colossal confection, you also put away a significant amount of cancer-fighting antioxidants plus a potent, naturally occurring chemical, eugenol, that will help prevent heart disease. Or you certainly would have if the cinnamon had been encased in a tad less fat.

Unfortunately, unless you used Anita's recipe (Whole Wheat Cinnamon Buns, p. 201), there's a good chance that the amount of fat in your bun blew the cinnamon's health benefits to smithereens. And that's not something you want

---

CINNAMON

BEST FOR HELPING YOU:

Prevent heart attacks and strokes

Ward off stomach ulcers

Kill mouth microbes that cause infection

Fight respiratory viruses

Lower cholesterol

Stabilize diabetes

CILANTRO AND CORIANDER BASICS

HOW TO BUY: Fresh cilantro leaves are available in the produce section of many supermarkets. Look for firm, green leaves with no signs of brown on the edges. Coriander seed, both whole and crushed, is available in the spice section of most supermarkets. Pick the whole seed if you have a choice. It'll give you maximum flavor and potency when it's used in cooking.

HOW TO STORE: Fresh cilantro should be covered with a damp cloth, placed in a plastic bag and stored in the refrigerator for no more than a day or two. Coriander seeds should be kept in tightly closed containers. Stored out of sunlight, they'll stay potent for up to a year.

HOW TO USE: If you've got somebody in the family with a delicate stomach, try adding either cilantro or coriander to family meals on a regular basis. Just keep in mind that cilantro has a distinctive flavor. If you like real Mexican food, you've probably tasted it in a number of dishes, including salsa. But it can be an acquired taste for some people. So start with just a small leaf here or pinch here and there, then increase the amount as your family gets used to it.

Cilantro works well in sauces and salads, while coriander seeds can be used to accent fish, rice, potatoes, cookies, and gingerbread.

to do. When cinnamon is used to spice up low-fat foods, its eugenol may help reduce the tendency of artery-clogging blood clots to form and lower cholesterol.

What's more, says David Fitzpatrick, Ph.D., a researcher at the University of South Florida, plant chemicals in cinnamon stimulate the cells lining blood vessels to release nitrous oxide, a substance that causes arterial walls to relax—an important factor in preventing heart attacks.

It gets even better. Preliminary reports from around the globe hint that cinnamon may actually be a kind of international white knight: It slays whatever virus, fungi, or bacteria are currently on the prowl. Consider:

- A Japanese study indicates that an acid in Chinese cinnamon fortifies the stomach's natural defenses and helps prevent bacteria from forming stomach ulcers.
- A Moroccan study finds that cinnamon prevents the formation of toxic molds that grow on foods such as

peanuts.
- A British study reveals that the spice kills five different types of infectious microbes.
- A study at the Veterans Affairs Medical Center in Brooklyn, New York, found that Ceylon cinnamon reduced much of candidiasis, a yeast that frequently infects the mouths of those infected with HIV.
- A study at India's Centre for Biochemical Technology found that

CINNAMON BASICS

HOW TO BUY: Avoid supermarket cinnamon. Instead, search out a gourmet store, farmer's market, or specialty merchant who offers a freshly ground spice. Use your nose to guide you. If the scent of a just-opened tube or jar of cinnamon practically makes your eyes water, there's a good chance that it's rich with the oils that carry the tree's therapeutic properties. If the scent is just kind of ho-hum, don't buy it. It probably won't do you much good as either a flavoring or a healing agent.

HOW TO STORE: In a tightly capped glass bottle, out of the sunlight.

HOW TO USE: Many of us think of cinnamon as that spice we use with apple dishes and ciders during the fall. But other cultures use it to spice up couscous (a Middle Eastern grain dish), meats, stews, and vegetables.

How much you should use is another question. Nobody really knows, although at least one scientist feels that as little as one-eighth of a teaspoon of cinnamon triples insulin efficiency. Whatever you do, however, stick with the powdered variety. Cinnamon oil is highly toxic.

The Spice Rack • 175

inhaling the aroma of Ceylon cinnamon may actually kill many of the infectious agents that cause respiratory disease.

At the United States Department of Agriculture, research into cinnamon's therapeutic abilities has also revealed that cinnamon helps people with Type 2 diabetes metabolize sugar. Since those with this type of diabetes frequently have a problem either getting or using the insulin their bodies make to break down simple sugars in their diet, substances that help them do so can frequently decrease or eliminate the need for medication.

Which cinnamon should you use?

That's hard to say. There are over 100 varieties of cinnamon. And although each of the spices you find in markets have been ground from the bark of a tree, most of them will fall into at least one of two categories: Chinese cinnamon, a sharply flavored spice that has enough of an edge to work well in flavoring even robust coffees, and Ceylon cinnamon, a soft, rich cinnamon that works best weaving together the delicate flavors of a cinnamon bun. Whether or not all varieties have the same pharmaceutical potency is unknown. But given the fact that both seem to have similar chemical properties, scientists suspect that they do.

Cloves: A Heart-Warming Spice

When your mother told you to hold a clove on an aching tooth, she was advising you to use one of the most effective toothache remedies known.

That's because cloves are the most potent source of eugenol, the substance that kills bacteria and viruses, soothes digestion, and relieves pain.

When used as a spice in food, eugenol helps prevent heart attacks by reducing the tendency of red blood cells to clump together and by lowering cholesterol levels. When used topically as an oil, it fights fungal infections in the ears, vagina, and on the skin—plus it relieves toothache pain and the itch of insect bites. When

CLOVE BASICS

HOW TO BUY: Since ground cloves quickly lose both flavor and potency, buy whole cloves.

HOW TO STORE: In a tightly capped jar out of sunlight.

HOW TO USE: Don't try to make your own homemade oils and extracts. Both can be toxic even in small amounts. Instead, add cloves to your cooking whenever and wherever you can. Traditionally, cloves have been used to flavor hams, gingerbread, and pumpkin pie, but they also add a piquant note to fruit compotes, stews, soups, vegetables, and just about anything that contains dried fruit.

A poultice of ground cloves can stop the itch in minutes. Just mix a half-teaspoon of ground cloves with enough warm water to make a paste, spoon the mixture onto the freshly washed bite, and cover with a clean cloth.

If any redness develops, you may be sensitive to the cloves. So toss the poultice into your compost, rinse your skin with clear water, and don't use cloves again.

To grind cloves, just drop a teaspoonful of whole cloves into an electric coffee mill and grind. One tip: If you'd like a cup of really great-tasting coffee, don't clean the mill afterward. Let the clove residue hang around to mix with the coffee beans next time you make a pot of coffee.

used as an extract, however, a laboratory study at the University of Iowa's Dows Institute for Dental Research revealed that it also killed the bacteria that cause tooth decay and gum disease.

Clearly it's a powerful herb. A laboratory study at Toyama Medical and Pharmaceutical University in Japan reveals that an extract made from cloves may also boost the therapeutic effects of an antiviral drug frequently used to treat cold sores. In that study, researchers gave mice infected with the cold sore virus a dose of the drug acyclovir. Other mice received a clove extract, while still others received a combination of both acyclovir and the extract.

The result? The mice who took oral doses of both acyclovir and the clove extract had significantly fewer of the painful skin lesions characteristic of the virus than other mice.

Dill: A Natural Digestive Aid

Dill can do much more than preserve your pickles and add a fresh garden taste to Dilly Bread (as well as Anita's delicious Dill and Onion Biscuits on page 203). For centuries, Egyptians have used it to prevent intestinal gas, Romans have chewed it to settle an upset stomach, and North Americans have used it to soothe colic in their children.

It's an all-around digestive aid that relaxes the muscles that move food through the digestive tract. It also prevents the formation of gas bubbles and inhibits growth of four of the most common bacteria associated with infectious diarrhea and stomach upset.

Fenugreek Seeds: A Woman's Best Friend

A favorite of India's Ayurvedic physicians and a staple in many curries, fenugreek seeds can help prevent hot flashes, lower cholesterol, stabilize diabetes, relieve constipation, and aid digestion.

The seeds contain several substances with therapeutic ability: plant estrogens,

CLOVES

BEST FOR HELPING YOU:

Take the itch out of insect bites

Prevent heart attacks and strokes

Fight herpes

Eliminate gum disease

Soothe a toothache

Lower cholesterol

Kill fungal infections

Aid digestion

DILL

BEST FOR HELPING YOU:

Settle your stomach

Soothe colic

which counteract a woman's diminishing stores of estrogen at menopause; saponins, which grab hold of cholesterol and send it to the body's trash dump for disposal; and mucilage, a gummy substance that absorbs water and soothes irritated tissues—the perfect combination to relieve constipation and soothe a cranky digestive tract.

All in all, fenugreek is pretty powerful stuff. In one Indian study, just four ounces of ground seeds a day was enough to significantly lower artery-clogging LDL cholesterol while preserving the beneficial effects of artery-scrubbing HDL cholesterol. And that's tough to do. Most LDL lowering substances—both natural and pharmaceutical—lower HDL cholesterol as well.

How much these seeds can lower cholesterol will likely vary from person to person. One animal study found that cholesterol levels dropped a whopping 18 percent; those involving humans have yet to be done.

As for its effect on diabetes, scientists are both amazed and puzzled. In one study there was some indication that fenugreek seeds helped those with insulin-dependent diabetes improve chemical measures of their condition by 50 percent. How much of this translates into better symptom control has yet to be determined.

Garlic: Your Kitchen's Most Powerful Medicine

If I had just one spice to choose for my kitchen, garlic would be it. That's because the powerful chemicals that occur naturally in garlic can prevent heart attacks and strokes, stop the damaging effects of cholesterol on artery walls, reduce cholesterol, lower blood pressure, fight infectious agents, and stop cancer cells from both getting a foothold and growing into a life-threatening tumor. What's more, garlic even seems to stop the heart from aging.

If that sounds incredible, look at the evidence. There are whole file cabinets full of studies indicating that three major substances in garlic—diallyl disulfide, diallyl trisulfide, and S-allylcysteine—are pretty much responsible for these life-saving effects.

Diallyl disulfide seems to prevent red blood cells from clumping together into the artery-blocking blood clots that trigger heart attacks. It also stops the growth of cancer cells in their tracks. S-allylcysteine

---

FENUGREEK

BEST FOR HELPING YOU:

Prevent hot flashes

Lower cholesterol

Control diabetes

Relieve constipation

Aid digestion

DILL BASICS

HOW TO BUY: As seeds in your supermarket. Fresh dill leaves have the best flavor, but they wilt so quickly that unless you grow them yourself and use them immediately after picking or direct from the freezer, it's best to stick with the dried seed.

HOW TO STORE: In a tightly capped bottle, out of sunlight.

HOW TO USE: Sprinkle dill seeds in marinades you plan to use for fish and vegetables, over potatoes or slaw, or in flavored vinegars headed for your salad.

disrupts the metabolic activity involved when a healthy cell turns into a cancerous one. And allicin, a naturally occurring chemical created when garlic is chewed or chopped, kills the bacteria that cause a wide array of bacterial and fungal infections. In fact, allicin is so strong that scientists say one single clove of garlic is packed with as much antibacterial firepower as 100,000 units of penicillin—or about one-sixth the dose your physician might prescribe for an infection.

Triple Heart Protection

Most amazing to me is garlic's effect on the heart. For years, scientists have suspected that people who regularly consume several cloves of garlic a day are less likely to die of heart disease or a heart attack. But nobody could figure out why. Now, however, one study after another is discovering the secrets of garlic's amazing power.

A study at Loma Linda University in California found, for example, that S-allylcysteine liter-

ally stopped LDL cholesterol from tucking itself inside the walls of cells lining your heart's arteries. Since a build-up of cholesterol in those walls is what narrows your heart's arteries, keeping as much of it away from those walls as possible will significantly reduce your chances of a heart attack.

But it usually takes more than narrowed arteries to trigger a heart attack; it also takes a bunch of red blood cells that have clumped together into a clot. The clot gets stuck in the narrowed artery, blood can't get through to the heart, and parts of the heart start to die.

But garlic seems to affect that process, too. In fact, when researchers at Brown University in Providence, Rhode Island, gave 45 men the equivalent of five or six cloves of garlic a day, they found that the tendency for the men's blood to form clots dropped anywhere from 10 to 58 percent. As a result, they were less likely to have a clot get stuck in their arteries and trigger a heart attack.

GARLIC

BEST FOR HELPING YOU:

Protect your heart from aging

Prevent heart attacks and strokes

Reduce cholesterol

Prevent cholesterol damage to arteries

Lower blood pressure

Eliminate the bacteria that causes ulcers

Fight infections

Block cancer

FENUGREEK BASICS

HOW TO BUY: This is one spice you will not find in a chain supermarket. Instead, look for small merchants in Indian neighborhoods or contact one of the spice merchants listed in "The Spice Chest" on page 188.

HOW TO STORE: In a tightly capped bottle out of the sun.

HOW TO USE: Fenugreek seeds have a bittersweet flavor reminiscent of maple syrup. In fact, many commercial manufacturers use the seeds to prepare imitation maple flavoring. So anything in which you enjoy maple syrup is a candidate for fenugreek. Try it cooked in oatmeal or use it to add flavor to soups and stews.

And that's not all garlic does for our hearts. As we age, another factor that sets us up for a heart attack is stiffening of the blood vessels. The stiffness is due partly to increased deposits of cholesterol and partly to other factors such as hormones that ebb and flow as we get older. Think of an old rubber garden hose that's been left out in the backyard for a few years and you've got the general picture. It's dry. It's tough. And it's very likely to crack under pressure.

Your arteries are much the same. They aren't as elastic as they used to be. A clot is far more likely to get stuck in a stiffened artery than in one that stretches to let the clot ease its way through.

Researchers at the Centre for Cardiovascular Pharmacology in Mainz, Germany, set up a study to determine whether or not garlic—which has proved so amazingly helpful in other matters of the heart—could possibly offset the loss of arterial elasticity during aging.

GARLIC BASICS

HOW TO BUY: Buy fresh garlic wherever and whenever you can. Look for plump heads with an intact papery cover over a cluster of 12 to 16 cloves. Avoid heads that have sprouts or spots. There's some evidence that Australian garlic may have more of the compounds that give garlic its healing abilities, so if you find a bag of the stuff marked "Product of Australia," grab it quick. Garlic powder is easily purchased in your local market.

HOW TO STORE: Fresh garlic will keep for six months in a cool corner of your kitchen counter. Powdered garlic will keep for up to a year if you put it in a tightly capped bottle on your spice rack.

HOW TO USE: Pull off the papery covering on the head. Put however many cloves you need on a cutting board and, one by one, rest the flat side of a broad-bladed kitchen knife on each clove and press. The peel will split so you can easily remove it. Remove any green sprouts you find in the center by simply slicing it out of the clove. The sprout sometimes appears as garlic matures, and it can occasionally lend a slightly bitter flavor.

Chop or crush the clove, then drop it into whatever you're cooking. Garlic works particularly well with soups, stews, pastas, and anything tomato. Use low heats. High heats will cause some of the therapeutic substances in garlic to vaporize.

Keep in mind that garlic is a powerful plant. If you're taking any medication, check with your doctor before you start increasing the amount you eat. Here are other ways to work more garlic into your life:

Rub. Rub two to four peeled cloves on a loaf of whole wheat French bread. Brush the bread with olive oil and pop it under the broiler until lightly browned. Serve warm.

Wipe. Wipe your salad bowl with a couple of peeled cloves before you throw in the green stuff.

Toss. Use a salad dressing that has fresh, chopped garlic infused into its oil. "Newman's Own" is my husband's favorite. Or make your own. (See "Two Quick Ways to Get Garlic's Healthy Benefits" on next page.)

Sliver. Make tiny slits under the surface of any meat and slip tiny slivers of garlic into the slits before roasting.

Specifically, the researchers took 200 healthy men between the ages of 50 and 80, measured the flexibility of their main heart arteries, then split the men into two groups. One group took 300 milligrams a day of garlic powder—the equivalent of one or two fresh cloves—while the other group did not.

After two years, researchers found that the main heart arteries of those who had not taken garlic had steadily gotten stiffer. The arteries of those who had taken garlic remained significantly more elastic.

The researchers' conclusion?

Garlic counteracts the effect of aging on old hearts.

Triple Protection against Cancer

The garlic sitting innocently on your kitchen counter has shaken up the cancer world as well. Laboratory studies have found that the S-allylcysteine in garlic stops healthy cells from turning into cancerous ones. The diallyl disulfide stops already existing cancers from spreading, and diallyl trisulfide kills lung cancer cells outright.

The practical implications are astounding. Diallyl trisulfide is being investigated as a chemotherapy agent, and researchers throughout the world are wondering what garlic will prove to do next.

One therapeutic use on the horizon:

TWO QUICK WAYS TO GET GARLIC'S HEALTHY BENEFITS

I love garlic. My family loves garlic. But on most weeknights, we're far too (check one) exhausted, busy, or stressed to stand patiently by the stove peeling and chopping garlic.

So how do we get the protective benefits of *Allium sativum*?

Two ways: Powdered garlic seems to retain just as many disease-fighting nutrients as the peeled stuff, so we always keep it handy in the spice rack. You just whip off the cap and shake to your heart's content. But we also keep a bottle of olive oil infused with garlic oil right next to the spice rack on the kitchen counter. The oil has every single one of garlic's precious nutrients—plus it retains the decadently robust flavor of fresh garlic that characterizes fine Italian cooking. A splash in this pot, a splash in that, and my whole kitchen smells like the Via Veneto.

Unfortunately, store-bought garlic-infused oil tends to be expensive—about $7.99 for 6.75 fluid ounces, or 200 milliliters. So whenever I have a Saturday morning free, I buy a liter of a good, extra-virgin olive oil and a fresh braid of garlic. I get out a few empty pint jars that I normally use for canning, or a couple of those fancy, long-necked bottles that once held the imported stuff. I sterilize the bottles in boiling water. When dry, I fill each bottle half full with oil. I peel and chop the garlic, then drop four cloves worth into each container. I top the containers with oil, cap them tightly, shake, and store them in the back of my refrigerator. I bring them out as needed over the next couple of weeks—or I tie a square of fabric over the top with some raffia and use them as hostess gifts for friends.

One caveat: Homemade oils can harbor botulism. So always refrigerate the oils, use them up quickly, and check with your local state extension service for up-to-the-minute home canning safety guidelines.

garlic may actually cancel out the fertilizing effects of a high-fat diet on cancer.

In a study presented at the 16th International Congress of Nutrition in Montreal, John A. Milner, Ph.D., head of the nutrition department at Penn State University, showed that when laboratory rats were fed a high-fat diet and then exposed to a cancer-causing agent, most of them developed cancer. Curious about the effects of garlic on the cancer-initiation process, the researchers decided to feed the rats garlic along with their fats. They found that the garlic prevented the carcinogens from doing any damage.

It will take a few years before researchers know whether or not this holds true for humans as well, says Dr. Milner. "But when garlic is present in a fatty meal, it looks as though the fat's ability to trigger cancer is blocked."

Ginger: The Keystone of Good Health

Ginger has been prescribed by Chinese physicians for more than 3,000 years to cure everything from motion sickness to headaches. And medical research has spent much of the past two decades proving that those ancient healers knew what they were doing.

More than 400 different chemicals have been identified in ginger. Zingibain, an enzyme that digests proteins, makes up a full 2 percent of the fresh root—or rhizome, as this underground stem is more accurately called. Zingiberene is a constituent that helps your body heal stomach ulcers and expel gas, and gingerol,

---

GINGER

BEST FOR HELPING YOU:

Stimulate sluggish digestion

Reduce arthritic aches and pains

Heal stomach ulcers

Stop migraine headaches

Prevent motion sickness

Reduce nausea from chemotherapy

Prevent heart attacks and strokes

Move gas

GINGER BASICS

HOW TO BUY: Both powdered and fresh varieties are available in your local market. If buying the fresh root, look for a firm, heavy rhizome. Younger rhizomes, which tend to have soft, pinkish skin, have fewer therapeutic constituents. Avoid anything that looks moldy or shriveled.

HOW TO STORE: Put powdered ginger in the spice rack and use it within a year. Wrap fresh rhizomes in a paper towel, tuck them in a plastic bag and store in your refrigerator. They'll keep for about two weeks.

HOW TO USE: We have to get beyond gingerbread. Try adding a teaspoon of powdered ginger or a few thin slices of fresh ginger to anything with fruit—fruit salads, fruit pies, or berry cobblers, for example. Or pop a few slices of fresh ginger into a whole chicken. I recommend Anita's "Hot and Spicy Ginger Carrot Soup," p. 207, a rich, warm brew of antioxidants and healing ginger. You could even mix a glaze of soy sauce, honey, garlic, and ginger, then brush it on your Thanksgiving turkey. No one will be bored with the traditional feast when that baby hits the table.

an oily substance that represents about 5 percent of the rhizome, is responsible for ginger's ability to prevent the blood clots that lead to heart attacks.

It's a powerful little rhizome. Scientists are just beginning to sort out all the therapeutic values associated with its myriad constituents. But while some researchers are up to their elbows in petri dishes, other researchers have already documented the relationship between ginger and various conditions and diseases.

In a Danish study, for example, researchers asked 56 people who had either rheumatoid arthritis, osteoarthritis, or general muscular discomfort to add ginger to their diets on a regular basis. More than 75 percent of the participants—including all of those who had muscular discomfort—reported they felt better.

A second Danish study, this one of Danish naval cadets, revealed that those sailors-to-be who took ginger were significantly less like to get seasick than those who didn't.

And in a study of cancer patients at the University of Alabama, those who ingested ginger reported that the nausea associated with chemotherapy was significantly less intense and lasted a shorter time after chemotherapy than when they didn't take ginger.

Various other studies indicate that ginger effectively stops migraine headaches and speeds the transport of food through the digestive system—a big plus for the elderly. In older folks, the delayed movement of food from one part of the digestive system to another is a common problem. It can result in chronic nausea, stomach upset, excess gas, and a general sensation of just not feeling up to par. It makes older folks feel miserable. Yet a study at Kyoto Pharmacological University in Japan indicates that relatively small amounts of ginger are as effective at igniting a sluggish digestive system as some of the heavy-duty drugs doctors frequently prescribe. You don't have to eat

---

THE CALIFORNIA COLD REMEDY

While interviewing a researcher at one of California's fabulous state universities, I came down with the worst cold of my life. By the end of our discussion, my head was so stuffy I could hardly see straight. As he handed me into a cab, the researcher—a serious immunologist with a national reputation—paused for a moment, then asked if I'd mind a suggestion for my cold.

Expecting to hear of some incredibly potent new drug that would turn my sinuses inside out or separate my nose from my face, I gamely nodded my head. "Sure," I replied miserably. "Anyding to ged rid of dis congestin."

"Well," he said, "when you get back to your hotel, call room service. Ask for two slices of toast, a small pot of olive oil, and four freshly chopped cloves of garlic. Spread the oil on your toast, top with garlic, and eat. Alternate bites with a hot cup of tea. Your head will be clear within minutes."

Suspecting that the cold had affected my hearing, I nevertheless followed what I thought were his instructions. Thank God I did. Less than 30 seconds after I started eating, my head was clear. I didn't have that hyped-up-but-dopey feeling I frequently get from an over-the-counter decongestant. And instead of spending the night miserably in bed, I tripped off to watch whales dancing past La Jolla in the moonlight.

a lot of ginger to get its healing effects, either. Most studies use less than one teaspoon of powdered or freshly ground ginger a day. If you're taking any medication, however, common sense dictates that you should check with your doctor before you use it. And even though some studies indicate that ginger may be a help in preventing morning sickness, don't start chowing down on rhizomes if you're pregnant. Ginger does alter your body's complex hormone structure. And one day scientists may find out that using more than a sprinkle to spice up your stir-fry once in a while may affect your baby.

Oregano: The Italian Antiseptic

Visit a pizza parlor and there's not a pie that hits the table without oregano. But visit your drugstore and you'll find that there's not a bottle of mouthwash without it either.

Hard to believe?

It's true. Oregano is not just that quintessential Italian spice that we all know and love. It also contains thymol, a naturally occurring substance that mows down bacteria. And that's what it does whether it's being swished through our mouths in the form of Listerine or tossed over our pizza in the form of dried leaves.

Oregano may have some other uses, as well. A preliminary study at the USDA's Beltsville Human Nutrition Research Center reveals that oregano increased the activity of insulin in the body several times over. If human studies verify what's going on in the lab, the regular use of oregano may help diabetics maintain better control of their condition.

OREGANO

BEST FOR HELPING YOU:

Freshen your breath

Kill oral bacteria

Parsley: A Handful of Pure Vitality

Parsley is the most frequently used herb in my kitchen. It adds a contrasting touch of green when my nouvelle pasta gets too light and white, plus it adds a hidden boost of mineral power to every dish in which it appears. In fact, when used with stronger flavors like tomato or garlic, parsley's slightly bitter note is muted enough that it can be slipped into toddler-sized vegetable haters without fuss.

A single ounce of the fresh herb—not much when it's chopped and buried in a plate of spaghetti or rolled into a serving of meatloaf—has nearly as much calcium as a glass of milk. It has a nice chunk of

---

OREGANO BASICS

HOW TO BUY: Oregano is so easy to grow that it begs to be planted in a windowsill herb garden. If you prefer the dried leaves, however, oregano is available in just about every supermarket on the planet.

HOW TO STORE: Dried leaves should be kept in a tightly capped bottle on your spice rack.

HOW TO USE: Try it in everything you cook. Oregano works particularly well with anything tomato, but there's rarely a salad, soup, stew, vegetable, or piece of meat that isn't improved by the addition of oregano.

---

muscle-maintaining potassium, a smidgen of iron to build healthy red blood cells, and just enough vitamin C to improve iron absorption. It also has enough folic acid to keep your DNA repair squad on the job—an important activity if you want to stay cancer-free.

Parsley's a particularly good herb for women. It has a diuretic effect that helps you unload excess fluid both premenstrually and during menopause. And its folic acid helps your body fight off the ravages of various sexually transmitted viruses—including the ones that can lead to cervical cancer.

The folic acid content of parsley also helps prevent spina bifida, a deadly birth defect that affects babies during the first few weeks of pregnancy—frequently before a woman even knows she's pregnant. And it may offset high homocysteine levels—a byproduct of metabolizing meat—that set the stage for heart disease.

Rosemary: A Potent New Weapon against Cancer

Looking at the amazingly delicate sprigs of dried rosemary hanging from the spice rack in my kitchen, I'm absolutely amazed at what scientists are discovering about this ancient herb.

"There's a whole bag of phytochemicals in rosemary," says Keith Singletary, Ph.D., associate professor of food science at the University of Illinois. "It's a potent antioxidant." It can grab hold of disease-causing molecules called free radicals and neutralize their harmful effects before they can damage cells.

"In rosemary," explains Dr. Singletary, "the compound most responsible for its antioxidant

PARSLEY
BEST FOR HELPING YOU:
Prevent sexually transmitted viruses
Build red blood cells
Drain extra fluid that causes bloating
Build strong bones
Maintain muscle function
Prevent birth defects
Ward off cervical cancer
Prevent heart disease

PARSLEY BASICS

HOW TO BUY: When buying fresh parsley, choose either the milder, curly type or the flat-leafed kind with a more pungent taste. Look for dark green bunches that are crisp and perky. Avoid anything yellow or wilted. Dried parsley should be purchased in large, sealed containers—large because an intelligent cook is going to use a lot.

HOW TO STORE: Wash fresh parsley, trim its stems, plunk it into a glass of cold water and stick it in the refrigerator. Put dried parsley in a tightly capped container in the spice rack.

HOW TO USE: In everything. Add fresh, chopped parsley to any dish just before you serve it. Or sprinkle a tablespoon or two of dried parsley over the top. It's the finishing touch to just about every entrée that comes out of my kitchen.

One caveat: Once a woman knows she's pregnant, some doctors feel that she should avoid eating more than half an ounce of parsley every day. Although not yet proven, some feel that more than that can cause uterine contractions.

properties is carnosic acid. It seems to have a number of beneficial effects on the early stages of breast cancer. And in studies with human lung cancer cells, it seems that rosemary is able to activate certain enzymes in the body to protect itself."

Exactly how rosemary works—how much it takes to have a therapeutic effect and exactly what it does—is still something of a mystery, says Dr. Singletary. When carnesol, a byproduct of carnosic acid, is injected into lab animals, for example, it works quite well at preventing cancer. But when carnosol is present in the diet, it doesn't seem as effective. "We're not sure what's going on," adds Dr. Singletary, "but it may be that carnosol is more available to the body when phytochemicals from other foods are also present in the diet."

His suggestion?

Eat rosemary with a wide variety of foods—particularly fruits and vegetables.

ROSEMARY

BEST FOR HELPING YOU:

Slash your risk
of breast cancer

Slash your risk
of lung cancer

Tarragon: A Cancer-Fighting Gift from St. Catherine of Siena

Anyone who's spent time in the French countryside generally comes away with a love of tarragon. That's because the herb is used, grown, and worshipped throughout the area. St. Catherine of Siena brought it from Asia in the 14th century, and it's safe to say that French cooking hasn't been the same since.

But now the French have discovered that there are other reasons for blending tarragon into their famous cream sauces. Scientists have found that this innocuous green herb contains at least 72 different substances that have the potential to block cancer. And the most powerful of them—caffeic acid—has the ability to zap maverick molecules that damage cellular DNA and trigger the cancer process.

If you're not familiar with tarragon's peppery taste, now might be the time to try it.

ROSEMARY BASICS

HOW TO BUY: Buy a *Rosmarinus officinalis* plant at your local gardening supply store, bring it home, and put it in a place of honor on your kitchen windowsill. Or buy the dried herb in your supermarket.

HOW TO STORE: A rosemary plant sometimes produces more leaves than you can use. So I simply snip off long branches, tie them in bunches and hang them upside down from my kitchen spice rack, away from direct sun. Dried rosemary from the store should be kept in tightly capped containers out of the light.

HOW TO USE: If you've got the fresh plant, just snip several inches off a branch, crush the leaves, and sprinkle them over meat, fish, or poultry toward the end of cooking. You can also trim a couple of extra branches and lay them alongside as a garnish. If you prefer using the dried herb, just sprinkle it over the food right before serving. Scientists don't know whether or not high temperatures destroy some of the herb's therapeutic constituents, so common sense dictates that it won't hurt to avoid exposing the herb to super-high temperatures.

Thyme: Respiratory Relief

Like oregano, thyme is probably found as often in your medicine chest as on your kitchen spice rack. That's because it contains thymol, a major antibacterial ingredient found in mouthwashes such as Listerine.

But thymol may have other benefits in addition to fresher breath. When the plant's oils are ingested or inhaled, some studies indicate that thymol can relieve cold symptoms. It can break up congestion in the respiratory system and relax muscles associated with it that frequently go into spasms when you cough.

Turmeric: Nature's Most Powerful Antioxidant?

For 3,000 years, Ayurvedic physicians in India have prescribed turmeric as frequently as American physicians have said, "Take two aspirin and call me in the morning."

HOMEMADE TARRAGON VINEGAR

Bottles of herb vinegar allow you to whimsically change the flavor of a salad at a moment's notice. And they make wonderful inexpensive—or last minute!—hostess gifts.

One of my favorites is tarragon vinegar. To make it, heat two cups of white vinegar just to a boil. Drop a handful of fresh washed-and-air-dried tarragon into a clean glass pint jar, pour in the hot vinegar, and cap tightly. Make sure you use a heavy glass jar that will withstand heat.

Then store your vinegar out in plain sight where everyone can enjoy the natural beauty of your tarragon. The vinegar will be ready for use in one week.

Yet most of us know turmeric only as a yellow coloring agent frequently used in butter, margarine,

TARRAGON BASICS

HOW TO BUY: Pick up a bottle of the dried leaves in your local supermarket, or buy a plant of French tarragon and add it to your kitchen windowsill. Make sure you buy the French kind, not the Russian. Russian tarragon has little flavor.

HOW TO STORE: The dried herb should be kept in tightly capped bottles in your spice rack. If you decide to grow the fresh plant, it grows so fast that you may want to occasionally snip a bunch, tie it into a bundle and hang it upside down in a dark place to dry. I thumbtack the bundle onto my spice rack and just snip whatever dried herbs I need as I cook.

HOW TO USE: Tarragon is great for flavoring chicken, fish, eggs, and soups. Experiment with just a pinch, then increase the amount as you become more comfortable with its flavor. If you use too much, its peppery, slightly bitter taste will overwhelm the flavors of subtler herbs.

Here's a list of spice merchants who will send freshly ground herbs to you through the mail:

Adriana's Bazaar
2152 Broadway
New York, NY 10023

Frontier Herbs
P.O. Box 118
Norway, IA 52318 (dried turmeric rhizomes)

Penzeys, Ltd.
P.O. Box 1448
Waukesha, WI 53187

Sultan's Delight
P.O. Box 253-H
Staten Island, NY 10314

cheese, jelly, and mustard. Or as an ingredient that adds bite to Worcestershire sauce.

But turmeric is also a powerful antioxidant that contains curcuminoids, a group of chemical substances that may protect the

liver from the damaging effects of alcohol and over-the-counter pain relievers. What's more, curcuminoids may also aid digestion, reduce arthritic symptoms, lower cholesterol, help prevent the blood clots that can cause heart attacks, and help prevent cancer—particularly cancers of the colon, mouth, esophagus, and skin. And one of the curcuminoids—curcumin—has been found to interfere with the replication of a number of viruses, including the hepatitis virus and HIV.

It's a pretty remarkable package. Some scientists even claim that the curcuminoids in turmeric are more powerful antioxidants than vitamin E or resveratrol. (See "Grapes" on page 44.)

Keith Singletary, Ph.D., an associate professor of food science and nutrition at the University of Illinois, has investigated the therapeutic effects of curcumin for some time. And his conclusion is that "there's

---

TURMERIC

BEST FOR HELPING YOU:

Protect the liver

Reduce arthritic symptoms

Prevent cancer

Lower cholesterol

Prevent a heart attack or stroke

Fight viral invaders

THYME BASICS

HOW TO BUY: Either buy the live plant and grow it on a sunny windowsill, or purchase the dried herb at your supermarket. The whole leaves have more therapeutic ability and flavor than the ground herb. Do NOT buy the oil. It's toxic.

HOW TO STORE: If you have the dried herb, simply keep it in a tightly capped bottle on your spice rack.

HOW TO USE: Sprinkle the dried or fresh herb into sauces, soups, stews, and stocks. As they simmer, the resulting vapors will help relieve your cold symptoms—as will eating the food you've cooked. You may want to consider Anita's "Golden Apple Soup with Wine and Thyme" (p. 212) as a cold remedy as well as a luscious lunch or appetizer before the main meal. As a flavoring agent, thyme works particularly well with tomato-based dishes and chicken. It's also a key ingredient in bouquet garni, a traditional bouquet of herbs that is used in French cooking.

enough evidence to suggest that there's something there.

"We don't know exactly how that evidence translates to our diet," he adds, "but there's a strong promise that it does."

TURMERIC BASICS

HOW TO BUY: As a freshly ground powder in Middle Eastern or Asian grocery stores, or directly from spice merchants. (See "The Spice Chest" on previous page.)

HOW TO STORE: In a tightly capped container, away from sunlight.

HOW TO USE: Turmeric's warm yellow hue and slightly bitter note make it a versatile spice. It's too pungent to do more than add color and bitterness on its own, but it provides nuances and subtle undertones in a dish when combined with other spices. It particularly works well with stronger herbs such as dill or thyme, bolder spices such as fenugreek, and sweet spices such as cinnamon or cloves. It's also the major ingredient in curry powder. (See "Learning to Use New Herbs: A Visit with the Spice Lady" on page 190.)

I use it to color brown rice and, with thyme, to make various chicken dishes. Turmeric also works well with sautéed cauliflower and fish.

Keep in mind that turmeric is powerful. If you're taking any medication, common sense says that you should talk with your doctor before ingesting large quantities of turmeric—especially if you have a heart or thyroid condition.

LEARNING TO USE NEW HERBS:
A VISIT WITH THE SPICE LADY

A late autumn sun pushed its way through the bare branches of oaks and hickory lining the twisting country road as I followed Betsy Jacob's directions across a meadow, over a brook, around a bend, and, finally, up to the door of her Bucks County herb barn in Pennsylvania.

A giant black dog bounced out of the barn to peer at me over the hood of my station wagon, closely followed by a laughing woman with cropped gray hair.

I didn't know who the dog was, but the human had to be Betsy. As indeed it was, I found out, when Betsy—probably 100 pounds dripping wet!—was finally able to tug the dog back far enough for me to open the car door. Two minutes later, amid introductions, apologies, and laughter, I had fallen in love with both Rufus and Betsy.

Aside from meeting these two wonderfully centered creatures, I had come to Betsy's herb barn because I wanted to learn more about the culinary herbs we keep on our kitchen spice racks—both the newer ones that we're just beginning to play with and the old ones that we now know have some amazing health benefits. I figured that as chairperson of the New York branch of the American Herb Society—and former director of children's education at the Brooklyn Botanical Garden—Betsy was the person to ask.

I was particularly interested in spices like turmeric, an herb that although rarely found in American spice racks, has been found to be one of the most powerful antioxidants ever measured.

Cloves, which contain eugenol, a substance that keeps artery-blocking blood clots from forming, and ginger, which contains gingerol, a substance that does everything from preventing nausea to preventing heart attacks, were also spices that I needed to know more about. As far as I was concerned, cloves and ginger were reserved for making pumpkin pie at Thanksgiving and gingerbread men at Christmas. And if I was to avail myself of their therapeutic abilities year-round, clearly I needed more information.

Helping me dissuade Rufus from slathering my face with kisses, Betsy escorted me inside the dim interior of the herb barn and gave me a tour. The first floor was an herbalist's delight. Dried flowers, grasses, roots, leaves, branches, stalks, and whole plants hung from low rafters and walls or overflowed baskets, wheelbarrows, and boxes on the floor. Some she was drying to make her own spices, others were reserved for workshops she taught on making dried wreaths.

Following her up a narrow, wooden stairway to the floor above, I saw an incredible array of Betsy's craft. Finished decorations—wreaths, swags, nosegays, door-toppers, and wall hangings, among others—lined part of the stairwell and extended onto the east wall of the floor above. The effect was so stunning that it was only slowly that I realized I had emerged into a two-story room that was filled with light—most of it coming from a bank of windows looking out over the raised beds in which Betsy grows her herbs. Some of those herbs went into the crafts decorating the stone and plaster walls, but many also went into the spices that she had stacked on counters and shelves under the windows in the kitchen area.

It was the spices that drew my attention, of course, and Betsy was kind enough to open their containers, shake some into my hand, let me taste to my heart's content, and explain how each herb is grown and used. She even told me how she makes her own spice blends—including curry powder, an Indian spice blend that can contain anywhere from 3 to 12 of the most potent disease-fighting antioxidants known to man.

"I like to throw a bunch of the herbs I grow into the blender with those I buy and make my own curry powder," says Betsy.

Some days she makes it one way, other days another. "It varies tremendously," she adds. "It's an infinitely variable kind of thing. You can leave out any one ingredient, substitute almost any other, and it would still taste great."

Here's her basic blend. Try it and you'll have enough for nearly three pounds of curry powder—enough for your own kitchen spice rack, and to give as hostess gifts when you visit friends.

Betsy Jacob's Basic Curry Powder

Toss everything in a blender; put the cover in place and process on "grind," says Betsy. When the mix seems to be smooth, let it sit for a few moments while the spice dust settles, or sprinkle a few drops of vinegar in to settle it for you. If you take off the blender cover too soon, cautions Betsy, you'll inhale the potent spice dust and irritate your entire respiratory system.

Once the dust has settled, slowly pour the mixture into bottles, cap tightly and store away from light. Your curry powder will stay fresh for a year.

"You can curry practically anything

INGREDIENTS

8 ounces turmeric powder
8 ounces coriander seeds
8 ounces cumin seeds
4 ounces ginger, dried and ground
4 ounces peppercorns
2 ounces cardamom pods
2 ounces fennel seeds
2 ounces dried red chiles (or cayenne pepper)
2 ounces mace
1 ounce cloves, whole
1 ounce poppy seeds
cinnamon (to taste)

with this mix," says Betsy. "You can use it with strong tastes like goat to mask the flavor, or you can use it with bland stuff like squash to give it flavor. And if the curry taste is too strong by itself, you can soften it with yogurt or sweeten it with raisins."

Jamaican Chicken Thighs with Red Lentils and Rice

This recipe takes about one hour to prepare. It can easily be adapted to serve a large group.

Remove the skin from the chicken and set aside. In a large pot, heat the oil, add the fenugreek and stir a few seconds. Add the onion, celery and garlic and sauté five minutes or until softened. Add the chicken, ginger, allspice, chicken broth and parsley. Bring to a boil, turn down the heat, cover and allow to simmer for 45 minutes.

About 20 minutes before the chicken is done, bring 2¼ cups of water to a boil.

Add the rice, turn the heat to medium-low, cover and cook for 10 minutes. After 10 minutes, add the red lentils, stir to combine, cover pot and allow to cook for 5 more minutes.

Serve the lentil and rice mixture with the chicken pan gravy. Top the chicken with chopped parsley and freshly ground black pepper.

INGREDIENTS

YIELD: 6 SERVINGS

6 chicken thighs (about 3 lbs with bone)
2 teaspoons olive oil
½ teaspoon fenugreek
1 onion, chopped
1 celery stalk, chopped
2 cloves garlic, minced
2 teaspoons fresh chopped ginger
½ teaspoon ground allspice
1 cup defatted chicken broth
2 tablespoons chopped fresh parsley
1 cup long grain white or brown rice
½ cup uncooked red lentils
1 tablespoon chopped fresh parsley (garnish)
Dash black pepper

PER SERVING

Calories 368
Carbohydrates .... 31 g
Fat.. 12 g
Monounsaturated Fat .... 5 g
Dietary fiber.. 3 g
Cholesterol .... 9 mg
Sodium.. 120 mg

Chocolate Allspice Cookies

*P*reheat the oven to 400 F.

In a bowl combine the margarine, honey, and egg. Stir in the yogurt and vanilla.

In a medium bowl combine the flour, soda, salt, cocoa, cinnamon, allspice, and cloves. Add the wet ingredients to the dry ingredients and mix well. The mixture should be firm. Add more flour if needed. Add half of the finely chopped walnuts.

Using a heaping tablespoon of dough, drop the cookies on a lightly greased or oiled cookie sheet. Top the cookies with some chopped walnuts. Bake for 8 to 10 minutes.

INGREDIENTS

YIELD: 36 COOKIES

¼ cup trans fat–free soft light margarine
½ cup honey
¼ cup egg substitute or 1 egg
¾ cup nonfat or low-fat plain yogurt
1 teaspoon vanilla
1¾ cups unbleached or half whole wheat and
    half unbleached flour
½ teaspoon baking soda
½ teaspoon salt
½ cup unsweetened cocoa powder
½ teaspoon cinnamon
1 teaspoon allspice
½ teaspoon ground cloves
2 to 4 tablespoons finely chopped walnuts

PER COOKIE

Calories	53
Carbohydrates	10 g
Fat	1 g
Saturated fat	0.3 g
Dietary fiber	1 g
Cholesterol	6 mg
Sodium	72 mg

Pork Loin Chops with Spicy Fruit and Rice

*P*reheat oven to 350 F.

In a large heavy skillet, heat the olive oil over medium-high heat and quickly brown the chops on both sides. Remove the pan from the heat.

In a deep casserole with a lid, mix together all the other ingredients. Add the browned meat to the casserole. Cover and bake in oven for 45 minutes or until the pork is tender. Serve chops with hot cooked rice and the fruited pan juices.

Recipe adapted from original, courtesy the National Pork Producers Council.

INGREDIENTS

YIELD: 6 SERVINGS

6 pork loin chops (1½ inches thick)
2 teaspoons olive oil
1 cup dried apricots
¾ cup golden raisins
½ cup slivered almonds
3 cups orange juice (juice from 8 oranges)
1 teaspoon grated orange zest
1 tablespoon grated fresh ginger root
½ teaspoon ground cinnamon
½ teaspoon ground allspice

PER SERVING

Calories	386
Carbohydrates	48 g
Fat	11 g
Saturated fat	3 g
Dietary fiber	5 g
Cholesterol	65 mg
Sodium	44 mg

Anise-Spiced Biscotti

This is a firm cookie that won't wilt if you dunk it in a hot beverage, but it's just as tasty with a cold one, too—like skim milk.

Preheat oven to 375 F.

In a large bowl, combine the sugar and crushed anise seed. Beat in the margarine until well blended. Add the egg and beat well.

In another bowl, combine the flour, baking powder, and salt. Add to the sugar mixture and combine well. The dough will be sticky. With floured hands, divide the dough in two parts. Form one part into a flat loaf on a nonstick sprayed baking sheet. The loaf will be about 11 inches long and 3 inches wide. Shape the other half of the dough on the baking sheet along side the first.

Bake for 20 minutes. Remove the baking sheet from the oven. Cut each loaf into 10 slices. Turn the slices over and bake for 5 more minutes so that the sides will be browned. After 5 minutes, remove the pan from the oven and turn each biscotti so the other side will be browned. Return to the oven for another 5 minutes. Cool.

INGREDIENTS

YIELD: 20 BISCOTTI

1 cup packed light brown sugar
2 teaspoons anise seed, crushed
⅔ cup trans fat–free soft light margarine
¼ cup egg substitute or 1 egg
2¼ cups all-purpose flour
2 teaspoons baking powder
¼ teaspoon salt

PER BISCOTTI

Calories	122
Carbohydrates	23 g
Fat	2.6 g
Saturated fat	0.6 g
Dietary fiber	0.4 g
Cholesterol	0 mg
Sodium	125 mg

Fruit Compote with Anise

Remove the skin from the peaches by dipping into boiling water for several seconds. Peel and halve peaches. Remove the pit.

In a saucepan, bring the apple juice, anise seed, and honey to a boil. Turn the heat to medium-low and add the dried apricots, pears, and prunes. Simmer the mixture for 10 minutes. Add the prepared peaches, cover, and simmer for 5 more minutes.

Serve warm.

INGREDIENTS

YIELD: 8 SERVINGS

2 peaches
2 cups apple juice
1 teaspoon anise seed
1 tablespoon honey
12 dried apricots
12 dried pears
12 prunes

PER SERVING

Calories	140
Carbohydrates	36 g
Fat	0.3 g
Saturated fat	0 g
Dietary fiber	4 g
Cholesterol	0 mg
Sodium	4 mg

Tummy Soother Tea

When added to black tea these spices are all proven to be tummy soothing: allspice, anise, fennel, clove, and coriander. Make a batch to have on hand in the spice rack.

Combine the tea and spices in an airtight jar. To make the tea add two teaspoons of the mix to a cup of boiling water. Sweeten with honey if desired.

INGREDIENTS

YIELD: ENOUGH FOR
18–20 CUPS OF TEA

1 cup black tea leaves
2 tablespoons anise seeds
1 tablespoon whole allspice
1 tablespoon fennel seeds
1 tablespoon coriander seeds
1 teaspoon whole cloves

PER SERVING

Calories 0

Spicy Spaghetti with Tomatoes and Cayenne

Heat oil in a large skillet. Add garlic and sauté for 30 seconds. Add the tomatoes, tomato paste, oregano, and cayenne. Cook on medium-low about 10 minutes. Add the olives and capers and heat another few minutes until heated through.

Toss with cooked spaghetti. Top with freshly ground black pepper and Parmesan cheese if desired.

*NOTE: To peel the tomatoes, dip them into boiling water for 1 minute. Remove them from the boiling water with a spoon and transfer them quickly to a bowl of ice water. As soon as they are cool enough to handle, simply peel off the skins. Cut the tomatoes into chunks.

INGREDIENTS

YIELD: 4 SERVINGS

1 tablespoon olive oil
2 cloves garlic, finely chopped
3 cups peeled, seeded, and chopped tomatoes*
1 tablespoon tomato paste
1 tablespoon fresh oregano or 1 teaspoon dried oregano
¼ teaspoon cayenne
4 Kalamata olives, pitted and chopped
1 tablespoons capers
8 ounces spaghetti, cooked
Freshly ground black pepper (optional)
Freshly ground Parmesan cheese (optional)

PER SERVING

Calories 301
Carbohydrates .... 53 g
Fat.. 6 g
Saturated fat .... 0.8 g
Dietary fiber... 5 g
Cholesterol .... 0 mg
Sodium.. 158 mg

Cajun Pork Roast Sandwiches

If you've ever tasted a po'boy, the New Orleans–style hero sandwich, you'd swear there's no way to make it low-fat and healthy. But this is it. Use thinly sliced meats roasted with health-giving herbs and spices and place them between slices of crusty French bread.

Preheat oven to 350 F.

Combine all seasonings and rub well over all surfaces of roast. Place roast in shallow pan and roast in oven for about an hour or until internal temperature of the roast is 160 F. Remove from oven and let rest 5 to 10 minutes before slicing.

Each sandwich should have about 3 ounces of meat. A great way to serve is to provide shredded lettuce, sliced veggies, and coarsely ground mustard so everyone can top their own sandwich.

Recipe adapted from original, courtesy of the National Pork Producers Council.

INGREDIENTS

YIELD: 8–12 SERVINGS
(1 SANDWICH EA.)

2 pounds boneless single loin pork roast
3 tablespoons paprika
1 teaspoon cayenne
1 tablespoon garlic powder
2 teaspoons oregano
2 teaspoons thyme
½ teaspoon ground white pepper
½ teaspoon cumin
¼ teaspoon nutmeg
16 slices French bread or 8 rolls

PER SERVING

Calories	321
Carbohydrates	29 g
Fat	10 g
Saturated fat	3 g
Dietary fiber	3 g
Cholesterol	57 mg
Sodium	362 mg

Fresh Tomato Salsa

Combine all ingredients. It can be served immediately or refrigerated in a covered bowl or jar for up to a day. After one day, though, the quality can begin to deteriorate.

INGREDIENTS

YIELD: 3 CUPS

3 jalapeño peppers, seeded and finely chopped
4 teaspoons finely chopped cilantro
¾ cup finely chopped mild white onion
3 tomatoes, peeled, seeded, and chopped
3 tablespoons olive oil
⅓ cup white wine vinegar

PER ¼-CUP SERVING

Calories	43
Carbohydrates	3 g
Fat	4 g
Saturated fat	0.5 g
Dietary fiber	0.5 g
Cholesterol	0 mg
Sodium	4 mg

Caponata

Spice up your next party with caponata, a spread made from a combination of vegetables cooked together and used to top slices of toasted Italian bread. This flavorful appetizer also makes a nice light lunch or snack.

Preheat the oven to 375 F.

Slice the unpeeled eggplant vertically into long slices about ½-inch thick. Lay in one layer on a nonstick sprayed baking pan. Roast in the oven for 15 to 20 minutes or until tender and lightly browned. Cut into small cubes and reserve.

Place garlic cloves in a piece of aluminum foil and drizzle a bit of oil over them. Wrap securely in foil and bake in the oven at 375 F for 20 minutes or until garlic is soft and creamy. The garlic can be put in the oven at the same time as the eggplant to save time.

INGREDIENTS

YIELD: 3 CUPS

1½-pound eggplant
1 tablespoon olive oil
1 cup chopped onions
5 cloves garlic, peeled
1 teaspoon celery seed
2 large tomatoes, peeled, seeded, and
    chopped (2-2½ cups)
2 tablespoons drained capers
2 tablespoons golden raisins
12 Kalamata olives, pitted and chopped
1 tablespoon brown sugar
¼ cup red wine vinegar

PER 2-TABLESPOON SERVING

Calories	30
Carbohydrates	5 g
Fat	1 g
Saturated fat	0.2 g
Dietary fiber	1 g
Cholesterol	0 mg
Sodium	60 mg

In a large sauté pan, heat the oil and add the onions and celery seed. Sauté until the onions are softened. Add the tomatoes and roasted garlic and cook 2 to 3 minutes more, mixing until well combined.

Add reserved eggplant, capers, raisins, olives, brown sugar, and vinegar. Cook on low heat for 15 minutes until well blended. Stir occasionally. Store refrigerated in glass jars for up to 2 weeks.

Celery Seed Salad Dressing

Combine all ingredients in a jar. Refrigerate for 15 minutes to allow flavors to blend. The dressing can be made a day before serving.

INGREDIENTS

YIELD: ¾ CUP

2 tablespoons honey
2 tablespoons vinegar
¼ cup chopped fresh parsley
1½ teaspoon celery seed
½ cup light mayonnaise

PER 1-TABLESPOON SERVING

Calories	46
Carbohydrates	4 g
Fat	3 g
Saturated fat	0.7 g
Dietary fiber	0 g
Cholesterol	0 mg
Sodium	75 mg

Creamy Vegetable Soup

*H*eat the oil in a skillet. Add the garlic, onion, and pepper and sauté until softened. Add the carrot, corn, water, and celery seed and cook about 20 minutes or until vegetables are tender.

Combine cold milk and cornstarch in a medium bowl. Slowly add the milk mixture to the soup and cook until the milk is warmed and the soup is slightly thickened.

Garnish with fresh or dried dill leaves.

INGREDIENTS

YIELD: 6 SERVINGS (1 CUP EA.)

1 tablespoon olive oil
1 teaspoon minced garlic
1 small onion, chopped
½ green pepper, chopped
1 carrot, shredded
3 cups corn
2 cups water
½ teaspoon celery seed
2 cups low-fat milk (1% or 2%)
2 tablespoons cornstarch
1 tablespoon chopped fresh parsley
Fresh or dried dill leaves for garnish

PER SERVING

Calories	145
Carbohydrates	26 g
Fat	4 g
Saturated fat	0.9 g
Dietary fiber	3 g
Cholesterol	3.3 mg
Sodium	51 mg

Soybean, Corn, and Macaroni Salad

*B*oil the macaroni until tender.

Meanwhile, in a large bowl mix together the remaining ingredients.

Drain the macaroni and rinse with cold water. Add to remaining ingredients and mix well.

*NOTE: Canned soybeans can be purchased in health food stores. The Westbrae Natural and American Prairie brand names are two that are available.

INGREDIENTS

YIELD: 8–16 SERVINGS OR 8 CUPS

1 cup uncooked macaroni
1 can (15 ounces) soybeans, rinsed and drained*
1 can (15 ounces) unsalted corn, drained or
    10-ounce package frozen corn or 1½ cups
    cooked corn
1 cup chopped green pepper
1 cup chopped red pepper
1 teaspoon celery seed
1 green onion, finely chopped
1 teaspoon minced garlic
¼ cup light mayonnaise
1 teaspoon prepared mustard

PER 1-CUP SERVING

Calories	220
Carbohydrates	29 g
Fat	8 g
Saturated fat	1 g
Dietary fiber	5 g
Cholesterol	0 mg
Sodium	68 mg

Tomato Bulgur Salad

Tabouleh

Pour warm water over the bulgur. Warm water from the tap is perfectly fine. Allow to set for 15 minutes. Any remaining water should be drained and squeezed out.

Combine the tomatoes, green onions, parsley, cilantro, and garlic.

Add the drained bulgur, lemon juice, and olive oil to the tomato mixture and combine well.

INGREDIENTS

YIELD: 6 SERVINGS

½ cup bulgur
1 cup seeded and diced tomatoes
8 thinly sliced green onions, including green tops
½ cup minced fresh parsley
¼ cup minced fresh cilantro
1 clove garlic, minced
3 tablespoons lemon juice
2 tablespoons olive oil

PER SERVING

Calories	93
Carbohydrates	12 g
Fat	5 g
Saturated fat	0.6 g
Dietary fiber	3 g
Cholesterol	0 mg
Sodium	9 mg

Thai Shrimp and Coriander

Bring 2 cups water to a boil. Add coriander and rice. Stir, lower heat to medium and cook for 10 to 15 minutes or until water is absorbed.

Combine the green onion, soy sauce, canola oil, lime juice, and lime peel in a bowl. Add shrimp and cooked rice. Mix well, cover, and chill.

When ready to serve, line plates with romaine, fill with the shrimp mixture, and garnish with a dash of cayenne.

INGREDIENTS

YIELD: 4 SERVINGS

1 teaspoon ground coriander
1 cup long grain rice
⅓ cup chopped green onion
2 tablespoons low-sodium soy sauce
2 tablespoons canola oil
3 tablespoons lime juice
1½ teaspoons minced lime peel
¾ pound medium shrimp, cooked, shelled and deveined
Dash cayenne pepper (optional)
Romaine

PER SERVING

Calories	335
Carbohydrates	41 g
Fat	9 g
Saturated fat	0.9 g
Dietary fiber	2 g
Cholesterol	129 mg
Sodium	431 mg

Chilled Artichoke and Rice Salad

Combine water and artichoke hearts in a saucepan and bring to a boil. Add the rice, cover, turn heat to low, and cook for 15 minutes or until water is absorbed by rice.

Meanwhile, combine all other ingredients in a bowl. Finally, add rice mixture and combine well. Cover and chill.

*NOTE: Drained, canned artichokes (14½ ounces) can be substituted for the frozen artichokes. Add the canned artichokes with the ingredients that are combined in a bowl. The canned artichokes do not have to be cooked with the rice.

INGREDIENTS

YIELD: 6 SERVINGS

1 cup water
1 package (10 ounces) frozen artichoke hearts*
⅔ cup long grain rice
2 tablespoons olive oil
2 tablespoons lemon juice
½ teaspoon grated lemon rind
1 clove garlic, minced
¼ cup finely sliced green onions, including green tops
¼ cup chopped cilantro
Dash of cinnamon

PER SERVING

Calories	139
Carbohydrates	22 g
Fat	5 g
Saturated fat	0.7 g
Dietary fiber	3 g
Cholesterol	0 mg
Sodium	42 mg

Blueberry and Yogurt Breakfast

In an ovenproof or microwavable individual serving bowl, spoon in the yogurt and top with the blueberries. Cover with the oats and then the maple syrup. Finally dust with the cinnamon.

Heat in the microwave on high for about 40 to 50 seconds or until the mixture is warmed. Serve.

INGREDIENTS

YIELD: 1 SERVING

½ cup low-fat or nonfat vanilla yogurt
½ cup fresh blueberries
2 tablespoons rolled oats
1 tablespoon maple syrup

PER SERVING

Calories	243
Carbohydrates	52 g
Fat	1 g
Saturated fat	0.3 g
Dietary fiber	3 g
Cholesterol	2 mg
Sodium	91 mg

Whole Wheat Cinnamon Buns

In a large bowl, combine the whole wheat flour, yeast, and salt.

In a saucepan, add the milk, sugar, and margarine. Heat on low just until the margarine melts and the milk is warmed. Remove the pot from the stove.

Add 1 cup of the whole wheat flour mixture to the milk mixture and combine with a wooden spoon. Add the egg to the mixture and beat well. Then add the remaining cup of whole wheat flour and combine well. The dough will be sticky. Now add ¼ cup of unbleached flour and turn the dough out onto a floured board.

Knead the dough for 5 minutes, adding all-purpose flour if necessary. Pour canola oil in the bottom of a large bowl. Add the dough to the bowl, making sure to coat the bottom of the dough with the oil. Once the bottom is coated, turn the dough over to coat the other side. Cover the bowl with a clean dish towel or saran wrap and allow to rise for an hour in a warm place.

Meanwhile, combine the maple syrup, raisins, nuts, and cinnamon in a small bowl. Spray an 8-inch x 8-inch square pan with nonstick spray and spread half the mixture over the bottom of the pan.

When the dough is doubled in bulk, punch the dough down and roll it out on a floured board to a 9-inch x 5-inch rectangle. Spread the soft margarine over the surface. Then spread the remaining maple syrup mixture over the margarine. Roll up the dough like a jelly roll, and pinch to secure the edges. Then cut the roll into 1-inch slices.

Lay the slices in the bottom of the pan in rows, three to a row. Cover and allow to rise until doubled in bulk, about 20 minutes.

Preheat the oven to 375 F.

Bake for 20 minutes. Turn over onto a wire rack covered with foil and allow to cool. Serve.

INGREDIENTS

YIELD: 9 CINNAMON BUNS

2 cups whole wheat flour
2 packages dry yeast or 2¼ teaspoons
½ teaspoon salt
¾ cup low-fat or skim milk
¼ cup sugar
2 tablespoons trans fat–free soft margarine
¼ cup egg substitute or 1 egg
½ to 1 cup unbleached flour
½ teaspoon canola oil
¾ cup maple syrup
⅓ cup raisins
¼ cup finely chopped walnuts
2 teaspoons cinnamon
1 tablespoon trans fat–free soft margarine

PER BUN

Calories	306
Carbohydrates	56 g
Fat	8 g
Saturated fat	1 g
Dietary fiber	4 g
Cholesterol	1 mg
Sodium	209 mg

Peach and Blackberry Crunch

*T*here's something comforting about cinnamon and nutmeg mixed with cooked fruits. This dish makes a wonderful dessert as well as a nutritional breakfast.

Preheat the oven to 350 F and spray a nonstick 8-inch x 8-inch baking pan.

Combine the cooked rice, blackberries, fresh peaches, and 2 tablespoons of the brown sugar in the baking pan.

Mix the flour, cinnamon, nutmeg, and remaining 2 tablespoons of brown sugar in a small bowl. Cut in the margarine. Cover the rice/fruit mixture with the flour mixture. Sprinkle the finely chopped walnuts over the flour mixture.

Bake for 20 to 25 minutes or until slightly browned.

INGREDIENTS

YIELD: 6 SERVINGS

2 cups cooked rice (white or brown)
1 cup blackberries, fresh or frozen
2 cups fresh peach slices (about 4 peaches)
¼ cup firmly packed brown sugar
¼ cup whole wheat or unbleached flour
½ teaspoon cinnamon
¼ teaspoon ground nutmeg
2 tablespoons trans fat–free soft light margarine
2 tablespoons chopped walnuts

PER SERVING

Calories	208
Carbohydrates	37 g
Fat	6 g
Saturated fat	0.9 g
Dietary fiber	4 g
Cholesterol	0 mg
Sodium	56 mg

Apricots Preserved with Honey and Cloves

*C*ombine in a stainless steel pot the honey, water, and vinegar. Bring to a boil. Add the apricots and return to a boil, lower heat, and cook for 3 minutes. Remove from heat.

In 4 sterilized half-pint canning jars, add 1 inch of cinnamon stick and ½ teaspoon whole cloves each. Divide the apricots evenly among the 4 jars. Reserve liquid.

Continue cooking the liquid until it is boiled down by half, leaving about 1½ cups. Pour the boiling syrup over the apricots. Cover jars with metal lids and screw bands. Allow to cool and then refrigerate.

INGREDIENTS

YIELD: 4 HALF-PINT JARS

1 cup honey
1 cup water
¾ cup cider vinegar
2 pounds apricots, peeled, halved, and pitted*
1 cinnamon stick (4 pieces about 1 in long)
2 teaspoons whole cloves

PER SERVING
(ABOUT 2 APRICOTS AND JUICES)

Calories	247
Carbohydrates	65 g
Saturated fat	0.1 g
Fat	0.4 g
Dietary fiber	0 g
Cholesterol	0 mg
Sodium	4 mg

*NOTE: Apricots should be firm, not soft. To peel easily, apricots can be blanched. Dip the apricot in boiling water for not more than one minute, then dip in icy cold water and peel.

Black Tea with Cloves

ring water and cloves to a boil, turn heat to simmer and continue cooking for 10 minutes. Strain out cloves and pour water into cups or teapot and prepare tea as usual.

INGREDIENTS

YIELD: 4 SERVINGS OR 8 CUPS

6 whole cloves
1 quart water
4 black tea bags or enough black or herbal tea for 4 servings

PER CUP

Calories 0

Dill and Onion Biscuits

reheat oven to 425 F.

In a medium bowl, beat onions, egg substitute, and yogurt together. In another bowl, combine flours, baking powder, dill, and salt. If using fresh dill, combine with the wet mixture. Combine dry and wet mixtures.

Pat or roll out the dough onto a floured board. Press or roll into a rectangle about 1 inch high. Using a biscuit cutter or glass about 2½ inches in diameter, cut 8 to 12 biscuits from the dough.

Bake for 10 to 15 minutes.

INGREDIENTS

YIELD: 8–12 BISCUITS

3 medium onions, grated or finely blended
½ cup egg substitute
½ cup nonfat yogurt
1 cup whole wheat flour
2 cups unbleached flour
2 teaspoons baking powder
2 tablespoons dried dill leaves or
    4 tablespoons fresh chopped dill
½ teaspoon salt

PER BISCUIT

Calories 205
Carbohydrates ....40 g
Fat...1 g
Saturated fat ....0.2 g
Dietary fiber...4 g
Cholesterol ....0.4 mg
Sodium...311 mg

Pickled Beets with Vidalia Onions

*W*ash beets. Remove green ends down to about ½ inch from the beet. Add the beets to a pot and cover with water. Bring the water to a boil, lower heat to medium, cover the pot with a lid, and cook the beets for 30 minutes or until they are tender. Test tenderness by inserting the point of a sharp knife into the beet. It should easily reach the center of the beet with little pressure. Drain the beets, saving a cup of liquid.

Peel and slice the beets into a bowl or storage container. Cover with the sliced Vidalia onion. Add the cup of reserved beet liquid, the vinegar, honey or sugar, and dill. Cover and refrigerate until serving time. These will keep at least a week in the refrigerator.

INGREDIENTS

YIELD: 6 SERVINGS

4 medium raw beets (about 2 pounds) or 2 pounds canned beets, drained, and saving 1 cup liquid
1 Vidalia onion, thinly sliced
½ cup cider vinegar
2 tablespoons honey or sugar
2 teaspoons chopped fresh dill or 1 teaspoon dried dill weed

PER SERVING

Calories	87
Carbohydrates	21 g
Fat	0 g
Saturated fat	0 g
Dietary fiber	0 g
Cholesterol	3 mg
Sodium	108 mg

Turkey Sausage Patties with Fennel

*C*ombine ground turkey, egg, and bread crumbs in a bowl. In a mortar and pestle or electric coffee grinder, grind herbs and spices together. Add to ground turkey mixture. Form into 5 patties. Cook in a lightly oiled, medium-size nonstick skillet for 5 minutes on each side or until patties are cooked through. Serve.

INGREDIENTS

YIELD: 5 PATTIES

1 pound skinless ground turkey
¼ cup egg substitute or 1 egg, lightly beaten
⅓ cup dried bread crumbs
½ teaspoon ground coriander
½ teaspoon fennel seeds
¼ teaspoon salt
½ teaspoon whole marjoram
½ teaspoon dried thyme
⅛ teaspoon turmeric
⅛ teaspoon ground black pepper
Dash of ground red cayenne pepper

PER SERVING

Calories	160
Carbohydrates	6 g
Fat	5 g
Saturated fat	1 g
Dietary fiber	0.3 g
Cholesterol	50 mg
Sodium	248 mg

Spicy Vegetarian Minestrone

*H*eat oil in a large heavy pot. Add celery, carrot, onion, and garlic. Sauté for 10 minutes on medium-low heat. Add the stewed tomatoes, water, canned soybeans, herbs, spices, parsley, and dry pasta and bring to a boil, then lower heat, cover, and simmer for 20 minutes.

Garnish with fresh parsley or grated Parmesan cheese and serve.

INGREDIENTS

YIELD: 6 SERVINGS (1 CUP)

1 tablespoon olive oil
½ cup chopped celery
½ cup chopped carrot
½ cup chopped onion
1 clove garlic, minced
1 can (14½ ounces) no-salt added, sliced, stewed tomatoes
2 cups water
1 can (16 ounces) soybeans
1 can (16 ounces) kidney beans
1 tablespoon chopped fresh parsley
1 teaspoon fresh oregano or ½ teaspoon dried
¼ teaspoon crushed red pepper
½ teaspoon crushed fennel seed
¼ teaspoon ground black pepper
½ cup dry small pasta, such as shells, elbows, fusilli, or rotini
1 tablespoon chopped fresh parsley
Chopped parsley or grated Parmesan cheese for garnish

PER SERVING

Calories	243
Carbohydrates	31 g
Fat	8 g
Saturated fat	1 g
Dietary fiber	8 g
Cholesterol	0 mg
Sodium	427 mg

Potato and Lentil Curry

Since fenugreek is a pulse (an edible seed), it needs to be softened before using. When you add it to the heated oil, it softens enough to flavor the food.

Bring the water to a boil and add lentils. Lower heat, cover, and cook for 30 minutes. Add the potatoes and cook for 15 minutes more or until both are tender.

Meanwhile, heat the canola oil in a skillet. Add the fenugreek and heat for several seconds. Add the garlic and onion and cook for 10 minutes or until soft. Add the coriander, turmeric, cumin, cayenne, and black pepper. Stir. Remove from the heat.

When the lentils and potatoes are tender, add them and any liquid to the onion and spice mixture. Return to heat, cover, and cook on medium-low for 5 minutes or until the vegetables are hot and the flavors blend.

INGREDIENTS

YIELD: 6 SERVINGS (½ CUP EA.)

2 Idaho potatoes, peeled and cubed
1 cup brown small lentils*
4 cups water
2 teaspoons canola oil
½ teaspoon fenugreek
1 teaspoon minced garlic
1 onion, sliced
½ teaspoon ground coriander
½ teaspoon turmeric
1 teaspoon ground cumin
¼ teaspoon cayenne
Freshly ground black pepper

PER SERVING

Calories	206
Carbohydrates	38 g
Fat	2 g
Saturated fat	0.2 g
Dietary fiber	12 g
Cholesterol	0 mg
Sodium	10 mg

*NOTE: Small lentils can be purchased in an Indian grocery store.

Kale with Spicy Yogurt

Heat olive oil in a large skillet and sauté fenugreek seeds for a few minutes. Add the cayenne pepper and cumin and for heat a few seconds. Add kale and stir well. Remove from heat and set aside to cool. Stir in the yogurt and top with paprika.

Serve over a baked potato.

INGREDIENTS

YIELD: 6 SERVINGS (½ CUP EA.)

2 teaspoons olive oil
⅛ teaspoon fenugreek seeds
¼ teaspoon cayenne pepper
½ teaspoon ground roasted cumin
1 package (10 ounces) frozen chopped kale or spinach, cooked and drained
2 cups plain nonfat yogurt or low-fat yogurt
Pinch paprika
1 baked potato

PER SERVING

Calories	73
Carbohydrates	—
Fat	2 g
Saturated fat	0.3 g
Dietary fiber	1 g
Cholesterol	2 mg
Sodium	70 mg

Grilled Turkey with Ginger Couscous

Place the turkey breast in a glass pan. In a small bowl, combine the soy sauce, chopped ginger, honey, and black pepper. Pour over the turkey and let marinate for 15 minutes, turning occasionally.

Preheat broiler.

Bring chicken broth to a boil. Add the couscous, cover, and remove from heat. After 5 minutes, fluff and put in a bowl. Add carrots, cilantro, rice wine vinegar, sesame oil, and grated ginger. Stir to combine.

Remove turkey from marinade and place on broiler pan. Broil for 10 minutes on a side. The turkey should be browned and cooked through. Use a meat thermometer to check temperature at 160 F. Allow to cool slightly and slice. Place slices over the couscous and serve.

INGREDIENTS

YIELD: 6–8 SERVINGS

1½ to 2 pounds skinned and boned turkey breast
¼ cup reduced-sodium soy sauce
2 tablespoons chopped fresh ginger
1 tablespoon honey
¼ teaspoon black pepper
2 cups chicken broth
1 cup couscous
2 medium carrots, shredded
¼ cup chopped cilantro
2 tablespoons rice wine vinegar
1 tablespoon sesame oil
2 teaspoons grated ginger

PER SERVING

Calories 209
Carbohydrates ....29 g
Fat..4 g
Saturated fat ....0.7 g
Dietary fiber...2 g
Cholesterol ....77 mg
Sodium...578 mg

Hot and Spicy Ginger Carrot Soup

Heat oil in a pan, add onions, and sauté until onions begin to soften. Add carrots, ginger, chicken stock, and tomato paste. Bring to a boil, lower heat, and simmer for ½ hour. Purée in blender or food processor. Pour back into pot, add milk, and heat just long enough to warm the milk, up to five minutes. Do not let it boil, or the milk will curdle. Serve.

INGREDIENTS

YIELD: 4 SERVINGS
(1 CUP EA.)

1 tablespoon olive oil
1 cup chopped onion
2 large carrots, cut into chunks
2 teaspoons chopped fresh ginger
1 quart low-sodium chicken stock or canned broth
1 tablespoon tomato paste
1 cup skim milk

PER SERVING

Calories 111
Carbohydrates ....12 g
Fat..6 g
Saturated fat ....2 g
Dietary fiber...3 g
Cholesterol ....6 mg
Sodium...159 mg

Oregano, Ziti, and Fresh Tomato Salad

Cook the ziti according to package directions. Meanwhile, in a medium bowl, combine the tomato, green onions, oregano, garlic, vinegar, olive oil, and Parmesan cheese.

When the ziti are tender, drain and add to the bowl with the tomato mixture. Combine well, coating the ziti.

INGREDIENTS

YIELD: 4 SERVINGS (1 CUP)

1 cup ziti, uncooked
1 large tomato, chopped
2 green onions, finely sliced
1 tablespoon fresh oregano
1 teaspoon minced fresh garlic
1 tablespoon cider vinegar
2 teaspoons olive oil
1 teaspoon grated Parmesan cheese

PER SERVING

Calories	130
Carbohydrates	22 g
Fat	3 g
Saturated fat	0.5 g
Dietary fiber	1 g
Cholesterol	0 mg
Sodium	15 mg

Easy Chicken Cacciatore

Heat oil in a nonstick skillet. Add onion and sauté for 1 minute on medium heat. Add the garlic, mushrooms, and green pepper and continue sautéing for a few minutes until the pepper begins to soften.

Cook the pasta according to package directions.

Drain and chop the tomatoes, saving the juice. Add the tomatoes, tomato paste, oregano, black pepper, and wine to the skillet. Bring the mixture to a boil, then turn the heat down to medium. Cover and simmer for about 5 minutes.

Finally, add the chicken, cover, and simmer for 5 more minutes or until the chicken is cooked throughout. Add any of the reserved tomato liquid that you need to give the sauce the consistency you prefer.

INGREDIENTS

YIELD: 4 SERVINGS

1 tablespoon olive oil
1 onion, chopped (about ½ cup)
2 garlic cloves, minced
8 ounces sliced mushrooms
1 green pepper, cut into chunks
8 ounces linguini
1 can (28 ounces) tomatoes, no salt added
2 tablespoons tomato paste
1 tablespoon fresh oregano or 1 teaspoon dried
½ teaspoon ground black pepper
¼ cup dry white wine
16 ounces skinless, boneless chicken breast, cut into bite-size chunks

PER SERVING

Calories	503
Carbohydrates	63 g
Fat	11 g
Saturated fat	3 g
Dietary fiber	8 g
Cholesterol	69 mg
Sodium	91 mg

Peach and Red Pepper Salsa

*C*ombine all ingredients in a small serving dish. Serve with poached fish.

INGREDIENTS

YIELD: ¾ CUP

1 peach, skinned and chopped
2 tablespoons finely chopped red pepper
2 tablespoons finely chopped zucchini
2 teaspoons balsamic vinegar
1 teaspoon olive oil
½ teaspoon minced peppermint

PER 2-TABLESPOON SERVING

Calories	16
Carbohydrates	2 g
Fat	0.8 g
Saturated fat	0.1 g
Dietary fiber	0.4 g
Cholesterol	0 mg
Sodium	0.5 mg

Mexican Chili Soup

*H*eat oil. Add garlic, celery, pepper, and onion. Sauté on medium-low heat for 10 minutes or until softened. Add ground turkey and sauté until cooked through. Add tomatoes, water, stock, parsley, cumin, and oregano. Bring to a boil, lower heat, cover, and cook for 30 minutes. Finally add kidney beans and heat through.

Serve with strips of tortillas and chopped parsley as garnish on top.

INGREDIENTS

YIELD: 6 TO 8 SERVINGS (2 CUPS EA.)

1 tablespoon canola oil
½ pound ground turkey breast
3 cloves garlic, minced
1½ cups diced celery
1 green pepper, chopped
1 medium onion, chopped
3 cups peeled, seeded, and chopped tomatoes
1 cup water
2 cups chicken stock
2 tablespoons chopped fresh parsley or 1
    tablespoon dried parsley
1½ teaspoons ground cumin
2 teaspoons fresh oregano or 1 teaspoon
    dried oregano
2 cups cooked kidney beans
3 flour or corn tortillas, warmed and cut into
    2-inch strips
Chopped parsley for garnish

PER SERVING

Calories	297
Carbohydrates	42 g
Fat	6 g
Saturated fat	0.9 g
Dietary fiber	10 g
Cholesterol	25 mg
Sodium	559 mg

Easy Rosemary and Garlic Roasted Potatoes

Preheat the oven to 425 F.
Peel and cut the potatoes into large chunks or wedges.

Place the garlic, rosemary, and olive oil in a 1-gallon plastic freezer bag. Add the potatoes to the bag. Close the bag and shake it so the oil and herb mixture is distributed evenly over the potatoes.

Open the bag and spread the potatoes on a sprayed nonstick baking pan. Bake for 15 minutes. Turn the potatoes and bake on the other side for 10 more minutes or until the other side is browned and the potatoes are soft on the inside.

INGREDIENTS

YIELD: 4 SERVINGS

4 Idaho potatoes
2 cloves garlic, minced
2 teaspoons rosemary
2 teaspoons olive oil

PER SERVING

Calories	169
Carbohydrates	35 g
Fat	3 g
Saturated fat	0.4 g
Dietary fiber	3 g
Cholesterol	0 mg
Sodium	8 mg

Herbed Turkey Burgers with Rosemary

Combine all ingredients in a bowl and form into four patties. Flatten as much as possible and place on broiler pan. Broil or grill for 6 to 8 minutes on each side, turning when nicely browned.

INGREDIENTS

YIELD: 4 BURGERS

1 pound ground turkey breast
¼ cup minced fresh parsley
2 tablespoons sunflower seeds or pine nuts, toasted and chopped
1 teaspoon rosemary, crushed
2 garlic cloves, minced
6 green pitted or stuffed olives, chopped

PER SERVING

Calories	169
Carbohydrates	2 g
Fat	4 g
Saturated fat	0.6 g
Dietary fiber	0.7 g
Cholesterol	82 mg
Sodium	194 mg

Parsnip Carrot Soup with Tarragon and Dill

*P*our chicken stock into a medium pot. Add the onion, fennel, carrots, parsnips, dill, and tarragon. Bring to a boil, turn heat to simmer, cover, and cook for 20 minutes or until the carrots and parsnips are soft. Allow to cool.

Purée the soup in a food processor. Pour the purée back into the pot and heat again. Whisk in the milk and lemon juice. Heat.

Serve. Garnish each bowl with pepper and allspice.

INGREDIENTS

YIELD: 4 SERVINGS (1 CUP)

2½ cups low-sodium chicken broth
1 medium onion, chopped (4 ounces or 1 cup)
½ cup chopped fennel or celery
2 carrots, sliced
2 parsnips, sliced
¼ cup chopped fresh dill
1 teaspoon dried tarragon
1 cup 1% low-fat milk
2 tablespoons lemon juice
Dash pepper
Dash ground allspice

PER SERVING

Calories	144
Carbohydrates	28 g
Fat	2 g
Saturated fat	1 g
Dietary fiber	6 g
Cholesterol	6 mg
Sodium	316 mg

Tarragon and Lemon Linguini

*C*ook linguini according to package directions. Drain.

In a bowl, combine the olive oil, tarragon, and lemon rind. Add the linguini and toss to coat.

In a large skillet, combine the stock, lemon juice, and cornstarch. Bring to a boil, mixing with a wire whisk and continue to mix until the stock thickens. Add to the linguini and toss.

Top with freshly ground black pepper and grated Parmesan cheese if desired. Serve.

INGREDIENTS

YIELD: 4 SERVINGS

8 ounces linguini
2 teaspoons olive oil
1 tablespoon chopped fresh tarragon or 1 teaspoon dried
1 teaspoon grated lemon rind
1 cup low-sodium, low-fat chicken stock
2 tablespoons lemon juice
2 teaspoons cornstarch
Freshly ground black pepper
Grated Parmesan cheese (optional)

PER SERVING

Calories	256
Carbohydrates	47 g
Fat	4 g
Saturated fat	0.7 g
Dietary fiber	5 g
Cholesterol	1 mg
Sodium	29 mg

Tarragon Vinegar

ring the vinegar to a boil. Allow to cool to lukewarm.

Place the tarragon in a bottle and pour the vinegar over it. Cool. The vinegar can be stored at room temperature.

INGREDIENTS

YIELD: 2 CUPS

2 cups rice wine vinegar
1 sprig (3 inches) fresh tarragon

PER TABLESPOON

Calories	0
Fat	0 g
Cholesterol	0 mg
Sodium	0 mg

Golden Apple Soup with Wine and Thyme

n a pot, combine broth with water, wine, chopped apples, sliced carrots, onion, celery, bay leaf, and thyme. Bring to a boil. Reduce heat, cover, and simmer for 20 minutes or until carrots are tender.

Remove bay leaf. Blend or purée soup in food processor or blender. Serve with a dash of pepper and a tablespoon of yogurt.

INGREDIENTS

YIELD: 4 SERVINGS

2 cups low-sodium chicken broth
1 cup water
½ cup white wine
2 Golden Delicious apples, peeled, cored, and chopped (3 cups)
1 large carrot, sliced
1 small onion, sliced
½ cup chopped celery
1 bay leaf
1 teaspoon thyme leaves, or ½ teaspoon dried thyme
Dash pepper
¼ cup plain low-fat yogurt

PER SERVING

Calories	94
Carbohydrates	15 g
Fat	1 g
Saturated fat	0.6 g
Dietary fiber	3 g
Cholesterol	3 mg
Sodium	88 mg

Flounder with Lemon Thyme Rice

Preheat oven to 350 F.

Cook rice following package directions, until tender.

Meanwhile, in a large ovenproof skillet, heat the 2 teaspoons of canola oil. Add the celery and onion and sauté on medium until celery is softened. When rice is cooked, add to the skillet along with the lemon rind and 1 teaspoon dried or 2 teaspoons fresh thyme. Combine well.

Cover the rice with the flounder fillets in one layer. Brush the flounder with the teaspoon of canola oil. Distribute lemon juice evenly over the fish. Then scatter the black pepper and the ½ teaspoon dried or 1 teaspoon fresh thyme and finally the fresh parsley over the fish.

Cover the skillet and bake for 20 minutes. The fish should be white and opaque and flake easily.

INGREDIENTS

YIELD: 4 SERVINGS

1 cup long grain white rice
2 teaspoons canola oil
½ cup finely chopped celery
½ cup finely chopped onion
2 teaspoons grated lemon rind
1 teaspoon dried thyme or 2 teaspoons fresh
12 ounces fresh flounder fillets (about 4 fillets)
1 teaspoon canola oil
1 tablespoon fresh lemon juice
Ground black pepper
½ teaspoon dried thyme or 1 teaspoon fresh
1 tablespoon chopped fresh parsley

PER SERVING

Calories	289
Carbohydrates	40 g
Fat	5 g
Saturated fat	0.6 g
Dietary fiber	2 g
Cholesterol	41 mg
Sodium	86 mg

Chile Bean Dip

This spicy dip is great with unsalted tortilla chips or toasted pita triangles. It can also be heated and served over hot cooked rice.

Combine ingredients in serving bowl. Serve.

INGREDIENTS

YIELD: 3 CUPS

2 cups cooked white beans
1 jalapeño pepper, seeded and chopped
1 tablespoon chopped cilantro
⅓ cup chopped mild onion
2 cups seeded and chopped tomatoes
2 tablespoons olive oil
2 tablespoons cider vinegar
1 teaspoon minced garlic
½ teaspoon turmeric

PER 2-TABLESPOON SERVING

Calories	36
Carbohydrates	5 g
Fat	1 g
Saturated fat	0 g
Dietary fiber	2 g
Cholesterol	0 mg
Sodium	2 mg

Sweet Potatoes and Cauliflower with Turmeric

Add water or chicken stock to a pot with turmeric and garlic. Mix well and bring to a boil. Add onion and sweet potato. Turn heat to medium, cover, and cook for 3 minutes. Add the cauliflower and cook another 10 minutes or until the vegetables are tender. Place in a serving bowl. Top with chopped parsley and black pepper and serve.

INGREDIENTS

YIELD: 4 SERVINGS

¾ cup water or chicken stock
½ teaspoon turmeric
1 clove garlic, minced
¼ onion, thinly sliced
2 sweet potatoes, peeled and coarsely chopped
2 cups cauliflower florets
1 tablespoon fresh chopped parsley
Dash black pepper

PER SERVING

Calories	97
Carbohydrates	22 g
Fat	0.4 g
Saturated fat	0 g
Dietary fiber	3.4 g
Cholesterol	0 mg
Sodium	26 mg

Stewed Garlic, Tomatoes, Mushrooms, and Green Beans

Lots of garlic in this recipe makes it delicious. I prepared this dish using fresh green beans given to me by a friend. They were great the next day, too, when reheated in the microwave.

In a large pot, heat the oil. Add the onion, green pepper, mushrooms, and garlic. Cook on medium heat for 10 minutes. Add the basil, parsley, tomatoes, and green beans. Cover and cook for 25 to 30 minutes or until the beans are tender.

INGREDIENTS

YIELD: 6 SERVINGS

1 tablespoon olive oil
2 medium onions, sliced
½ green pepper, sliced
8 ounces sliced mushrooms
4 garlic cloves, peeled and chopped
½ cup fresh, chopped basil
2 tablespoons chopped parsley
4 plum tomatoes, chopped
2 pounds green beans, washed, and stem ends trimmed

PER SERVING

Calories	105
Carbohydrates	19 g
Fat	3 g
Dietary fiber	6 g
Cholesterol	0 mg
Sodium	12 mg

The Snack Cupboard

✸✺✸

"No snacks! You'll ruin your supper."

"Don't you dare go near that cookie jar!"

"Eat your breakfast so you won't need a snack!"

"Do you really want that snack?"

"Aren't you afraid snacks will make you fat?"

Sometimes it seems as though the Food Police are everywhere. From cradle to grave, there's always someone who has a comment about what you're eating if you're anywhere but at a table that's set for breakfast, lunch, or dinner. Man, woman, or child—put something in your mouth between meals and at the least, you'll escape with a look of concern. On average, you'll get a comment that ostensibly reflects envy: "You're going to eat that? Wow! I wish I could eat snacks!" And once in a while, particularly if you carry a few extra pounds, complete strangers will feel morally compelled to run interference: "Isn't it almost lunchtime? You don't really need to eat that, do you?"

Clearly, snacking has a bad rep. Dietitians deplore it. Mothers campaign against it. Calorie-counters hold weekly meetings to figure out how to cope with

10

SNACK CUPBOARD

BEST FOR HELPING YOU:

Prevent anemia

Prevent cancer

Prevent childhood nutritional deficiencies

Prevent heart disease

Prevent obesity

Prevent osteoporosis

it. But despite all the buzz, there's nothing wrong with snacking. In fact, as my friend Anita—the most commonsensical dietitian on the planet—says with a shrug, "How else are you gonna get all the nutrients you're supposed to eat?"

Exactly. With a Food Pyramid that recommends 6 ounces of grains, 2½ cups of vegetables, 2 cups of fruits, 3 cups of milk or calcium-rich foods and 5½ ounces of meats and beans or protein-rich foods a day, you can either eat gargantuan meals that will leave you lying in the gutter and useless for the rest of the day—or you can snack.

And it isn't as though we don't have a precedent. Our ancestors, at least the ones who lived before supermarkets spanned the globe, did exactly that. They ate when they were hungry. They ate when food was available. They ate what they liked or found. And they didn't get fat or run stark raving mad through the bushes. So, unless we succumb to the artificially created snacks of hydrogenated shoe leather mixed with granulated purple slime and a squirt of fruit juice offered by the food industry—"If it's sweet or fat, they will come," is a maxim engraved on the hearts

215

of food industry executives everywhere—there's no reason to believe that we will get fat or go nuts either.

In fact, there's every reason to think that people who snack may avoid the kind of obesity that begins to plague both men and women as they pass their 30th birthday. A USDA study at Tufts University in Boston found, for example, that older women burn far fewer fat calories than younger women after eating a large meal, but burn pretty close to the same amount after eating a 250- or 500-calorie snack. As a result, the researchers suggest that getting a day's calories scattered throughout the day in several small snack meals rather than in a traditional 1,000-calorie dinner may help us avoid middle-age spread and the ballooning obesity that rides with it.

Other studies indicate that those smaller snack meals may also keep heart attacks at bay. After a meal that contains 50 grams of fat—a steak and baked potato with sour cream would do it—these studies show that your arteries can expand only half as much as they usually do. And the effect can last for hours. If a renegade blood clot just happens to wander through your coronary arteries during those after-meal hours, the artery may not be able to expand enough to let it pass. So it'll get stuck, block the flow of blood to your heart, and trigger a heart attack.

How high is the risk that this might happen? Too high. Unfortunately, scientists have also found that eating a big meal with 80 grams of fat—a steak and baked potato with sour cream followed by a piece of cake—triggers an increase in the release of a substance that promotes those very clots. And the increased clotting goes on for more than six hours following the meal.

So don't be afraid to reduce the traditional "three squares a day" and increase your snacks. Just make sure you select those snacks from the low-fat, nutrient-dense foods found in *The Healing Kitchen*. You could save your life.

After-School Snacks Can Reverse Childhood Deficiencies

Studies by the U.S. Department of Agriculture consistently show that children and adolescents, particularly preschoolers and teen girls, are deficient in the iron, calcium, and folic acid necessary to build red blood cells, strong bones, and healthy hearts. And that puts them at risk for anemia, heart disease, cancer, and osteoporosis.

Given what kids are eating, the deficiencies shouldn't be a surprise. A study of more than 3,000 young people between the ages of 2 and 19 by the National Cancer Institute in Bethesda, Maryland, found that only 1 percent of kids in the United States get the amounts of grains, vegetables, fruit, dairy, and poultry, fish, or beans that they need to maintain basic health. Sixteen percent of the kids don't get any of the foods they need.

That's tragic. And it's scary. Because if kids in the most well-nourished nation on the face of the earth aren't getting the nutrients they need, who is?

In some cases, the problem is ignorance. Parents just don't know what to feed their kids so they grab whatever's cheap, fast, and/or handy. In other cases, however, those loving parents simply can't afford fresh fruits and vegetables, much less fish or poultry. Here's how we can help both groups—as well as our own kids:

Get fresh. What kinds of snacks will help remedy nutritional deficiencies? "Fruits and vegetables, preferably fresh, preferably raw," says Marla Reicks, Ph.D.,

R.D., an associate professor of nutrition at the University of Minnesota. "A touch of low-fat dip if you need it." Whole grain crackers are also good, she adds, especially topped with a big fat smear of no-added-crap peanut butter.

Gale Frank, Ph.D., R.D., a professor of nutrition at California State University at Long Beach, agrees. She also suggests these nutritious and appealing treats:

- Fruit floats and slushies
- Milk shakes made with low-fat milk and fresh fruit
- Fruit kabobs
- Puddings made with low-fat milk and topped with fruit
- Oatmeal cookies
- Whole wheat pretzels
- Mini pizzas made with low-fat cheeses and tomato
- Cheese sticks
- A small bowl of cereal with fresh fruit or yogurt on top
- Whole grain sandwiches, cut with cookie cutters and layered with lean turkey, tomato, and lettuce

Be creative. One of the reasons that kids are so intrigued by high-fat, high-calorie snacks is the creative way in which foods are presented by advertisers. Now, no one expects you to compete with a New York ad agency. But instead of simply leaving a minimalist bowl of oranges on the table, melt a tablespoon of honey in the microwave, drizzle it over some mandarin orange slices, and top with a sprinkle of cinnamon before you slide it under a preschooler's nose. Or mix a half cup of tropical fruit with a quarter cup of yogurt and a handful of mini-marshmallows. Ten to one, any attempt you make to add a splash of excitement or a twinge of intrigue to an everyday snack will be re-

warded with an empty plate and a smile.

Dried is better than fried. Dried fruit isn't a bad choice, either, particularly as an alternative to potato chips, the deadly but undeniably number-one snack food among kids. Just make sure it's real dried fruit and not the high-sugar, low-fruit "fruit leathers" that line supermarket shelves. A handful of dried apricots, cranberries, apples, or raisins will contribute toward a healthy, well-run body. In fact, a study at the Health Research and Studies Center in Los Altos, California, found that both male and female soccer players ages 12 to 14 were able to maintain the blood glucose levels necessary to prevent fatigue during an entire game simply by eating 2 or 3 ounces—84 grams—of raisins at the half.

Munch freely. And if you're worried about encouraging obesity, forget it. Experts today advise that, as long as you keep to the foods mentioned above, just put the food on the table and walk away. The kids will eat what they need—and feed the rest to the dog.

Support community food banks. Those who live in the States can support Second Harvest, a national organization that opens the food pipeline between surplus food sources and local community food banks throughout the United States. Those who live outside the United States can support the United Nations Children's Fund, which sends food, medicine, clothes, and farming implements to communities where children are in need. In fact, a portion of the profits from this book will be divided between these two caring organizations.

Feed the neighborhood. We can also help by sharing nutrition information with our friends, neighbors, coworkers, and fellow parent/teacher organization members. And we can feed body-building snacks to every kid who comes through our door—our own, their friends, school-mates, church pals, playground buddies, and community league teammates. You can be the soccer mom who's always ready with a bag of ice-cold, freshly quartered oranges at the quarter, the homeroom dad who sends in double-trouble oatmeal cookies every Friday, or the baseball coach who pulls out chocolate-drizzled fresh strawberries after the game. And, yes, it can get expensive. But can you think of a better way to spend your money than to build happy, healthy kids?

A Generation at Risk

If you thought that once your kids got through a childhood filled with leafy greens, whole grains, and a glass of milk with every meal they'd know what to eat, forget it. Your kids haven't a clue. As a joint study between the Nestlé Research Center in Switzerland and the Universi-

ty of North Carolina at Chapel Hill indicates, the eating habits of kids ages 11 to 18 are going to hell in a handbasket.

The study showed that teens decreased milk consumption by 30 percent during adolescence and replaced it with soft drinks. Vegetable consumption dropped 25 percent in boys and 30 percent in girls. Fruit consumption decreased 27 percent in boys and 44 percent in girls. Bread consumption fell 33 percent in boys and 29 percent in girls. Fiber consumption was completely inadequate.

So what were the kids eating?

Low-fiber, high-sugar, ready-to-eat cereals.

It's enough to strike terror into the calmest parental heart. The one ray of hope is that the kids also reduced their fat intake from 39 percent to a healthier 34 percent. And the fat that they dropped was mostly the bad stuff that causes heart disease: saturated fat intake dropped from

---

DIP IT, DRIZZLE IT, DRIBBLE, OR DROP IT—CHOCOLATE IS HEALTHY!

Believe it or not, for most people, there's nothing wrong with chocolate. It doesn't cause acne. It doesn't raise your cholesterol levels. It doesn't make you hyper. It's not high in caffeine. It's not high in fat. What's more, it may actually do you some good. Studies at the University of California at Davis indicate that chocolate contains phenolics, which are powerful disease-fighting antioxidants that can help prevent the cell damage that leads to cancer and heart disease.

The key to using chocolate healthfully is to minimize sugar and use the chocolate with foods containing a smidgen of "good" monounsaturated fat like walnut oil rather than a "bad" saturated fat like butter. Not only will it contribute toward a healthy heart and cancer-free lifestyle, the combination of a small amount of sugar with a good fat and chocolate zips up your brain's production of endorphins and serotonin, two brain chemicals that make you feel happy and calm.

Both kids and adults love giant strawberries drizzled with semi-sweet chocolate chips that have been melted and made drizzle-able with the addition of a drop or two of canola oil. And they love just about any combination of fruit and nuts mixed into melted semi-sweet chocolate and allowed to harden in the refrigerator. So feel free to dip, drizzle, dribble, and drop chocolate on any group of fruits or nuts that takes your fancy.

15 to 13 percent, which almost brings it down to a healthier range.

Still, USDA consumption data indicates that 9 out of 10 teenage girls and 7 out of 10 boys do not get anywhere near the 1,300 milligrams of calcium recommended by the National Academy of Sciences—putting an entire generation at major risk for osteoporosis.

YOGURT DELIGHT

Another great snack for kids is to mix equal parts of unsweetened applesauce and some plain or vanilla nonfat yogurt and then top with a sprinkle of cinnamon. Kids love it, it's good for them, and it is a delicious way to introduce kids to yogurt. And you'll probably like it too. —Anita Hirsch

Healing Snacks for Women

Studies by the U.S. Department of Agriculture show that women, particularly those who diet, don't get enough calcium, vitamin E, folic acid, vitamin B6, magnesium, and zinc to build strong bones, a healthy heart, steady nerves, and an effective immune system. As a result, they're leaving themselves wide open to heart disease, irregular heartbeats, cancer, and every virus that piggybacks its way home on a child's backpack.

How did women get into so much trouble?

A study at the USDA's Beltsville Human Nutrition Research Center in Riverdale, Maryland, reveals that women are simply eating the wrong things. Barely half have even one serving a day of fruit or dairy. Only 45 percent have one serving of cereal or pasta. Only 10 percent have one serving of deep green or yellow veggies. So although women are managing to eat

roughly 1,600 calories a day, they're just not eating anything that has much of a nutritional punch. Or any fiber.

Fortunately, as Dr. Reicks points out, "You'd never have a nutrient deficiency if you snacked all day on the right kind of food." Here's what she means:

Get inventive with fruit, dairy, and whole grains. For women, the "right" kind of food means low-fat cultured yogurt with fresh fruit slices on top or a banana/strawberry or papaya smoothie, says Dr. Frank. It also means:

- Oatmeal bars
- Granola bars
- Cheese quesadilla on a whole wheat tortilla
- Low-fat and whole wheat crackers with mozzarella cheese
- Unsalted peanuts
- Raisins
- Coconut-free dried fruit mix
- A glass of milk
- A mini-salad tossed with spinach, two or three lettuces, an artichoke, mandarin oranges, almonds or walnuts, and drizzled with low-fat dressing

If you're pressed for time during the day, you could even make a peanut butter sandwich on whole wheat bread with strawberry jam before work and stuff it in your handbag or briefcase, says Dr. Frank. Eat half for a morning pick-me-up; half on the trip home after work.

Swear by soy. Two tablespoons of roasted soy nuts are enough to keep hot flashes and night sweats away for many menopausal women. The plant estrogens in soy—particularly an isoflavone called genistein—apparently fool your body into thinking it's making as much estrogen as it was before meno-

A handful of walnuts provides your body with as many heart-healthy omega-3 fatty acids as a three-ounce serving of salmon.

pause. What's more, genistein has also been found to lower cholesterol and discourage the formation of blood clots that can lead to heart attacks. One caveat: Since added estrogen can apparently make some hormone-dependent tumors grow, if you or a member of your family have a history of cancer, you should discuss using soy and other plant estrogens with your doctor before increasing the amount of soy in your diet. With soy, it's beginning to look as though a little is great, but a lot is not. (See "Soy" in The Bottom Cupboard" on page 235.)

Add crunch. Studies at Loma Linda University have found that a handful of nuts five days a week cut the risk of a heart attack in half. Yes, nuts are high in fat, researchers admit, but it's a "good" fat—the omega-3 kind that keeps your arteries clean. A study at the Health Research and Studies Center in California found that adding nuts to the diet lowered the artery-clogging LDL cholesterol by 15 percent. And significantly for those of us who watch calories, no one in the study who ate nuts gained weight!

Nuts also contain the antioxidant vitamin E to trap any disease-causing free radicals that may be wandering about, plus they contain calcium and magnesium to help maintain strong bones and a steady heartbeat. They also contain quercetin and kaempferol, two naturally occurring plant chemicals that have suppressed lung and prostate cancer cells in the lab. And they contain nitric oxide, a substance that your body converts into a potent compound that dilates arteries and lets more blood reach the heart.

Healing Snacks for Men

Studies indicate that men eat as badly as women. Except for calcium, of which most men seem to get enough, guys are lacking the same nutrients as women. That means they need to focus their snacking on foods that will boost their intake of vitamin E, folic acid, vitamin B6, magnesium, and zinc.

Following the suggestions given for women in the preceding section—crunching on nuts, finding time to eat fruit, feeding on whole grains—will help them do it. But guys really need to pay particular attention to the fiber in those whole grains—especially if they're prone to colon cancer, constipation, or diverticulitis—and selenium, a trace mineral that seems to help men prevent prostate cancer.

Reduce prostate cancer by a third. More than 40,000 men die from prostate cancer every year. Yet many scientists feel that if men were getting more selenium from whole grain foods in their diets, the disease might not be so deadly. Their thinking is based on a study at the University of Arizona that several years ago found that men with the highest levels of selenium were 63 percent less likely to develop prostate cancer, 58 percent less likely to develop colon or rectal cancer, and 45 percent less likely to develop lung cancer than those who had the lowest levels. More recently, a study of more than 33,000 men conducted at Harvard University found that men with the highest levels of selenium in their diets had about one-third the risk of developing advanced prostate cancer as those with the lowest.

Cut colon cancer by 40 percent. But

selenium is not the only thing in whole grains that protects men. Whole grains also contain the kind of fiber that can protect against diverticular disease and colon cancer as well. In another study at Harvard University, for example, researchers found that men who ate 32 grams of fiber a day had little more than half the risk of diverticular disease as men who ate less. And in a study of nearly 4,000 men at the University of Utah, researchers there found that men with higher levels of whole grain intake reduced their risk of colon cancer by a whopping 40 percent.

What kind of snacks can bring about this type of protection? Nothing horribly complicated: Whole wheat crackers. Whole wheat pretzels. Whole grain rice cakes. Air-popped popcorn. Individual boxes of whole grain cereals. Just make sure it's all low-fat as well.

Healing Snacks for Older Folks

Once past age 65, our bodies seem to have slightly different nutritional needs than they did in the preceding years. And they're more likely to be low in vitamins A, C, D, E, B1, B2, B6, and B12, as well as calcium, folic acid, magnesium, niacin, and zinc.

Low intakes of such a wide variety of nutrients can cause everything from itchy skin and dry hair to depression, mental confusion, and forgetfulness. But the key deficiency that stands out is zinc. At a recent nutrition conference in Montreal, Ranjit Chandra, M.D., director of the WHO Centre for Nutrition and Immunology, estimated that 12 to 15 percent of the world's seniors have evidence of a mild zinc deficiency—a deficiency that lowers their immune system's ability to fight off cancer and a wide variety of infectious diseases just when they need it most.

Complicating the problem, adds Dr. Frank, the nutrition professor at California State University, is the fact that the number of taste buds diminish over time—so older folks have less taste perception. They also have less stomach acid with which to digest what they eat, a problem that can mean more digestive upsets and a disinclination to eat a wide range of foods.

Other problems that discourage eating a well-balanced diet include sensitive teeth and digestive diseases or conditions such as diverticulitis, chronic constipation, or irritable bowel syndrome.

Fortunately, a number of snack foods that are easy for older people to keep on hand will boost a number of these low-level nutrients and help prevent digestive diseases.

Here are just a few.

Figure on figs. Figs have an intensely sweet taste that can not only overcome lessened taste perception in those over age 60, they can also relieve constipation, help reduce cholesterol, lower blood pressure, and prevent osteoporosis. That's because a single handful of these dried beauties, just 3½ ounces, or 100 grams, contains a whopping 12 grams of fiber—literally one-third of the all the fiber you need in a day. It also contains about 20 percent of the magnesium experts recommend, 14 percent of the daily amount of potassium, plus 18 percent of the calcium. There's also some evidence that figs contain benzaldehydes, a group of naturally occurring chemicals that fight cancer. And figs require no preparation at all. Just keep a container of them tucked in a drawer and nibble at will.

Find yourself some dates. Dried dates are another easy snack food that can boost necessary nutrients that beat back the diseases associated with aging and provide an intensely sweet taste experience. A 3½-ounce (100-gram) serving provides about 25 percent of the amount of fiber you need in a day, roughly 20 percent of the potassium, 12 percent of the iron, and 10 percent of the calcium. Scientists also suspect dates contain a natural form of aspirin that works like a laxative. Like figs, they can be kept nearby in a tightly capped container and nibbled at will. Transfer them to the refrigerator if you're intending to keep them around for more than a month. One caveat: Pitted dates may occasionally contain a pit. Check before you eat.

Pick prunes every day. Prunes are dried plums that retain every flavor nuance of their original fruit, with all the subtleties intensified and brought to fruition in one passionate burst of flavor. A handful will provide roughly 40 percent of the vitamin A you need for an entire day, 20 percent of the potassium, 13 percent of the magnesium, 12 percent of the riboflavin, and 10 percent of the fiber. What's more, prunes also contain diphe-nylisatin, a naturally occurring compound that is similar to one found in many over-the-counter laxatives. Keep them nearby in a tightly closed container. And, as with dates, watch out for pits!

Reach for an avocado. If you need to gain a couple of pounds as well as boost your nutrient level, give avocados a try. Yes, they're full of calories. But the fat they contain is the monounsaturated kind that contributes to a healthy heart, not clogged arteries. Avocados also contain roughly 20 percent of the potassium you need for an entire day and nearly the same amount of folic acid. Plus they have 15 percent of a day's supply of vitamin B6, 12 percent of the vitamin A, and 12 percent of the magnesium. (See "Avocados" on page 72.)

Grab a handful of nuts. Nuts are loaded with zinc, the one nutrient that really seems to power your immune system. One extra, added benefit: Studies have found that a handful five times a week is enough to reduce your risk of a heart attack by 50 percent. (See "Nuts" on page 240.)

Apple Raisin Breakfast Squares

A great after-school snack, these squares are high in flavor, fiber, and minerals. They contain protein for staying power and are low in fat.

Preheat oven to 350 F. Spray a 9-inch x 13-inch baking pan with nonstick spray.

With an electric mixer, combine the brown sugar and margarine in a large bowl. Beat until combined. The mixture will be crumbly. Add the applesauce, eggs, and vanilla and beat again.

In another bowl, combine the flour, baking soda, salt, spice, and oats. Stir in the raisins and half of the chocolate chips. Add the flour mixture into the applesauce mixture and stir to just combine. Spread the batter in the baking pan. Scatter the remaining chocolate chips over the top. Bake 30 minutes or until the sides are browned and a toothpick inserted in the center comes out clean.

Cool and cut unto 24 squares.

INGREDIENTS

YIELD: 24 SQUARES

1¼ cups brown sugar
6 tablespoons trans fat–free light soft margarine
1½ cups applesauce
½ cup egg substitute or 2 eggs
2 teaspoons vanilla
2 cups unbleached flour
¾ teaspoon baking soda
¼ teaspoon salt
1½ teaspoons pumpkin pie spice
1½ cups rolled oats
½ cup raisins
½ cup mini chocolate chips

PER SQUARE

Calories	163
Carbohydrates	29 g
Fat	4 g
Saturated fat	1 g
Dietary fiber	1 g
Cholesterol	0 mg
Sodium	116 mg

Popcorn and Roasted Soybeans

Not only does this snack provide dietary fiber, it also includes 50 milligrams of powerful isoflavones so vital for women. Most experts recommend 30 to 50 milligrams of isoflavones per day to beat hot flashes and protect against cancer. This snack is high in folate as well.

Combine the two ingredients in your snack bowl and enjoy the break with a cup of hot tea.

*NOTE: Unsalted soybeans can be purchased in your local health food store or often they are available in the produce section of the supermarket with other roasted nuts.

INGREDIENTS

YIELD: 1 SERVING

2 cups air-popped popcorn
¼ cup roasted unsalted soybeans*

PER SERVING

Calories	255
Carbohydrates	27 g
Fat	10 g
Saturated fat	1.5 g
Dietary fiber	6 g
Cholesterol	0 mg
Sodium	1 mg
Folate	92 mcg

Men's Power Shake

A Power Shake reminds me of the movie *Rocky* and Sylvester Stallone cracking whole eggs into his blender drink and gulping it down. Today we don't advise drinking raw eggs because they can contain dangerous bacteria. But a blender drink is a good idea, especially one that contains about one-quarter to one-third of the day's nutrients and calories and can be used as a breakfast replacement. It makes a good afternoon snack, too.

This drink contains about 532 calories and is high in zinc and magnesium, two of the nutrients that have been found lacking low in diets of American men. It contains 29 percent of the daily requirement for zinc and 41 percent of the daily requirement for magnesium. It also is an excellent source of vitamin C, vitamin A, riboflavin, protein, folate, calcium, and potassium.

Remember, though—this is a meal replacement. If you need to watch your calories, drink half or prepare half.

Combine all ingredients in a blender container and whiz until all is blended and smooth.

INGREDIENTS

YIELD: 1 SERVING (2 CUPS)

½ banana
2 tablespoons natural peanut butter
1 cup cantaloupe chunks
½ cup red raspberries (fresh or frozen)
1 cup nonfat plain yogurt
2 teaspoons cocoa mix powder

PER SERVING

Calories	532
Carbohydrates	75 g
Fat	18 g
Saturated fat	3 g
Monounsaturated fat	8 g
Dietary fiber	9 g
Cholesterol	0 mg
Magnesium	165 mg
Sodium	300 mg

Fruit Salad Refresher

Prepare this fruit salad and serve it over pound cake, sponge cake, yogurt, or ice cream. If it is finely chopped, it can be served as a salsa with tortilla chips or as a simple fruit salad.

Combine all the fruit and the honey and serve.

INGREDIENTS

YIELD : 4 CUPS

1 pink or red grapefruit, peeled and chunked
2 peaches, halved and cubed
4 kiwi, peeled, halved, and sliced
1 cup blackberries or blueberries
2 tablespoons honey

PER SERVING (½ CUP)

Calories	68
Carbohydrates	17 g
Fat	0.3 g
Saturated fat	0 g
Dietary fiber	3 g
Cholesterol	0 mg
Sodium	2 mg

Easy Bean-and-Turkey Enchiladas

*A*uthentic enchiladas are made with a tortilla that is fried, dipped in a sauce, and then filled and rolled. These enchiladas omit the frying step, so they are lower in fat—containing about five grams per enchilada. There's more zinc in the dark meat of turkey, so use all dark or a combination of light and dark for the best mineral content.

And if you eat two, you get 25 percent of a day's allowance of magnesium and 22 percent of a day's allowance of zinc, the two minerals that have been found lacking in the diet of men. And all for less than 400 calories—a great snack! See if you can eat just two. (They can be reheated in the microwave.)

Preheat oven to 350 F.

Spray a 10-inch nonstick skillet and heat. Add the onion and garlic and cook on medium heat for 5 minutes or until softened. Add the ground turkey and sauté until all the meat is cooked.

Add the tomato paste, salsa, chile powder, and pinto beans and mix well. Heat through for 5 minutes.

Place a tortilla on a work surface and spread ½ cup of the turkey mixture down the center. Top with about 1 tablespoon of the cheese. Roll so the opened side is down and place in a sprayed 9-inch x 13-inch baking pan. Continue with the remaining 9 tortillas. Cover the pan with a sheet of aluminum foil and bake for 10 minutes until all is hot and the cheese is melted inside.

Serve with favorite toppings, such as low-fat sour cream, guacamole, or red beans.

INGREDIENTS

YIELD: 10 ENCHILADAS

1 medium onion, chopped
2 cloves garlic, minced
1 pound ground turkey
2 tablespoons tomato paste
½ cup medium hot tomato salsa
1 tablespoon chile powder
1 can (15 ounces) pinto beans, drained and rinsed
10 small flour tortillas
4 ounces shredded low-fat Monterey Jack cheese

PER 3 ENCHILADAS

Calories	393
Carbohydrates	44 g
Fat	10 g
Saturated fat	4 g
Dietary fiber	8 g
Cholesterol	66 mg
Sodium	561 mg

Barbecue Sauce

Cold or hot, a barbecued chicken leg is an enjoyable and filling snack. Just brush on the sauce, throw the leg on the grill, and enjoy. Dark chicken meat is high in zinc—a mineral lacking in the diets of many American men—so keep that in mind when choosing the best barbecuing meat for your family.

Combine all ingredients in a small saucepan. Bring to a simmer and continue to cook and stir occasionally for 5 minutes.

Cool, pour into a glass jar, and refrigerate until ready to use. The sauce will keep for up to one week.

INGREDIENTS

YIELD: 1¼ CUPS

1 can (6 ounces) tomato paste
¼ cup apple cider vinegar
3 tablespoons molasses
2 tablespoons honey
2 tablespoons chopped onion
2 tablespoons chopped green pepper
1 tablespoons Worcestershire sauce
1 tablespoon prepared horseradish
1 clove garlic, minced
2 teaspoons Dijon mustard
Dash cayenne pepper

PER 2 TABLESPOONS

Calories 52
Carbohydrates .... 13 g
Fat .... 0.4 g
Saturated fat .... 0 g
Dietary fiber .... 0.8 g
Cholesterol .... 0 mg
Sodium .... 110 mg

Date and Honey Muffins

Set oven to 350 F. Spray a 12-muffin pan with nonstick spray.

Combine flours, baking powder, baking soda, and cinnamon in a large bowl. Mix thoroughly.

In another bowl, beat the egg. Beat in the milk, honey, oil, and dates. Pour over dry ingredients. Combine with a wooden spoon until just moistened. Spoon into prepared muffin pan, about ¼ cup of batter per muffin.

Bake for 20 minutes or until the edges are browned lightly and a toothpick comes out clean. Allow to rest for 5 minutes. Remove the muffins from the pan by loosening them with a table knife and gently lifting them out. Cool on a wire rack.

INGREDIENTS

YIELD: 12 MUFFINS

1 cup whole wheat flour
1 cup all-purpose flour
1½ teaspoons baking powder
½ teaspoon baking soda
1 teaspoon cinnamon
¼ cup egg substitute or 1 egg
1 cup nonfat milk
½ cup honey
3 tablespoons canola oil
1 cup chopped dates

PER MUFFIN

Calories 196
Carbohydrates .... 39 g
Fat .... 3.8 g
Saturated fat .... 0.3 g
Dietary fiber .... 2.8 g
Cholesterol .... 0.4 mg
Sodium .... 134 mg

Chai Tea Afternoon Soother

My daughter came home from Thailand with a love of a spiced tea with milk, called a Chai Tea Latté at Western coffee shops. Use your favorite loose black tea, and save yourself the trip to Starbucks.

In a saucepan, bring the water to a boil. Remove from the stove and add the tea, cloves, cardamom, and cinnamon. Simmer for 3 minutes and then strain. Add the milk, return the pan to the stove and reheat. Pour into a mug and serve. It can also be reheated by pouring it into the mug as soon as the milk is added and reheating it in the microwave.

INGREDIENTS

YIELD: 1 CUP

1 cup water
1 tablespoon Ceylon or Darjeeling tea
3 cloves
¼ teaspoon ground cardamom
¼ teaspoon ground cinnamon
1 teaspoon fat-free condensed milk
1 teaspoon brown sugar or honey

PER SERVING

Calories	45
Carbohydrates	10 g
Fat	0 g
Saturated fat	0 g
Dietary fiber	0.4 g
Cholesterol	0.9 mg
Sodium	22 mg

Fig Granola Bars

These bars are made using Toasted Almond Granola (page 254) and a fig purée prepared from dried figs.

Combine the figs, the maple syrup, and the orange juice in a small saucepan. Bring to a boil on medium-high heat. Cover and remove from heat. Let stand for 30 minutes. After soaking, blend or process the mixture until puréed. This should yield about 1 cup of purée.

Preheat oven to 350 F.

Combine the purée with the granola. Add the egg whites and fold in. Combine well.

Spray an 8-inch x 8-inch square pan with a nonstick spray. Spread the mixture in the pan and press flat. Bake for 15 minutes.

Cut into 16 bars. Allow to cool, wrap, and refrigerate to store.

INGREDIENTS

YIELD: 16 BARS

½ pound dried figs (about 12), stems removed
2 tablespoons maple syrup
¼ cup orange juice
2 cups Toasted Almond Granola or any granola
2 stiffly beaten egg whites

PER BAR

Calories	130
Carbohydrates	21 g
Fat	4 g
Monounsaturated Fat	2 g
Polyunsaturated fat	2 g
Saturated Fat	0 g
Dietary fiber	3 g
Cholesterol	0 mg
Sodium	10 mg

Chuck's Favorite Chocolate Chip-Walnut Bars

The version of this recipe I served to my children and my nephew Chuck when they were young contained a perfect amount of fat for growing kids. The version below, however, has been modified to appeal to today's moms: it's now lower in fat and high in folate and isoflavones, both of which are perfect for adult women. It still contains nuts and chocolate, though in smaller amounts. After all, moms do need some chocolate. And Chuck still enjoys them himself. I still serve them every time he and his own children come for a visit.

Preheat oven to 325 F and grease a 9-inch x 13-inch pan.

Beat egg whites until stiff. Set aside.

In a large bowl, beat the egg substitute until thickened. Add the ½ cup of brown sugar and the margarine and beat. Add the flours, baking powder, and salt and combine. Mixture may be crumbly. Press with fingers into pan, forming an even layer across the bottom.

To the beaten egg whites, add the ⅔ cup of brown sugar and mix well. Add the chocolate chips, walnuts, and vanilla. Combine well and spread over the mixture in the pan.

Bake for 20 minutes or until the top is golden brown. Cool in pan and cut into 35 bars.

INGREDIENTS

YIELD: 35 BARS

2 egg whites
¼ cup egg substitute
½ cup brown sugar
⅓ cup trans fat–free soft margarine
1¾ cup unbleached flour
½ cup soy flour
1 teaspoon baking powder
¼ teaspoon salt
⅔ cup brown sugar
⅓ cup semisweet mini-chocolate chips
¼ cup chopped walnuts
1 teaspoon vanilla

PER BAR

Calories	88
Carbohydrates	15 g
Fat	3 g
Saturated fat	1 g
Dietary fiber	0.5 g
Cholesterol	0 mg
Sodium	55 mg

Fruit Snow Cone

$\mathcal{S}$ ince kids enjoy frosties and slurpies (or whatever they call those chopped ice confections covered with brightly covered sugar syrups), why not give them a real fruit ice? The Steel Packing Council and Melanie Barnard, its spokesperson, came up with this unique idea.

Put an unopened can of fruit in the freezer, and after a minimum of 18 hours submerge the can in hot water for 1 minute. Then open the can and pour any syrup into a food processor. Cut it the fruit into chunks and then put it in the food processor. Purée until smooth and add liqueur (for adults only!) or other flavorings if desired, and process to blend.

There are many possible fruits and fruit combinations that can be used. Use your imagination.

INGREDIENTS

YIELD: VARIES

1 can (16 ounces) apricot halves in light syrup
1 can (20 ounces) crushed pineapple in light syrup
1 can (16 ounces) sliced or halved pears in light syrup
1 can (16 ounces) sliced or halved peaches in light syrup
1 can (11 ounces) mandarin oranges in light syrup

PER ½-CUP SERVING (APPROXIMATE)

Calories 72
Carbohydrates .... 17 g
Fat .... 0 g
Saturated fat .... 0 g
Dietary fiber .... 3 g
Cholesterol .... 0 mg
Sodium .... 0 mg

You will find it necessary to use canned fruit with light syrup or fruit juice. Unsweetened fruit tastes sour when frozen because, for some reason, our tongues often taste frozen foods as sour. Also, try to stay away from fruit in a heavy syrup since that means extra sugar.

For adults, 2 to 4 tablespoons of a liqueur can be added for a delightful sorbet dessert. Spices such as nutmeg and cinnamon can also be added: about ¼ to ½ teaspoon per can of fruit.

The sorbet can be served immediately or packed into a plastic freezer container and frozen until ready to serve, up to 8 hours.

YIELD: Servings vary slightly according to can size, but a 16-ounce size makes about 1½ to 1¾ cups of sorbet, or about 4 servings.

Steel Packaging Council
American Iron and Steel Institute
1101 Seventh St. NW
Washington, DC 20036 (202-452-7100)

Fresh Tomato Vegetable Soup

Gazpacho

A lycopene-rich snack, this quick cold soup is made from all fresh vegetables and herbs with a base of tomato juice. Let it chill and top with a spoonful of plain yogurt or light sour cream.

Combine the tomatoes, cucumber, onion, green pepper, garlic, and basil in a glass or non-reactive bowl. For chunkier gazpacho, mix in the remaining ingredients, garnish with yogurt or sour cream and green onions, and serve.

If you prefer a smoother soup, some or all of the vegetables can be puréed. After puréeing, mix in the other ingredients, garnish, and serve.

INGREDIENTS

YIELD: 6 CUPS

2 cups chopped fresh tomatoes
1 cucumber, peeled, seeded, and chopped (about 2 cups)
½ cup chopped mild onion
1 small green pepper, finely chopped (about ⅔ cup)
2 (or more) cloves fresh garlic, minced
1 tablespoon chopped fresh basil (about 10 leaves)
2 lemons, juiced, about ½ cup
1 tablespoon balsamic vinegar
2 cups tomato juice
Dash black pepper
Dash Tabasco, optional
Yogurt or light sour cream
Finely sliced green onion

PER CUP

Calories	50
Carbohydrates	12 g
Fat	0.4 g
Saturated fat	0 g
Dietary fiber	2 g
Cholesterol	0 mg
Sodium	300 mg

The Bottom Cupboard

꧁ ꧂

*A*n autumn wind swirls leaves past the lavender-trimmed windows of Vermont's Natural Foods Market in Bristol, then knocks a pot of purple chrysanthemums off the porch and into my path. Picking it up, I tuck the flowers safely behind a large pumpkin sitting in the sun, then run up the stairs and into the store. Like a squirrel storing up nuts against the coming winter cold, I've come to stock my bottom cupboard with a variety of dried beans, peas, seeds, grains, and oils that will make the rich soups, warm breads, and rib-sticking cereals that will nourish my family until the coming of spring. Grabbing a tiny cart from beside the door, I head for the back of the store where bin after bin is stocked with every kind of organically grown bean or grain I could want. A self-service honor system prevails, so I gather a stack of bags from a nearby shelf, some masking tape to seal them shut, and a marking pen to write the price per pound on each package. Then I open the first bin, pick up the scoop, and start shoveling.

Fifteen minutes later my cart is loaded with pounds and pounds of black beans, red beans, garbanzo beans, black-eyed peas, split peas, sunflower seeds, oats, walnuts, and brown rice. A quick trip up one aisle toward the front of the store, and the cart is overflowing with barley, wheat, and oat cereals, plus a whole wheat pancake mix that my husband loves. The store is small, but by the time I steer my overloaded cart toward the cash register, I have also managed to add a half-dozen boxes of soymilk and a quart of organically grown, cold-pressed olive oil.

I hold my breath as the cashier rings up my total. I know it's going to be a lot, but I also know that what's in this cart can single-handedly cut my family's risk of cancer, cholesterol, heart disease, high blood pressure, diabetes, and every digestive disease I can think of—by at least 50 percent.

So I let out my breath, open my wallet, and smile at the cashier. The total may be high in terms of dollars. But in terms of health, it's dirt cheap. Here's how you can get just as good a bargain.

Barley: A Blast of Antioxidants

Barley is a quadruple-threat grain: it contains lignans, selenium, vitamin E, and

---

BOTTOM CUPBOARD

BEST FOR HELPING YOU:

Stimulate a sluggish digestion

Fight diverticulitis

Prevent constipation

Beat high cholesterol

Sidestep diabetes

Prevent heart attacks

---

tocotrienols—four naturally occurring compounds that help prevent the oxidative process that turns cholesterol into artery-damaging molecules that can cause a heart attack and cost you your life. It's also a powerful source of beta-glucan, a soluble fiber that sops up cholesterol in the intestines and sends it to the nearest cellular trashcan.

Barley also makes a terrific hot breakfast cereal. Simmer the grain in water, then store in the refrigerator overnight. In the morning, reheat with skim milk, fruit, and nuts in the microwave. These five compounds make barley a powerful friend in the fight against heart disease.

But barley has a few other tricks up its sleeve. A joint study among several universities in Japan has found that barley may help prevent the after-meal blood-sugar spikes that are frequently associated with diabetes. And a study at the University of Minnesota found that barley speeded up the amount of time it took for a meal to move through the digestive tract. Given the fact that slow transit times, which cause nausea and "bloating," are common among those over age 60, barley may be an important part of maintaining a youthful gut.

Beans: The Number 1 Disease-Fighting Food in the World

Beans are nothing short of miraculous.

Originally they were prized as a source of cheap protein—inexpensive enough for most people to afford, but with a high protein content that powered the immune system, prevented constipation, and gave your body the raw materials it needs to build new cells.

But two decades ago, scientists began to realize that the fiber in beans absorbed water, bulked up the stool, and prevented digestive diseases like diverticulitis.

A few years later, they realized that the soluble fiber in beans grabbed hold

---

BARLEY

BEST FOR HELPING YOU:

Stimulate a sluggish digestion

Fight diverticulitis

Prevent constipation

Beat high cholesterol

Sidestep diabetes

Prevent heart disease

BARLEY BASICS

HOW TO BUY: Forget the pearled stuff. It's been refined so many times that there's little left you'd want to eat. Instead, look for hulled whole barley. That means the inedible outer hulls have been removed, but all of the inner nutrients have been retained. You may have to get it from a health food store, but so be it. It's definitely worth the trip.

You can also buy barley flour and substitute it for 1½ cups of the bread flour in your favorite bread recipe. It bakes up into the sweetest loaf you'll ever eat.

HOW TO STORE: In a tightly closed container in your bottom cupboard.

HOW TO USE: Barley is a remarkably versatile grain. Simmer it in soups, stews, and vegetable broths. You can add one-half to two cups of liquid, simmer for 90 minutes, then enjoy a dish with the subtle undertones that only this particular grain can add.

of cholesterol before the body absorbed it, then got rid of it before it could harm your heart. In a study at the University of Kentucky, 20 men with high cholesterol ate six ounces of pinto and navy beans a day. As a result, their total cholesterol dropped 19 percent in three weeks. And the artery-clogging LDL cholesterol dropped by 24 percent.

A few more years of study, and sci-

THE TOP 10 CEREALS AT YOUR MARKET

Whole grains are the foundation of a healthy diet. Loaded with fiber, vitamins, and minerals, they prevent cancer, fight diverticulitis, even out blood sugar, relieve chronic constipation, and stave off heart attacks. "In America, cereal fiber can reduce coronary heart disease by 30 to 40 percent," says Walter Willet, M.D., head of nutrition at Harvard School of Public Health.

An amazing study of 43,000 men between the ages of 40 and 75 done at the Harvard School of Public Health found, for instance, that just adding a couple of bowls per week of high-fiber cereal to your diet can significantly reduce your risk of a heart attack. In fact, for every 10-gram increase in cereal fiber, the study reported, you reduce your risk of a heart attack by 30 percent.

What's more, a Finnish study of more than 21,000 men found that, even among men who smoked, 35 grams of a good water-soluble fiber like oatmeal a day cut the men's risk of death from heart disease by a full 30 percent!

Just watch out for all the hype in the cereal aisle at your market. "Multigrain goodness" on the outside of a cereal box does not mean whole grains on the inside. In fact, so determined is the cereal industry to mislead you, the only way to be sure you're getting a product that will protect your family from disease is to ignore all the glitz on the front of the package and check the ingredient list on its side panel. The cereal you want lists the grain as its first ingredient—"whole wheat" or "oats" or "hulled barley." Good luck, because it's not as easy to find as you might think.

One of the easiest and fastest ways to integrate whole grains into your diet is to stock up on single-serving boxes of whole grain cereals from your local market, then use them as breakfast cereals, easy-to-grab snacks, and toppings for fruit desserts.

Which ones are best?

Based largely on fiber content, but with personal taste the wild card that rules, here are my top 10:

Granola or muesli (look for low-fat varieties)
McCann's Oatmeal
Grape Nuts
Oat Bran
General Mills Fiber One
Honey-Nut Cheerios
Raisin Bran
Shredded Wheat
Fantastic Foods Banana Nut Barley Hot Cereal
Fantastic Foods Wheat 'n Berry Hot Cereal

entist found that beans contain five different cancer-fighting compounds—isoflavones, lignans, phytic acid, protease inhibitors, and saponins—that fight cancer in two different ways. First, they prevent the cancer from getting a foothold to begin with; second, they prevent any cancer cells from growing.

And more recently, scientists have figured out that the soluble fiber in beans helped prevent adult-onset diabetes. According to Michael McBurney, Ph.D., a professor of nutrition at the University of Alberta in Edmonton, a high-fiber diet forces the gut to increase its production of GLP-1, a substance that tells the pancreas your body needs more insulin. More fiber means more insulin, says Dr. McBurney. And that means a lower risk of diabetes.

What's more, a study from the USDA's Arkansas Children's Nutrition Center in Little Rock reveals that small red beans, dried red kidney beans, and pinto beans have some of the highest levels of cancer-fighting antioxidants of any food on the planet.

As if that's not enough to get beans into your shopping cart, consider this: beans are also stuffed with folate, a B vitamin that counteracts the dangerous effects of homocysteine on the heart (See "Meat" on page 151)—and it prevents serious birth defects. Plus, folate is the fuel that powers the DNA repair squads that roam your body, trying to fix what cigarette smoke, insecticides, and cheeseburgers do to your insides.

Unfortunately, 90 percent of Americans don't get enough folate in their diets. And even if they eat breads and cereals that have been "fortified" with B vitamins, studies show that 75 percent of all adults will still not get enough folate to protect themselves and their children.

Is it any wonder that my bottom cupboard overflows with beans? Young or old, pregnant or postmenopausal, beans are one of the best things you can put in your body.

BEANS

BEST FOR HELPING YOU:

Drop cholesterol

Prevent heart disease

Lower homocysteine

Stop cancer

Prevent constipation

Sidestep diverticulitis

Avoid birth defects

Prevent adult-onset diabetes

Zap hot flashes

BEAN BASICS:

HOW TO BUY: Either canned or dried. Both are equally nutritious.

HOW TO STORE: In a dry bottom cupboard, away from the light.

HOW TO USE: Spice 'em up. Adding a teaspoon of ground ginger or summer savory to your beans can reduce the "explosive" effects in those who are full of beans.

Most beans can be used cold in a salad or hot as a side dish or mixed into a casserole or stew. My family's favorite recipe is based on the Southern dish "Hoppin' John." I simmer a ham bone, two onions, one bag of dried beans (that I soaked the night before), and a cup of brown rice in eight cups of water for maybe four hours or so. It's great on a cold winter's day. The aroma drives them crazy and whets their appetite, while the food itself has enough heft to satisfy even the toughest snow-shoveller.

Which bean is best? Pinto beans seem to have the most fiber (nearly 10 grams a cup); lentils have the most folate—a single cup has almost an entire day's supply. But I'd have to nominate the soybean for the "Best Bean" award. Its widespread consumption in the East may very well be why heart disease and cancer are thought of throughout the world as "Western" diseases.

Soy: A Hot Flash from the Beanfield

There is nothing a soybean can't do—especially when it comes to preventing the diseases that plague modern man and woman. Studies indicate that it can help prevent breast cancer, colon cancer, heart disease, high cholesterol, hip fractures, hot flashes, kidney disease, lung cancer, prostate cancer, and stroke. It is possibly the single most healing food in the world. But not all soy is created equal.

That's because most of soy's healthful benefits seem to be due to a naturally occurring chemical in the bean called genistein. And the problem is, the farther away from the basic soybean you get, the less genistein in what you're eating.

Soy foods that contain the most genistein include soy nuts (94 milligrams per 3½-ounce serving), roasted soybeans (87 mg), soy flakes (105-195 mg, depending on how they're prepared), soy flour (94 mg; essentially ground soybeans), dried soybeans (70 mg), and miso (34 mg).

Soy foods that contain the least are so-called "second generation" products such as soy hot dogs (8 mg), soy bacon (7 mg), tofu (4 to 42 mg), and soy cheeses (1–4 mg). Soy sauce contains virtually no genistein, by the way. And even though soybean oils do contain genistein, some doctors question their usefulness since they're loaded with omega-6 fatty acids, a fat that

---

BEAN BEAUTY: A NATURAL FACE SCRUB

Expensive face scrubs made of nuts, salt, or plastic particles and a squirt of fragrance at the cosmetic counter may promise to restore the glow of youth, but they're frequently too harsh for delicate skin. Especially if your skin has reached the point where it's a little drier and less elastic than it was when you lived on Clearasil. If commercial face scrubs tend to give you red, irritated skin that's ready to break out from sheer misery, here's an alternative from The Healing Kitchen. Used twice a week, it gives you the fresh-scrubbed glow of summers spent on the tennis court—and costs about one-tenth what you paid for the scrub at a cosmetics counter!

Steal two ounces of dried red kidney beans out of your bean jar.

Toss them into a coffee grinder and grind into a fine powder.

Pour into a small, deep bowl. Discard any chunks that escaped the grinder.

Add one tablespoon water and mix into a paste.

Add a few drops of olive oil—just enough to make the paste easy to work with.

Gently—gently!—rub the paste into your skin, using small, circular motions. Stay away from the eye area—skin there is too thin to take any kind of pushing and pulling. Nor do you want to irritate your eyes.

Rinse your face thoroughly with warm water.

Apply your usual moisturizer.

Admire your soft, beautiful skin!

has been associated with breast cancer (See "Healthy Oils" on page 242).

How much soy do you need?

Experts aren't sure. Researchers are experimenting with levels around 60 milligrams a day, but most doctors seem to be recommending that you stay between 30 and 50 milligrams a day—the amount commonly found in an ordinary, disease-preventing Asian diet. The reason is simple: too little genistein and you may as well be eating corn flakes. Too much genistein and in some cases you may very well encourage a hormonally dependent cancer like breast or ovarian cancer.

The explanation lies in the fact that genistein is actually a naturally occurring plant estrogen that your body will use pretty much as though it were the real thing. So in those instances where a little extra estrogen is good—hot flashes or clogged arteries, for instance—soy can work wonders. But in those instances where any extra estrogen is bad—an existing breast or ovarian tumor, for example—soy may be able to harm.

Complicating the issue still further is the fact that scientists suspect that small amounts of genistein can actually stop breast cancer from starting, but that large amounts may very well cause cell proliferation.

The jury is still out on soy's dangers. In any case, common sense dictates that if breast or ovarian cancer run in your family, if you have cancer, or if you've already experienced menopause, you should check with your doctor before adding large amounts of soy to your diet. Otherwise, stick to the 30–50 milligram range that doctors suggest—and look forward to a very long, very healthy life.

As for genistein supplements, many doctors suggest you steer way away—and get genistein only from the soybean.

BROWN RICE

BEST FOR HELPING YOU:
Reduce cholesterol

Brown Rice: A Quick and Easy Way to Control Cholesterol

Brown rice has been associated with healthy eating for a couple of decades. But nobody in our fast-paced lives has the extra 30 minutes or so it takes to cook it, so it rarely makes it to the table.

Now that excuse is gone. Quick brown rice, which takes only 10 minutes to make, is widely available, as is instant brown rice, a product that takes only five minutes from pot to table.

Why should you bother? Because brown rice is loaded with fiber, B vitamins, magnesium, vitamin E, copper, zinc, and a unique substance called oyzanol that re-

BROWN RICE BASICS

HOW TO BUY: Parboiled and dried. In box or bag.

HOW TO STORE: In an airtight canister, out of the light, in your bottom cupboard.

HOW TO USE: Simmered in chicken, vegetable, or fish broth as a side dish, mixed with any kind of vegetables, dropped in any soup, broth or stew. Sometimes I simmer rice in a fish broth, color it with curry powder or turmeric—thus boosting its antioxidant capabilities—then spread it over a dinner plate as a colorful backdrop for baked salmon.

The only reason to serve white rice is as a nondescript white background for more adventurous food—or because you like it. It has little nutritional value. In fact, it's made by stripping away all the things that make rice nutritious: fiber, magnesium, vitamins B6 and E, zinc, and oyzanol, the cholesterol-lowering substance that protects you from heart disease. So unless white is a necessity to your taste buds or your presentation, brown is a better choice.

duces the body's production of cholesterol.

Cholesterol levels are determined by two things, experts say: the amount of dietary cholesterol found in various foods, plus the amount of cholesterol made by the body itself. That's why reducing cholesterol in your diet doesn't always reduce the cholesterol levels in your blood—cutting back on high-fat and high-cholesterol foods only affects half the cholesterol equation.

Brown rice—or more accurately, the oyzanol in it—affects the other half. It actually lowers cholesterol levels by lowering the body's production of it. In a study at Louisiana State University, those who ate a single serving of brown rice—about 3½ ounces—a day, lowered their cholesterol levels by 7 percent within three weeks. What's more, they lowered the artery-clogging LDL cholesterol by a full 10 percent—without dragging down the artery-cleaning HDL cholesterol as well.

Buckwheat: A Vegetable that Works As a Grain

Strangely enough, buckwheat has no relation whatever to wheat. It's actually a "kissin' cousin" of rhubarb that works as well in the kitchen as a grain.

Usually ground into a flour and baked into pancakes, breads, and muffins, buckwheat contains quercetin and rutin, two naturally occurring substances that block cancer-causing agents from setting up camp in one of your cells. The rutin also helps prevent platelets from becoming excessively sticky and clumping together to form an artery-blocking clot that can trigger a heart attack.

Buckwheat has a sharp, nutty taste that can take some getting used to. But when you do, the flour can either be mixed with whole wheat flour or, if you have celiac disease, a condition in which you cannot process a protein called gluten, it can be used on its own as a replacement for wheat.

BUCKWHEAT

BEST FOR HELPING YOU:

Beat celiac disease

Dodge a heart attack

Block cancer

BUCKWHEAT BASICS

HOW TO BUY: Ground into flour. Look for the "light" buckwheat flour, which, because it's not diluted by the hull, is actually more nutritious than "whole" buckwheat flour.

HOW TO STORE: In your bottom cupboard.

HOW TO USE: As a substitute for wheat flour in any baked good that would benefit from a nutty taste.

Oats: Two Ounces a Day Will Keep the Doctor Away

Everything you've probably heard about oats in the past few years is true. Yes, they lower cholesterol. Yes, they help control diabetes. Yes, they lower your risk of heart disease. Yes, they lower your risk of cancer. Yes, they help you lose weight. No, they don't walk the dog—but that's about the only thing they don't seem to do.

Study after study has confirmed that oats are a gift from the earth. They contain three powerful antioxidants—caffeic acid, ferulic acid, and tocotrienols—that grab hold of maverick molecules called free radicals before they can damage your cells in ways that lead to heart disease and cancer. They also contain saponins, naturally occurring substances that put the cuffs on excess bile acids. Left unmolested, these acids can be converted by the body into substances that damage the intestine and set the stage for cancer. And they contain beta-glucan, a type of soluble fiber that lines your intestine with a sticky gel designed to trap cholesterol and move it out of the body.

How well do oats reduce cholesterol? In a study at Harvard Medical School in Boston, researchers found that those who included oats in a calorie-controlled diet lowered their artery-clogging cholesterol by a whopping 23 points in six weeks. And as an extra, added bonus, their blood pressure dropped 7 points as well.

Since the diets of those in the study were custom-designed for each individual, scientists can't say exactly how many oats you'd have to eat to get the same effect. One thing they are sure of, however, is that one bowl of oatmeal a day—that's roughly two ounces of pure oats—will lower the artery-clogging LDL cholesterol in your bloodstream by at least 14 percent.

Oats are also a boon to those who have celiac disease, a condition in which they cannot digest the gluten in wheat. Unfor-

---

OATS

BEST FOR HELPING YOU:

Prevent heart disease

Lower cholesterol

Fight cancer

Beat celiac disease

OAT BASICS

HOW TO BUY: As oat bran, oat groats, steel-cut oats, or rolled oats. The nutritional content is relatively the same. Oat bran contains the therapeutic elements of oats, and the same bran is in oat groats, rolled oats, and steel-cut oats as well. The difference? Primarily time. Oat groats are whole oat kernels that need to be soaked before they're cooked. Steel-cut oats, usually imported from Scotland or Ireland, are simply groats that have been sliced lengthwise. They also take a bit of cooking—usually around 35 minutes or so. Rolled oats are oats that have been heated and flatted by steel rollers so that they'll cook in five minutes or less.

HOW TO STORE: Tightly covered in a canister in the bottom cupboard.

HOW TO USE: As a hearty winter cereal, or in a quick summer breakfast muffin. You can also use oats in cookies, granola, and breads or, mixed with a little brown sugar, as a topping for cobblers and fruits.

tunately, people with this disease can't eat breads, pastas, cereals, baked goods, and even gravy for fear that the wheat it may contain will set off an explosive reaction in their intestinal tract. As a result, some people with this disease have trouble getting enough calories and keeping up their weight. They also tend to lack all of the vitamins and minerals that a well-balanced diet would provide.

Stine Storsrud, Ph.D., a researcher at Sahlgrenska University Hospital in Sweden, wanted to see if those with celiac disease could boost their nutrition—and their menu choices—by using oats in place of wheat. Her concern, says Dr. Storsrud, was that oats contain minute quantities of avenin, a substance that might cause trouble in those who couldn't tolerate wheat. To find out, Dr. Storsrud gave 16 people whose disease was in remission about three ounces of oats a day for two years.

The result was encouraging. Oats had no effect on the lining of the intestinal tract, says Dr. Storsrud. What's more, those who included oats on their daily menu tended to eat a more balanced diet—and they were a lot happier about eating in general.

Yup. And with nothing artificial in them, either. Just replace the water in any oatmeal pancake recipe with berry juice and watch your kids smile before they've even had their milk. There'll be no more pleas to buy those high-sugar cereals for breakfast anymore, either!

Nuts and Seeds: A Handful of Heart Health

Nuts and seeds are those high-fat little trimmings that most of us can do without, right?

Wrong. A 12-year study of more than 22,000 doctors at Harvard Medical School in Boston found that the more nuts those doctors ate, the less likely they were to die of heart disease. The study didn't measure how much it took to give doctors that protective effect, but an older study in California did. That study, conducted by researchers at Loma Linda University, discovered that a handful of nuts four times a week or more cut the risk of a fatal heart attack by 50 percent. So unless you're allergic to them, that makes nuts an important part of a healthy diet.

Which is the healthiest nut? Almonds, walnuts, peanuts—it doesn't seem to matter which ones you choose. Each has an important contribution to make to your health:

- Peanuts are loaded with resveratrol, a naturally occurring substance that fights cancer and cuts your risk of artery-blocking blood clots. (They're actually also technically a legume, although most of us think of them as nuts.) A study at Penn State University found that those who ate 1½ ounces of peanuts a day lowered their cholesterol as much as those who ate either a low-fat diet or a diet rich in olive oil.

- Walnuts are little resevoirs of linoleic acid, a substance that reduces cholesterol, and magnesium, a mineral that helps keep your heart on a steady beat.

NUTS AND SEEDS

BEST FOR HELPING YOU:

Prevent irregular heartbeats

Lower cholesterol

Avoid a heart attack

NUT AND SEEDS BASICS

HOW TO BUY: Vacuum-packed if you can, loose if you can't. Check that the nuts or seeds feel heavy for their size. Reject any nuts that rattle in their shell or that appear shrunken. They're too old to do you any good. You should also reject any nuts or seeds that look as though they're moldy. They may contain aflatoxin, a toxic substance that's been associated with liver cancer. Flaxseed is most often found at your local health food store.

HOW TO STORE: Tightly capped, out of the light. Put them in your bottom cupboard if you're going to use them up quickly; in the refrigerator if it's hot or if you're not going to use them for a while.

HOW TO USE: On and in everything. Particularly cereals and baked goods. Flaxseeds can be ground in a coffee mill before adding to dough—a process that releases their oil and produces moister baked goods.

- Almonds are stuffed with vitamin E, a natural oil that seems to prevent LDL cholesterol from turning deadly.

In one study, for example, California researchers gave a group of people 3½ ounces of almonds every day. Nine weeks later they found that the group's cholesterol levels had dropped 20 points.

In another study, researchers found that women who ate walnuts on a regular basis dropped their cholesterol by 22 percent.

With reports like that, it's no wonder that nuts are no longer being thought of as a decorating device. What many people don't realize, however, is that seeds are equally important. Here's why:

- Sunflower seeds are packed with vitamin E and the amino acid arginine—both of which protect your heart. When it occurs in food, vitamin E is everybody's favorite antioxidant, of course, and arginine is a substance that stimulates the body to produce nitric oxide, a substance that relaxes and dilates blood vessels. The more nitric oxide you have, the less likely you are to have a heart attack caused by blockage from a wandering blood clot.

- Pumpkin seeds are loaded with magnesium—in fact, a single ounce provides nearly half the amount your body needs every day to keep your muscles moving smoothly and your heart beating well.

- Flaxseeds are the single richest source of lignans on the planet. Lignans are a type of fiber found in plant cell walls that have 11 different ways of inhibiting or blocking breast cancer tumors and their spread, says Lillian Thompson, Ph.D., a researcher at the University of Toronto in Canada.

ARE WE GETTING THE MESSAGE?

If the message is that monounsaturated fats are good, we sure are. In the United States alone, olive oil consumption increased from 15 million gallons a year in 1986 to 32 million gallons in 1996. Contributing to the total is the fact that any restaurant that claims cutting-edge status now serves flavored olive oils with its bread rather than deadly butter.

HEALTHY OILS

BEST FOR HELPING YOU:

Zap heart disease

OIL BASICS

HOW TO USE: As a substitute for butter and margarine in every single recipe. Flaxseed oil should never be heated above 212 degrees, so it should be reserved for salad dressings and light sautéing. Canola oil is the workhorse of the kitchen. There's nothing it can't do.

HOW TO BUY: Unrefined or cold-pressed is best. That means no heat has been used in processing to destroy the good stuff in oils.

HOW TO STORE: Most oils can be stored for four to eight months when left in a cool, dark bottom cupboard. Flaxseed is one exception. It only lasts six to eight weeks. In fact, some scientists feel you should refrigerate it in warm weather.

A FAST, CHEAP EGG SUBSTITUTE

Next time a recipe calls for an egg, save yourself the cholesterol and actually reduce your cholesterol instead. Just substitute one tablespoon of ground flaxseed mixed with four tablespoons of water. Add the mixture to your batter, and it will bind ingredients just like an egg—plus it will add an extra touch of moisture, a whisper of nutty flavor, and a shot of heart-healthy omega-3s.

And flaxseeds contain 77 times more lignans than any other plant. What's more, flaxseeds are also packed with omega-3 fatty acids—those same fatty acids in fish that have been found to reduce your risk of heart disease, stroke, cancer, high blood pressure, arthritis, and maybe even Alzheimer's disease. Will they do the same thing in flax? Count on it, researchers say. And you don't need much to get a protective effect. According to Bruce Holub, Ph.D., another researcher at the University of Toronto, all you have to do is eat about 30 grams a day. That's less than an ounce—and it's easy to mix into baked goods as suggested in the recipes that follow.

Healthy Oils: Cut Heart Disease By 50 Percent

When Walter Willet, M.D., the tall, rangy head of nutrition at Harvard School of Public Health, hits his local supermarket, the trip is liable to end in frustration—especially when he's looking for an oil-based salad dressing.

"Salad dressings containing fat have almost disappeared overnight in the United States," says Dr. Willet. "And many of them were healthy."

The lack of full-fat salad dressings in Dr. Willet's market is just one consequence of the debate raging between scientists over fat. On one side is Dean Ornish, M.D., a California doctor who says that in order to reverse heart disease, people need to eat a diet that gets less than 10 percent of its calories from fat. That means no butter, no margarine, and no added oils.

On the other side is Dr. Willet and others who have studied the effects of an olive oil-rich diet on cardiovascular disease in the Mediterranean. They say that instead of eliminating all fats—which generally means replacing them with calorie-dense carbohydrates—you should simply replace bad fats with good. That means no butter and no margarine, but vegetable oils are fine. In fact, says Dr. Willet, they're so fine that replacing "bad" saturated and trans fatty acids with "good" vegetable oils could result in as much as a 50 percent reduction in your risk of heart disease.

Both sides can toss studies back and forth at one another for hours. Dr. Ornish did a study in which people who had advanced heart disease cut their risk of a heart attack by 50 percent when they exercised, meditated, and ate a super low-fat diet. Dr. Willet did a study of some 80,000 nurses in which he found that eating a diet that got 29 to 46 percent of its calories from fat did not make any difference at all to their hearts—and another study that found that the risk of heart disease dropped 19 percent when people increased the proportion of unsaturated fat in their diets by 5 percent.

But keep in mind the two things on which both Ornish and Willet seem to agree: Saturated fat—the kind found in meat and trans fatty acids—the kind found in hydrogenated oil-stuffed products like margarine and baked goods—is bad. Really, really bad.

So whether you decide, like Dr. Ornish, that you should eat a diet that gets 10 percent of its calories from fat, or, like Dr. Willet, that you should eat a diet that gets 30 or even 40 percent of its calories from fat, the bottom line is that whatever fat you eat should be from unsaturated vegetable oils.

Now, having said that, what are you supposed to do when you confront those great, gleaming rows of oil in your supermarket? Again, as science untangles one molecule's effects after another, there's no definitive answer. Both monounsaturated oils like olive, canola, and almond will reduce artery-clogging LDL cholesterol as well as polyunsaturated oils like corn and sunflower. But monounsaturated oils will not reduce the healthy artery-cleaning HDL cholesterol—as do polyunsaturated oils.

So score one for monounsaturated oils.

Plus, when a study at McGill University in Montreal examined the different responses 16 healthy men had to polyunsaturated corn oil and monounsaturated olive oil more closely than had others, they found that, yes, corn oil lowered cholesterol more than olive oil. But they also found that when other plant substances were mixed in with the olive oil, the olive oil lowered cholesterol as much as the corn oil—just as it probably would when you incorporated the oil into a balanced diet full of fruits and veggies.

So score another one for monounsaturated oils.

What's more, monounsaturated oils may protect your heart in more ways than one. In a laboratory study at the University of Oxford, for example, researchers have found that monounsaturated oils like olive oil stimulate substances that make it less likely that any circulating cholesterol will actually settle down and take up residence in your arteries. And in a lab study at Trinity Centre for Health Sciences in Dublin, Ireland, researchers found that monounsaturated oils are less likely to activate substances that manufacture the blood clots that can get stuck in clogged arteries and trigger a heart attack.

So score three for monounsaturated oils.

THE BOTTOM LINE ON MARGARINE

"Most margarine sold in the United States has trans fatty acids," says Walter Willet, M.D., head of nutrition at Harvard School of Public Health. A 14-year study of more than 80,000 nurses revealed that among nurses who ate the largest amounts of trans fatty acids, the risk of having a heart attack was 53 percent higher than among those who ate less. In fact, says Dr. Willet, tablespoon by tablespoon, the more trans fatty acids a woman ate, the more likely she was to develop heart disease.

So why are our doctors telling us to eat margarine?

For one thing, they're trying to get us away from heart-destroying saturated fats like butter. For another, until recently, nobody had any idea that trans fatty acids were so deadly. Not only do they increase your risk of heart disease, for instance, but a study at the University of North Carolina at Chapel Hill recently found that women who consumed trans fatty acids increased their risk of breast cancer by 40 percent.

Fortunately, some manufacturers are now making margarines without trans fatty acids. Read the labels to find out who really cares about your health.

But monounsaturated oils may not be the best choice for everyone. In a British study at the University of Surrey, researchers have found that northern Europeans—those from England and Ireland, for instance—may not get the same protective effect from monounsaturated oils as southern Europeans—those from Greece or Crete. That suggests that somewhere in our bodies is a genetic wild card that actually determines whether or not one oil is better than another. And if that's true, then until scientists can match our individual genetic heritage with the kind of oil that works for us, one unsaturated oil is as good as another.

But one other study keeps me from shrugging my shoulders and loading my grocery cart with whatever unsaturated oil's on sale. That study, conducted at Wake Forest University School of Medicine in North Carolina, examined the effects of various oils on a group of mice that were genetically rigged to have high levels of artery-clogging LDL cholesterol.

The result?

Animals fed polyunsaturated oils that were rich in omega-3 fatty acids—flaxseed and canola oil, for example—had the healthiest hearts with the least amount of cholesterol stuffing their arteries.

Need I say that, until more research reveals some other miraculous molecules in the future, these are the two oils in my bottom cupboard?

Three-Bean Salad

Combine all ingredients in a bowl. Cover and refrigerate and allow to marinate to blend ingredients.

INGREDIENTS

YIELD: 10 TO 12 SERVINGS

1 can (15 ounces) green canned unsalted lima beans or 10 ounces frozen lima beans
1 can (15 ounces) small white beans
1 can (15 ounces) black soybeans
¼ cup chopped celery
½ cup chopped red pepper
½ cup thinly sliced red onion
½ cup red wine vinegar
2 tablespoons fruity olive oil
1 tablespoon Worcestershire sauce
1 teaspoon sugar
1 garlic clove, minced

PER SERVING

Calories	125
Carbohydrates	18 g
Fat	4 g
Monounsaturated Fat	6 g
Dietary fiber	5 g
Cholesterol	0 mg
Sodium	198 mg

Oatmeal and Flax Breakfast Cereal

Bring the water to a boil in a saucepan. Add the oats, flaxseed and raisins. Lower the heat, stir the mixture and allow to boil for 1 minute. Stir at least once. After a minute, remove the pan from the heat, cover and allow to set for a few minutes.

Turn out into a serving bowl. Top with brown sugar and milk and serve.

INGREDIENTS

YIELD: 1 SERVING

1 cup water
½ cup oats
2 to 3 teaspoons flaxseed
2 tablespoons raisins
2 teaspoons brown sugar
2 tablespoons skim milk

PER SERVING

Calories	287
Carbohydrates	54 g
Fat	5 g
Polyunsaturated Fat	2 g
Monounsaturated Fat	1 g
Dietary fiber	7 g
Cholesterol	1 mg
Sodium	33 mg

Wheat and Barley Pastry

This quick dough can be prepared and frozen so it is ready when you have a strong urge to make a fresh peach or apple pie. It is easy to make and much healthier than the commercial crusts you'd find in your grocery store.

Preheat oven to 475 F.

Combine all ingredients in the food processor and blend. Remove from the processor, press into a ball, and then flatten slightly. Roll between two pieces of plastic wrap.

Peel the dough from the plastic wrap and place on an aluminum pie plate—pricked to prevent bubbles from forming—and bake for 8 to 10 minutes.

If not needed immediately, the dough can be folded in the plastic wrap into quarters and frozen. Or it can be placed in the aluminum pan, wrapped in aluminum foil or a Ziploc bag and frozen. The recipe can be doubled.

INGREDIENTS

YIELD: 1 SINGLE PIE SHELL (8 SERVINGS)

1 cup pastry flour
⅓ cup barley flour
¼ cup canola or peanut oil
¼ cup skim milk

PER SERVING

Calories	125
Carbohydrates	15 g
Fat	7 g
Saturated Fat	0.5 g
Dietary fiber	2.5 g
Cholesterol	0 mg
Sodium	4 mg

Refried Beans

Mattie, the daughter of a friend, did some cooking when she moved into Grad House at Purdue University in her senior year. She was always looking for ways to cut back on calories, fat especially, so this was one recipe that she made quite a bit.

This recipe tastes great as a dip, over rice, or served in a soft flour tortilla with lettuce, tomato, onion, and salsa.

Sauté onion in oil until soft. Add garlic and cumin and sauté, stirring, about 1 to 2 minutes more. Add drained beans and begin mashing and stirring. Slowly add bean liquid if necessary until the mixture is of desired consistency.

Add the salt, pepper, and cilantro (if desired) and serve.

INGREDIENTS

YIELD: 2 SERVINGS

1 medium onion, chopped
2 teaspoons olive oil
1 clove garlic, minced
2 teaspoons cumin seed, crushed or ground
1 can (15 ounces) pinto beans, drained (save liquid)
Salt and pepper to taste
1 tablespoon chopped cilantro (optional)

PER SERVING

Calories	243
Carbohydrates	38 g
Fat	5 g
Polyunsaturated Fat	0.7 g
Dietary fiber	12 g
Cholesterol	0 mg
Sodium	31 mg

Red Lentils and Bulgur

*W*hat I like about red lentils is that they are so quick to cook—they only take about five minutes. The combination of red lentils with a precooked grain like bulgur is a working woman's dream. This recipe can be served immediately or refrigerated and served as a cold salad the next day.

Red lentils and golden bulgur can be purchased in an Indian or Middle Eastern grocery store.

Into a medium saucepan, pour the chicken stock and bring to a boil. Add the lentils, lower the heat, cover, and simmer for 5 minutes.

Uncover, add the bulgur and raisins and stir. Recover. Turn off heat and allow to stand for 10 minutes. Add the parsley, olive oil, lemon juice, and capers. Combine well and serve.

INGREDIENTS

YIELD: 6 SERVINGS

2 cups chicken stock or broth
½ cup dried red lentils
1 cup golden bulgur
¼ cup raisins
¼ cup chopped parsley
2 tablespoons olive oil
1 tablespoon lemon juice
1 tablespoon chopped capers

PER SERVING

Calories	222
Carbohydrates	36 g
Fat	5 g
Saturated Fat	0.8 g
Dietary fiber	8 g
Cholesterol	0 mg
Sodium	122 mg

Rice Cakes

*T*hese cakes are adapted from a description of a rice cake that a friend of mine ate while he was in Holland and Belgium. He is a cyclist and enjoys eating one of these rice cake wedges while he riding because they are firm, easy to eat, and delicious when cold. When warm, the dish is more familiar as a rice pudding, but when baked in a round cake pan and sliced into wedges, it can be eaten as a cold snack.

Preheat oven to 350 F.

Place cooked rice in a medium bowl and add honey. Mix well. Beat the egg substitutes in another bowl and add to the rice. Add cinnamon, lemon zest, and raisins and combine.

INGREDIENTS

YIELD: 8 SERVINGS

2½ cups cooked long grain brown rice (1 cup raw)
2 tablespoons honey
1 cup egg substitute
½ teaspoon cinnamon
1 teaspoon lemon zest
½ cup seedless raisins

PER SERVING

Calories	144
Carbohydrates	30 g
Fat	0.7 g
Saturated Fat	0.2 g
Dietary fiber	1 g
Cholesterol	0 mg
Sodium	53 mg

Spray an 8-inch round cake pan with nonstick spray. Add the rice mixture and bake for 45 minutes to an hour until golden brown. Cut into 8 slices and serve or cool and refrigerate.

Indian Spiced Rice with Peas and Onions

In a large saucepan, heat the oil or butter. Add the onion, cumin, coriander, and turmeric and cook about 10 minutes, or until the onions begin to soften. Add the vegetable or chicken broth and bring the mixture to a boil. Add the rice, lower the heat, cover, and cook for 5 minutes. Add the peas and cook another 5 minutes. Let stand 5 minutes, fluff the rice, and serve.

INGREDIENTS

YIELD: 6 SERVINGS

2 teaspoons canola oil or butter
1 onion, finely chopped
2 teaspoons cumin
½ teaspoon coriander
¼ teaspoon turmeric
2 cups vegetable or fat-free chicken broth
2 cups quick brown rice
1 cup peas

PER SERVING

Calories	209
Carbohydrates	39 g
Fat	3 g
Saturated Fat	0 g
Dietary fiber	4 g
Cholesterol	0 mg
Sodium	82 mg

Honey-Ginger Salad Dressing

This sweet and sour dressing has a little canola oil in it, but the base is mainly honey and ginger.

Combine all the ingredients in a jar. Shake and serve.

*NOTE: Olive oil can be used as well.

INGREDIENTS

YIELD: 1 CUP

4 teaspoons canola oil*
4 teaspoons minced fresh ginger
½ cup honey
¼ cup freshly squeezed lemon juice

PER 1-TABLESPOON SERVING

Calories	87
Carbohydrates	18 g
Fat	2 g
Saturated Fat	0.2 g
Dietary fiber	0 g
Cholesterol	0 mg
Sodium	1 mg

Blueberry-Barley Crisp

This dessert can be prepared in one nine-inch by nine-inch pan or in individual custard cups. It can be served with ice cream, yogurt, or milk. The taste is very much like that of a rice pudding, and it can be prepared in the microwave. Since the barley is already cooked, it only needs to be heated.

Spray 6 individual serving dishes or custard cups with a nonstick spray. Combine the cooked barley, blueberries, and brown sugar in a bowl and divide the blueberry mixture among the dishes.

In another bowl, combine the almond granola and the cinnamon and divide this topping evenly over the dessert dishes.

Microwave the individual dishes for 40 to 60 seconds on high. Let stand 1 minute before eating. Serve with milk, yogurt, or ice cream if desired.

This dessert can also be prepared in a 1½-quart baking dish. Preheat the oven to 375°F and spray the dish with nonstick spray. Fill it with the blueberry mixture and then cover with the topping. Bake for 15 to 20 minutes or microwave on high for 4 to 5 minutes.

INGREDIENTS

YIELD: 6 SERVINGS

2 cups cooked barley*
2 cups fresh or frozen blueberries
2 tablespoons packed brown sugar
⅓ cup toasted almond granola*
2 teaspoons cinnamon

PER SERVING

Calories	170
Carbohydrates	35 g
Fat	3 g
Saturated Fat	0 g
Dietary fiber	7 g
Cholesterol	0 mg
Sodium	6 mg

*NOTE: Add 3 cups of water to a saucepan with 1 cup whole raw organic hulled barley. Bring the water to a boil. Then turn the heat off, cover the pot, and let the barley soak for about 1 hour. After 1 hour, bring the water to a boil again, cover, turn the heat to simmer, and let the barley cook for 45 to 55 minutes or until tender. If necessary, add more water if all the water is absorbed before the barley is cooked to the desired tenderness. Yields 3 cups.

*NOTE: If you do not have a granola ready and available, you can combine 2 tablespoons flour, 2 tablespoons slivered almonds, 1 tablespoon brown sugar, and ½ teaspoon cinnamon. Then cut into it: 2 tablespoons of a trans fat–free light margarine.

Barley Flour and Dried Cranberry Scones

To keep these scones as moist as possible, don't add too much flour and don't handle the dough too much. Flour your hands and then form the scones.

Preheat the oven to 400°F and spray a nonstick baking sheet.

Combine the barley flour, sugar, baking powder, baking soda, and salt in a small bowl. In another larger bowl, beat the oil and egg. Add the yogurt and combine well.

Add the dry ingredients and cranberries to the wet mixture and combine just until all is moistened. With floured hands, pick up half the dough and place on a floured board. Pat the dough to a circle about ¾ inches thick. With a floured knife, cut the circle into 6 to 8 triangular portions.

With a spatula or turner, carefully transfer the triangles to the baking sheet. Repeat with the other half of the dough.

Bake for 15 minutes or until golden brown.

INGREDIENTS

YIELD: 12–16 SCONES

1½ cups barley flour
1 tablespoon sugar
1 teaspoon baking powder
1 teaspoon baking soda
½ teaspoon salt
2 tablespoons canola oil
¼ cup egg substitute or 1 egg
½ cup nonfat plain yogurt
3 tablespoons dried cranberries
1 tablespoon barley flour for shaping

PER SCONE

Calories	76
Carbohydrates	13 g
Fat	3 g
Saturated Fat	0 g
Monounsaturated Fat	1 g
Dietary fiber	2 g
Cholesterol	0.2 mg
Sodium	256 mg

Ground Turkey and Rice-Stuffed Peppers

The combination of beef and peppers reminds me of home, specifically of a baked dish that my mother made. To make it healthier, I used only a half-pound of ground turkey and combined it with three cups of white rice and a small can of rinsed sauerkraut. I par-baked the peppers while I was preparing the filling so that the dish would not take so long in the oven.

Preheat the oven to 400°F.

Prepare peppers by cutting in half lengthwise and removing the seeds and stem. Place in a 9-inch x 13-inch baking dish with the cut side facing up. Add 1 cup of water to the pan and cover with a sheet of aluminum foil. Place the pan in the oven and bake for 15 to 20 minutes.

Meanwhile, heat the olive oil in a skillet. Add the chopped onion and minced garlic. Cook on medium until softened. Add the ground turkey and sauté until cooked through. Add the rice, sauerkraut, herb or spices, and tomatoes. Combine.

Remove the peppers from the oven. They should be softened and the bright green color changed to a dull green. Stuff with the filling.

Re-cover with the foil. Place in the oven and bake for another 15 minutes. Serve.

Any peppers that are left over can be reheated for another night, or they can be frozen.

INGREDIENTS

YIELD: 14 SERVINGS

7 to 8 small green peppers, about 3 inches long
1 tablespoon olive oil
1 medium onion, chopped
3 cloves garlic, minced
½ pound lean ground turkey or turkey breast
3 cups cooked long grain brown or white rice
1 can (8 ounces) sauerkraut, rinsed and drained
½ to 1 teaspoon allspice, thyme, or dill
1 can (15 ounces) diced tomatoes

PER SERVING

Calories	102
Carbohydrates	15 g
Fat	3 g
Saturated Fat	0.6 g
Dietary fiber	2 g
Cholesterol	13 mg
Sodium	119 mg

Buckwheat, Ground Turkey, and Bow Ties

This recipe was developed to taste like an old family recipe for beef pot roast which, when prepared in the oven, takes two hours or more depending on the size of the roast. This recipe, luckily, only takes 25 minutes. The meat is roasted with carrots, onions, celery, and tomato sauce and then sliced and served with the gravy, buckwheat, and bow-tie noodles.

But instead of pot roast, I used just eight ounces of lean ground turkey, which I combined with chopped onions, sliced mushrooms, and shredded carrots. After sautéing in a little olive oil, the meat and vegetables are combined with the cooked buckwheat and served over the prepared noodles. It can all be done in about 25 minutes.

Heat the olive oil in a large skillet. Add the onions, mushrooms, and carrots and sauté until the onions are softened. Add the ground turkey and continue to sauté until it is cooked through.

Meanwhile to a 3-quart to 4-quart pot add the tomato sauce, water, and celery seed. Bring to a boil. Turn the heat to simmer.

Cook the bow-tie noodles according to package directions. Drain.

When the ground turkey is cooked, add it and the vegetables to the simmering tomato sauce.

Beat the egg in a bowl. Add the buckwheat and stir until all the buckwheat is coated with egg. Add this mixture to the still-hot skillet. Stir the buckwheat until the egg is dried and the buckwheat is separated into individual grains again.

Add the buckwheat to the tomato mixture. Stir. Let the mixture simmer for about 8 minutes, covered, or until the buckwheat is tender.

Add the drained bow ties to the buckwheat mixture. Serve immediately. Any leftovers can be reheated.

INGREDIENTS

YIELD: 10 SERVINGS

2 teaspoons olive oil
1 cup chopped onion
1 cup sliced mushrooms
1 carrot, shredded
8 ounces lean ground turkey
1 can (8 ounces) low-sodium tomato sauce
2 cups water
½ teaspoon celery seed
4 ounces uncooked bow-tie noodles
1 egg
1 cup coarse buckwheat

PER SERVING (ABOUT 1 CUP)

Calories	149
Carbohydrates	21 g
Fat	4 g
Saturated Fat	0 g
Dietary fiber	3 g
Cholesterol	45 mg
Sodium	37 mg

Buckwheat Risotto with Wild Mushrooms

*R*isotto is really an Italian word for rice, and a term that has come to mean a type of rice that is cooked slowly by adding the liquid a little at a time until the rice reaches a creamy consistency. This recipe uses buckwheat in a similar cooking method. The egg in the recipe keeps the buckwheat from sticking together and becoming that creamy, cooked-cereal consistency. If you would prefer that texture, omit the egg.

Heat the olive oil in a 3-quart pot. Add the onions and mushrooms and sauté for about 10 minutes or until softened.

In a saucepan, bring the chicken stock to a boil and keep the stock hot.

INGREDIENTS

YIELD: 6 SERVINGS

1 tablespoon olive oil
1 cup chopped onion
3 cups sliced wild mushrooms (any variety, such as oysters, portobellos, or crimini)
3 cups chicken stock
¼ cup egg substitute or 1 egg
1 cup whole buckwheat

PER SERVING

Calories	150
Carbohydrates	24 g
Fat	3 g
Saturated Fat	0 g
Dietary fiber	3 g
Cholesterol	0 mg
Sodium	163 mg

Beat the egg in a bowl. Add the buckwheat and combine. Add the buckwheat mixture to the mushroom mixture. Add a cup of the hot stock and stir in to mix. Continue cooking the buckwheat until all the stock is absorbed. Then add more stock, about ½ cup at a time, until the buckwheat is tender to your liking. Add more stock if necessary, but only add hot stock.

This is best served as a side dish with roasted chicken or turkey or roasted pork.

Toasted Almond Granola

Most granolas taste healthy, kind of grainy, and earthy. This granola tastes delicious, with its roasted almond flavor. The recipe yields four cups, which can be stored in the refrigerator and used as needed. It will keep for several months.

Wheat, rye, soy or barley flakes can be substituted for the oats. I substituted barley flakes for the oats and cashews for the almonds, which also made a delicious granola.

Preheat the oven to 250°F.

Combine the oats, sunflower seeds, soybeans, almonds, and sesame seeds in a large bowl. In a measuring cup or small bowl, combine the water, oil, and honey. Mix well. Pour over the oat mixture and stir to combine.

Spread the granola mix evenly onto a nonstick sprayed jelly roll pan or baking sheet with sides and bake for about an hour. Stir every 15 minutes and remove from oven when the mixture is toasted and golden brown. Stir in the raisins and allow to cool.

Store in glass jars, storage containers, or plastic bags in the refrigerator. Will keep for several months.

INGREDIENTS

YIELD: 4 CUPS

2 cups rolled oats or quick oats
½ cup sunflower seeds
½ cup roasted unsalted soybeans
½ cup sliced almonds
3 tablespoons sesame seeds
¼ cup water
2 tablespoons canola oil
¼ cup honey
½ cup raisins

PER SERVING (¾ CUP)

Calories	159
Carbohydrates	19 g
Fat	8 g
Saturated Fat	0 g
Monounsaturated Fat	3 g
Dietary fiber	3 g
Cholesterol	0 mg
Sodium	2 mg

Oatmeal-Pumpkin Muffins

Applesauce can be substituted for pumpkin in this recipe. Either way, the results are delicious.

Preheat the oven to 375°F and grease a 12-muffin tin with nonstick spray.

Combine the oats, whole wheat flour, brown sugar, baking powder, baking soda, cinnamon, nutmeg, and salt in a large bowl.

In another bowl, beat together the egg, puréed pumpkin, canola oil, and yogurt.

Add the wet ingredients to the dry and combine just until all the flour is moistened.

Pour about ½ cup of the batter in each muffin section. Bake for 20 minutes or until a toothpick inserted in the center of a muffin comes out clean.

Cool and remove from pan.

INGREDIENTS

YIELD: 12 MUFFINS

1 cup oats
1 cup whole wheat flour
½ cup brown sugar
1 teaspoon baking powder
½ teaspoon baking soda
½ teaspoon cinnamon
¼ teaspoon nutmeg
¼ teaspoon salt
¼ cup egg substitute or egg
¾ cup puréed pumpkin
¼ cup canola oil
½ cup yogurt
2 tablespoons oats for topping

PER SERVING

Calories	152
Carbohydrates	24 g
Fat	5 g
Saturated Fat	0 g
Monounsaturated Fat	3 g
Dietary fiber	3 g
Cholesterol	0 mg
Sodium	163 mg

Cinnamon-Pumpkin Pancakes

Pumpkin is an easy and tasty way to add nutrients and fiber to a popular breakfast food. Using a commercial pancake mix makes this breakfast recipe quicker and hopefully more useful. Any leftover pumpkin can be saved or frozen in half-cup portions for another meal.

Heat a pancake grill to medium-hot. In a bowl, add the pancake mix, pumpkin, and milk. Beat the egg whites until foamy and add the eggs and the cinnamon to the pancake mixture. Combine well.

Add 2 teaspoons of canola oil to the pan. Spread over the surface. Place about ½ cup of batter on the hot pan for each pancake. Cook on one side until lightly browned and then turn and brown the other side.

Serve with maple syrup and pass the nutmeg.

INGREDIENTS

YIELD: 8 PANCAKES

2 cups commercial pancake mix
½ cup canned pumpkin puree
1 cup skim milk
2 egg whites
¼ teaspoon cinnamon
Freshly grated nutmeg for topping (optional)

PER SERVING (¾ CUP)

Calories	136
Carbohydrates	27 g
Fat	1 g
Saturated Fat	0 g
Dietary fiber	1 g
Cholesterol	0.6 mg
Sodium	517 mg

Sweet Squash and Onion Stew

This is a sweet, high-fiber mixture of cubed squash, onions, and dried fruit that can be served over couscous, orzo, or rice.

To soften the squash, wash it and then make small knife cuts all over the surface. Then place the squash in the microwave on a double layer of paper towels. Microwave on high for 3 minutes. Turn and microwave the other side on high for 3 more minutes. Carefully remove from the oven and allow to cool.

Meanwhile, in a large soup pot, heat the olive oil, add the onions, and let cook slowly on medium-low heat. Stir occasionally.

Peel the squash and cut into large chunks. Add to the pot with the onions. Add the water, the dried fruit, the molasses, and the honey. Bring to a boil, lower the heat to medium, cover, and cook for 15 minutes or until the squash is tender.

Add the chickpeas, stir to combine, cover again, and cook another 5 minutes. Serve hot over couscous, orzo, or rice.

INGREDIENTS

YIELD: 8–10 SERVINGS

1 Hubbard squash (about 2 pounds)
1 tablespoon olive oil
2 onions, thinly sliced
1½ cups water
¾ pound dried fruit (a mixture of apricots, cranberries, and prunes or your favorite)
1 tablespoon unsulphured or dark molasses
1 tablespoon honey
1 can (15 ounces) chick peas and the liquidl)

PER SERVING

Calories	242
Carbohydrates	50 g
Fat	4 g
Saturated Fat	0 g
Monounsaturated Fat	2 g
Dietary fiber	11 g
Cholesterol	0 mg
Sodium	127 mg

Chilled Watermelon Soup with Ginger

The grated ginger gives this soup a coolness and freshness. Top it with some yogurt and it looks beautiful, too.

Combine the watermelon, lemon juice, orange juice, and ginger in a blender or food processor. Purée.

Serve in soup bowls with a dollop of yogurt.

INGREDIENTS

YIELD: 4 SERVINGS (¾ EA.)

4 cups watermelon chunks
2 tablespoons lemon juice
⅓ cup orange juice
1 teaspoon grated ginger
¼ cup nonfat plain yogurt

PER SERVING

Calories	60
Carbohydrates	18 g
Fat	0 g
Saturated Fat	0 g
Dietary fiber	1 g
Cholesterol	0 mg
Sodium	17 mg

Under the Sink—
The Cleaning Cupboard

❧✖❧

Watching a friend rinse pesticides and fungicides from fresh vegetables, then place them on a countertop freshly wiped with a chemically based cleaning solution, I began to realize the paradoxical absurdity of my own kitchen.

On the one hand, I bend over backward to find chemical-free foods harvested at the peak of nutrition and flavor. On the other, I wipe my counters down every day with assorted chemical weapons that promise to terminate anything that moves. And then, of course, I prepare food on those very same counters.

How much would you bet that a few parts-per-million of my cleaning solution are sliding down my throat along with the food?

I guess some days I'm just slow. But although 437 scientists will probably swear that even gargling with cleaning solution won't hurt you, I've decided that any kitchen painstakingly filled with organic foods ought to be cleaned with organic substances. Not only are toxic chemicals less likely to get into my family's food supply and create cancer-causing free radicals, but the natural scents of citrus, soda, vinegar, and the other products I use are far less likely to fill my lungs with irritating and destructive vapors.

So just in case you'd like to join my naturally healthy kitchen, here's what's in the cleaning cupboard under my sink:

Citrus cleaner. A variety of citrus-based products like Citra-Solv are now widely available through health stores and grocery stores. You can buy citrus cleaners pre-mixed in a spray bottle or as a concentrated liquid that you shake up yourself. The spray bottles cost a for-

WHERE TO BUY NATURAL CLEANING PRODUCTS

If you have difficulty finding natural cleaning products at your local supermarket, contact either manufacturer listed below for the distributor nearest you. Or jot down the information on a separate piece of paper and hand it to the store manager of your local grocery. Then suggest he stock it on a regular basis.

Citra-Solv
Shadow Lake, Inc.
P.O. Box 2597
Danbury, CT 06813
(800-343-6588)

Ecover, Inc.
P.O. Box 5145
Huntington Beach, CA 92615

tune. The liquid concentrate works out to pennies per spritz.

I keep some of the concentrate mixed up in a spray bottle I bought empty at a local nursery, and I use it frequently on kitchen counters and appliances. It even cleans and shines stainless steel sinks. A tablespoon of the stuff in a bucket of warm water cleans the floor, and another tablespoon dumped into the washing machine freshens even the doggiest-smelling throw rugs—yes, even those that have been misused by puppies in training.

Citrus pet shampoo. Available in most pet shops, citrus-based pet shampoos clean your pet thoroughly and naturally while discouraging fleas (especially if you groom your pet with a flea comb after it's bathed). They are related to citrus cleaners, but are far gentler. Do not substitute a citrus cleaner for a citrus pet shampoo.

And keep both away from your pet's eyes.

Vinegar. Your grandmother probably used it, too. A quarter-cup in a gallon of water can keep tile and glass sparkling.

Lemons. You could keep them in the refrigerator, I suppose, but storing them under the sink keeps the area smelling fresh. I slice one in half to scrub down a cutting board after I cut up fish or to scrub stains—like the kind corn makes when it simmers—out of stainless steel pots.

Baking soda. To clean silver and other utensils, sprinkle baking soda into a damp cloth, rub well, then rinse thoroughly under warm water.

Vegetable cleaners. Vegetable-based cleaners such as Ecover, which are available in health food stores, are perfect for washing dishes, whether you wash by hand or use an automatic dishwasher.

Selected Bibliography

Adachi, Y., N. Ohno, M. Ohsawa, S. Oikawa, and T. Yadomae. 1990. "Change of biological activities of (1—>3)-beta-D-glucan from Grifola frondosa upon molecular weight reduction by heat treatment." Chem Pharm Bull 38:477–481.

Adachi, Y., M. Okazaki, N. Ohno, and T. Yadomae. 1994. "Enhancement of cytokine production of macrophages stimulated with (1—>3)-beta-D-glucan, grifolan (GRN), isolated from Grifola frondosa." Biol Pharm Bull 17:1554–1560.

Adler, A. J., and B. J. Holub. 1997. "Effect of garlic and fish-oil supplementation on serum lipid and lipoprotein concentrations in hypercholesterolemic men." Am J Clin Nutr 65:445–450.

Aeschbach, R., J. Loliger, B. C. Scott, A. Murcia, J. Butler, B. Halliwell, and O. I. Aruoma. 1994. "Antioxidant actions of thymol, carvacrol, 6-gingerol, zingerone and hydroxytyrosol." Food Chem Toxicol 32:31–36.

Agudo, A., M. G. Esteve, C. Pallares, I. Martinez-Ballarin, X. Fabregat, N. Malats, I. Machengs, A. Badia, and C. A. Gonzalez. 1997. "Vegetable and fruit intake and the risk of lung cancer in women in Barcelona, Spain." Eur J Cancer 33:1256–1261.

al Somal, N., K. E. Coley, P. C. Molan, B. M. Hancock. "Susceptibility of Helicobacter pylori to the antibacterial activity of manuka honey." J R Soc Med 87 (1): 9–12 (Jan 1994).

Albert, C. M. 1994. "Protection from sudden cardiac death in women may be linked with a diet rich in alpha-linolenic acid." Poster 3604. American Heart Association Meeting. November 8, 2004. New Orleans, LA.

Aldoori, W. H., E. L. Giovannucci, E. B. Rimm, A. L. Wing, D. V. Trichopoulos, and W. C. Willett. 1994. "A prospective study of diet and the risk of symptomatic diverticular disease in men." Am J Clin Nutr 60:757–764.

Asano, Y., S. Okamura, T. Ogo, T. Eto, T. Otsuka, and Y. Niho. 1997. "Effect of (-)-epigallocatechin gallate on leukemic blast cells from patients with acute myeloblastic leukemia." Life Sci 60:135–142.

Aukema, H. M., and J. M. Rawling. 1997. "Protein reduction on a soy protein based diet slows disease progression to a greater extent in female compared to male pcv mice with polycystic kidney disease." 16th International Congress of Nutrition. July 27–August 1, 1997. Montreal, Canada.

259

Bernstein, J. E., N. J. Korman, D. R. Bickers, M. V. Dahl, and L. E. Millikan. 1989. "Topical capsaicin treatment of chronic postherpetic neuralgia." J Am Acad Dermatol 21:265–270.

Birt, D. F., and E. Bresnick. 1991. "Chemoprevention by nonnutrient components of vegetables and fruits." Hum Nutr: A Compr Treatise 7:221–260.

Breithaupt-Grogler, K., M. Ling, H. Boudoulas, and G. G. Belz. 1997. "Protective effect of chronic garlic intake on elastic properties of aorta in the elderly." Circulation 96:2649–2655.

Cai, L., and C. D. Wu. 1996. "Compounds from Syzygium aromaticum possessing growth inhibitory activity against oral pathogens." J Nat Prod. Oct;59(10):987–990.

Colditz, G. A., L. G. Branch, R. J. Lipnick, W. C. Willett, B. Rosner, B. M. Posner, and C. H. Hennekens. 1985. "Increased green and yellow vegetable intake and lowered cancer deaths in an elderly population." Am J Clin Nutr 41:32–36.

Craig, W. J. 1997. "Phytochemicals: guardians of our health." J Am Diet Assoc 97:S199–S204.

Curhan, G. C., W. C. Willett, E. B. Rimm, and M. J. Stampfer. 1993. "A prospective study of dietary calcium and other nutrients and the risk of symptomatic kindey stones." N Engl J Med 328:833–838.

Deal, C. L., T. J. Schnitzer, E. Lipstein, J. R. Seibold, R. M. Stevens, M. D. Levy, D. Albert, and F. Renold. 1991. "Treatment of arthritis with topical capsaicin: a double-blind trail." Clin Ther 13:383–395.

Djuric Z., et al.1998. "Oxidative DNA damage levels in blood from women at high risk for breast cancer are associated with dietary intakes of meats, vegetables, and fruits." J Am Diet Assoc. 98:524–528.

Efendy, J. L., D. L. Simmons, G. R. Campbell, and J. H. Campbell. 1997. "The effect of the aged garlic extract, 'Kyolic,' on the development of experimental atherosclerosis." Atherosclerosis 132:37–42.

Ellison, N., C. L. Loprinzi, J. Kugler, A. K. Hatfield, A. Miser, J. A. Sloan, D. B. Wender, K. M. Rowland, R. Molina, T. L. Cascino, A. M. Vukov, H. S. Dhaliwal, and C. Ghosh. 1997. "Phase III placebo-controlled trial of capsaicin cream in the management of surgical neuropathic pain in cancer patients." J Clin Oncol 15:2974–2980.

Engelhardt, U. H., A. Finger, and S. Kuhr. 1993. "Determination of flavone C-glycosides in tea." Z Lebensm Unters Forsch 197:239–244.

Fabris, N. 1997. "Dietary zinc and the aging of neuro-immune networks." 16th International Congress of Nutrition. July 27–August 1, 1997. Montreal, Canada.

Ferenci, P., B. Dragosics, H. Dittrich, et al. 1989. "Randomized controlled trial of silymarin treatment in patients with cirrhosis of the liver." J Hepatology. 9:105–113.

Ferguson, P. J. 2004 "Flavonoid fraction from cranberry extract inhibits proliferation of human tumor cell lines." J Nutr. Jun;134(6):1529–35.

Fitzpatrick, D. F., S. L. Hirschfield, T. Ricci, P. Jantzen, and R. G. Coffey. 1995. "Endothelium-dependent vasorelaxation caused by various plant extracts." J Cardiovascular Pharmacol 26:90–95.

Freudenheim, J. L., J. R. Marshall, J. E. Vena, R. Laughlin, J. R. Brasure, M. K. Swanson, T. Nemoto, and S. Graham. 1996. "Premenopausal breast cancer risk and intake of vegetables, fruits, and related nutrients." J Natl Cancer Inst 88:340–348.

Fung, T. T. 2004. "Dietary patterns, meat intake, and the risk of type 2 diabetes in women." Arch Intern Med. Nov 8;164(20):2235–40.

Goodman, M. T. et al. 1997. "Association of soy and fiber consumption with the risk of endometrial cancer." Am J Epidemiology Aug 15;146(4):294–306.

Guh, J. H., F. N. Ko, T. T. Jong, and C. M. Teng. 1995. "Antiplatelet effect of gingerol isolated from Zingiber officinale." J Pharm Pharmacol 47:329–332.

Gylys, K. et al. 2004. "Synaptic changes in Alzheimer's disease: increased amyloid-beta and gliosis in surviving terminals is accompanied by decreased PSD-95 fluorescence." Am J Pathol. 2004 Nov;165(5):1809–17.

Hallfrisch, J., V. N. Singh, D. C. Muller, H. Baldwin, M. E. Bannon, and R. Andres. 1994. "High plasma vitamin C associated with high plasma HDL- and HDL2 cholesterol." Am J Clin Nutr 60:100–105.

Hautkappe, M., M. F. Roizen, A. Toledano, S. Roth, J. A. Jeffries, and A. M. Ostermeier. 1998. "Review of the effectiveness of capsaicin for painful cutaneous disorders and neural dysfunction." Clin J Pain 14:97–106.

He, Y., M. M. Root, R. S. Parker, and T. C. Campbell. 1997. "Effects of carotenoid-rich food extracts on the development of preneoplastic lesions in rat liver and on in vivo and in vitro antioxidant status." Nutr Cancer 27:238–244.

Hertog, M. G., E. J. Feskens, P. C. Hollman, M. B. Katan, and D. Kromhout. 1993. "Dietary antioxidant flavonoids and risk of coronary heart disease: the Zutphen Elderly Study." Lancet 342:1007–1011.

Hili, P., C. S. Evans, and R. G. Veness. 1997. "Antimicrobial action of essential oils: the effect of dimethylsulphoxide on the activity of cinnamon oil." Microbiol 24:269–275.

Holub, B. J. 1997. "Recent advances on dietary omega-3 fatty acids in the prevention of cardiovascular disease." 16th International Congress of Nutrition. July 27–August 1, 1997. Montreal, Canada.

Howell T. J., et al. 1998. "Phytosterols partially explain the difference in cholesterol metabolism caused by corn or olive oil feeding." J Lipid Res 39(4):892–900.

Hung, H. C. 2004 "Fruit and vegetable intake and risk of major chronic disease." J Natl Cancer Inst Nov 3;96(21):1577–84.

Ide, N., and B. H. Lau. 1997. "Garlic compounds protect vascular endothelial cells from oxidized low density lipoprotein-induced injury." J Pharm Pharmacol 49:908–911.

Jenkins, D. J., D. G. Popovich, C. W. Kendall, E. Vidgen, N. Tariq, T. P. Ransom, T. M. Wolever, V. Vuksan, C. C. Mehling, D. L. Boctor, C. Bolognesi, J. Huang, and R. Patten. 1997. "Effect of a diet high in vegetables, fruit, and nuts on serum lipids." Metabolism 46:530–537.

Ji, B. T., W. H. Chow, A. W. Hsing, J. K. McLaughlin, Q. Dai, Y. T. Gao, W. J. Blot, and J. F. Fraumeni, Jr. 1997. "Green tea consumption and the risk of pancreatic and colorectal cancers." Int J Cancer 70:255–258.

Joe, B., U. J. Rao, and B. R. Lokesh. 1997. "Presence of an acidic glycoprotein in the serum of arthritic rats: modulation by capsaicin and curcumin." Mol Cell Biochem 169:125–134.

Kalmijn, S., et al. 1997. "Dietary fat intake and the risk of incident dementia in the Rotterdam Study." Ann Neurol 42(5):776–782.

Katiyar, S. K., R. Agarwal, and H. Mukhtar. 1992. "Green tea in chemoprevention of cancer." Compr Ther 18:3–8.

Kearney, J., E. Giovannucci, E. B. Rimm, M. J. Stampfer, G. A. Colditz, A. Ascherio, R. Bleday, and W. C. Willett. 1995. "Diet, alcohol, and smoking and the occurrence of hyperplastic polyps of the colon and rectum (United States)." Cancer Causes Control 6:45–56.

Key, T. J., M. Thorogood, P. N. Appleby, and M. L. Burr. 1996. "Dietary habits and mortality in 11,000 vegetarians and health conscious people: results of a 17 year follow up." British Medical Journal 313:775.

Key, T. J., P. B. Silcocks, G. K. Davey, P. N. Appleby, and D. T. Bishop. 1997. "A case-control study of diet and prostate cancer." Br J Cancer 76:678–687.

Ko, F. N., T. F. Huang, and C. M. Teng. 1991. "Vasodilatory action mechanisms of apigenin isolated from Apium graveolens in rat thoracic aorta." Biochim Biophys Acta 1115:69–74.

Kobayashi, M., Y. Ishida, N. Shoji, and Y. Ohizumi. 1988. "Cardiotonic action of [8]-gingerol, an activator of the Ca++pumping adenosine triphosphatase of sarcoplasmic reticulum, in guinea pig atrial muscle." J Pharmacol Exp Ther 246:667–673.

Kono, S., K. Shinchi, K. Wakabayashi, S. Honjo, I. Todoroki, Y. Sakurai, K. Imanishi, H. Nishikawa, S. Ogawa, and M. Katsurada. 1996. "Relation of green tea consumption to serum lipids and lipoproteins in Japanese men." J. Epidemiol 6:128–133.

Kubo, K., H. Aoki, and H. Nanba. 1994. "Anti-diabetic activity present in the fruit body of Grifola frondosa (Maitake)." Biol Pharm Bull 17:1106–1110.

Kurashige, S., Y. Akuzawa, and F. Endo. 1997. "Effects of Lentinus edodes, Grifola frondosa and Pleurotus ostreatus administration on cancer outbreak, and activities of macrophages and lymphocytes in mice treated with a carcinogen, N-butyl-N-butanolnitrosoamine." Immunopharmacol Immunotoxicol 19:175–183.

Kurokawa, M., et al. 1995. "Efficacy of traditional herbal medicines in combination with acyclovir against herpes simplex virus type 1 infection in vitro and in vivo." Antiviral Res May;27(1–2):19–37.

Kurokawa, M., et al. 1998. "Purification and characterization of eugeniin as an anti-herpesvirus compound from Geum japonicum and Syzegium aromaticum." J Pharmacol Exp Ther Feb;284(2):728–735.

Ladas, S. D., D. N. Haritos, and S. A. Raptis. 1995. "Honey may have a laxative effect on normal subjects because of incomplete fructose absorption." Am J Clin Nutr 62:1212–1215.

Landgren, F., et al. 1995. "Plasma homocysteine in acute myocardial infarction: homocysteine-lowering effect of folic acid." J Intern Med 237:381–8.

Le Marchand, L., J. H. Hankin, L. R. Wilkens, L. N. Kolonel, H. N. Englyst, and L. C. Lyu. 1997. "Dietary fiber and colorectal cancer risk." Epidemiology 8:658–665.

Levine, G. N., M.D., B. Frei, Ph.D., S. N. Koulouris, M.D., M. D. Gerhard, M.D., J. F. Keaney, Jr., M.D., and J. A. Vita, M.D. 1996. "Ascorbic acid reverses endothelial vasomotor dysfunction in patients with coronary artery disease." Circulation 93:1107–1113.

Lipworth, L., et al. 1997. "Olive oil and human cancer: an assessment of the evidence." Prev Med 26(2):181–90.

Longnecker, M. P., P. A. Newcomb, R. Mittendorf, E. R. Greenberg, and W.

C. Willett. 1997. "Intake of carrots, spinach, and supplements containing vitamin A in relation to risk of breast cancer." Cancer Epidemiol Biomarkers Prev 6:887–892.

Matsui, T., C. Yoshimoto, K. Osajima, T. Oki, and Y. Osajima. 1996. "In vitro survey of alpha-glucosidase inhibitory food components." Biosci Biotechnol Biochem 60:2019–2022.

Matsuo, N., K. Yamada, K. Shoji, M. Mori, and M. Sugano. 1997. "Effect of tea polyphenols on histamine release from rat basophilic leukemia." Allergy 52:58–64.

Micozzi, M. S., G. R. Beecher, P. R. Taylor, and F. Khachik. 1990. "Carotenoid analyses of selected raw and cooked foods associated with a lower risk for cancer." J Natl Cancer Inst 82:282–285.

Mobarok, Ali A. T. 1995. "Natural honey exerts its protective effects against ethanol-induced gastric lesions in rats by preventing depletion of glandular nonprotein sulfhydryls." Trop Gastroenterol 16:18–26.

Moran, John P., Leslie Cohen, Jane M. Greene, Guifa Xu, Elaine B. Feldman, Curtis G. Hames, and Daniel S. Feldman. 1993. "Plasma ascorbic acid concentrations relate inversely to blood pressure in human subjects." Am J Clin Nutr 57:213–217.

Moriguchi, T., H. Saito, and N. Nishiyama. 1997. "Anti-ageing effect of aged garlic extract in the inbred brain atrophy mouse model." Clin Exp Pharmacol Physiol 24:235–242.

Morrison, J. I., et al. 1996. "Serum folate and risk of fatal coronary heart disease." JAMA June 26, 1996. 275(24):1893–1896.

Moshfegh, A.J., et al. 1997. "What we eat in America: Food and nutrient intakes in 1994–95." 16th International Congress of Nutrition. July 27–August 1, 1997. Montreal, Canada.

Mucsi, I., Z. Gyulai, and I. Beladi. 1992. "Combined effects of flavonoids and acyclovir against herpes viruses in cell cultures." Acta Microbiol Hung 39:137–147.

Munoz, K. A., et al. 1997. "Food intakes of US children and adolescents compared with recommendations." Pediatrics Sep 1;100(3):323–329.

Nakamura, K., et al. 1997. "Suppression of postprandial blood glucose elevation by barley-rice mixed diet in humans and rats." 16th International Congress of Nutrition. July 27–August 1, 1997.

Neuschwander, D., D. Drez, Jr., and S. Heck. 1996. "Pain dysfunction syndrome of the knee." Orthopedics 19:27–32.

Nygard, O., et al. 1997. "Plasma homocysteine levels and mortality in patients with coronary artery disease." N Engl J Med 1997 Jul 24;337(4):230–236.

Obi, C. L., E. O.Ugoji, S. A. Edun, S. F. Lawal, and C. E. Anyiwo. 1994. "The antibacterial effect of honey on diarrhea causing bacterial agents isolated in Lagos, Nigeria." Afr J Med Med Sci 23 (3): 257–260 (Sep 1994).

Okello, E. 1994. "In vitro anti-beta-secretase and dual anti-cholinesterase activities of Camellia sinensis L. (tea) relevant to treatment of dementia." Phytother Res Aug;18(8):624–7.

Orekhov, A. N., and J. Grunwald. 1997. "Effects of garlic on atherosclerosis." Nutrition 13:656–663.

Orekhov, A. N., and V. V. Tertov. 1997. "In vitro effect of garlic powder extract on lipid content in normal and atherosclerotic human aortic cells." Lipids 32:1055–1060.

Parazzini, F., et al. 2004. "Selected food intake and risk of endometriosis." Hum Reprod Aug;19(8):1755–9. Epub Jul 14, 2004.

Pietinen, P., et al. 1996. "Intake of dietary fiber and risk of coronary heart disease in a cohort of Finnish men. The Alpha-Tocopheral, Beta-Carotene Cancer Prevention Study." Circulation Dec 1;94(11):2720–2727.

Quale, J. M., D. Landman, M. M. Zaman, S. Burney, and S. S. Sathe. 1996. "In vitro activity of Cinnamomum zeylanicum against azole resistant and sensitive Candida species and a pilot study of cinnamon for oral condidiasis." M J Chin Med 24:103–109.

Rabinkov, A., T. Miron, L. Konstantinovski, M. Wilchek., D. Mirelman, and L. Weiner. 1998. "The mode of action of allicin: trapping of radicals and interaction with thiol containing proteins." Biochim Biophys Acta 1379:233–244.

Rachtan, J., and A. Sokolowski. 1997. "Risk factors for lung cancer among women in Poland." Lung Cancer 18:137–145.

Refsum, H., et al. 1998. "Homocysteine and cardiovascular disease." Annu Rev Med 49:31–62.

Rimm, E. B., et al. 1996. "Vegetable, fruit and cereal fiber intake and risk of coronary heart disease among men." JAMA Feb 14;275(6):447–451.

Rimm, E. B., et al. 1998. "Folate and vitamin B6 from diet and supplements relation to risk of coronary heart disease among women." JAMA. 1998 Feb 4;279(5):359–64.

Roche, H. M., et al. 1998. "Effect of long-term olive oil dietary intervention on postprandial triaglycerol and factor VII metabolism." Am J Clin Nutr 68(3):552–60.

Rudel, L. L., et al. 1998. "Dietary monounsaturated fatty acids promote aortic atherosclerosis in LDL receptor-null, human ApoB100-overexpressing transgenic mice." Arterioscler Thromb Vasc Biol 18(11):1818–1827.

Russell, R. M. 1997. "Soy protein and nutrition." JAMA. June 18;277(23): 1876–1878.

Salmi H. A., Sarna S. 1982. "Effect of silymarin on chemical, functional, and morphological alterations of the liver." Scan J Gastroenterol 17:517–20.

Sartippour, M. R. 2004. "cDNA microarray analysis of endothelial cells in response to green tea reveals a suppressive phenotype." Int J Oncol. Jul;25(1):193–202.

Schulick, P. 1992. "Ginger (Zingiber officinale) in rheumatism and musculoskeletal disorders." Medical Hypotheses 39:342–348.

Selhub, J., et al. 1995. "Association between plasma homocysteine concentrations and extracranial carotid-artery stenosis." N Engl J Med 332:286–291.

Selhub, J., et al. 1997. "Total plasma homocysteine and vitamin status." 16th International Congress of Nutrition. July 27–August 1, 1997. Montreal, Canada.

Shalev, E., S. Battino, E. Weiner, R. Colodner, and Y. Keness. 1996. "Ingestion of yogurt containing Lactobacillus acidophilus compared with pasteurized yogurt as prophylaxis for recurrent candidal vaginitis and bacterial vaginosis." Arch Fam Med 5:593–596.

Shinchi, K., H. Ishii, K. Imanishi, and S. Kono. 1997. "Relationship of cigarette smoking, alcohol use, and dietary habits with Helicobacter pylori infection in Japanese men." Scand J Gastroenterol 32:651–655.

Sigounas, G., J. Hooker, A. Anagnostou, M. Steiner. 1997. "S-allylmercaptocysteine inhibits cell proliferation and reduces the viability of erythroleukemia, breast, and prostate cancer cell lines." Nutr Cancer 27:186–191.

Simon, J. A., M.D., M.P.H. 1992. "Vitamin C and Cardiovascular Disease: a review." J Am Coll Nutrition 11:107–125.

Singh, H. B., et al. 1995. "Cinnamon bark oil, a potent fungitoxicant against fungi causing respiratory tract mycoses." Allergy 50(12):995–999.

Sivam, G. P., J. W. Lampe, B. Ulness, S. R. Swanzy, and J. D. Potter. 1997. "Helicobacter pylori—in vitro susceptibility to garlic (Allium sativum) extract." Nutr Cancer 27:118–121.

Slattery, M. L., et al. 1997. "Plant foods and colon cancer: an assessment of specific foods and their related nutrients." Cancer Causes Control. Jul;8(4)575–590.

Somal, N., K. E. Coley, P. C. Molan, and B. M. Hancock. 1994. "Susceptibility of Helicobacter pylori to the antibacterial activity of manuka honey." J R Soc Med 87:9–12.

Spiller, G. A., et al. 1992. "Effect of a diet high in monounsaturated fats from almonds on plasma cholesterol and lipoproteins." J Am Coll Nutrition, Vol. 11, No.2, 126–130.

Srivastava, K. C., Malhotra N. 1991. "Acetyl eugenol, a component of oil of cloves (Syzygium aromaticum L.) inhibits aggregation and alters arachidonic acid metabolism in human blood platelets." Prostaglandins Leukot Essent Fatty Acids Jan;42(1):73–81.

Steinmetz, K. A., Ph.D., R.D., and J. D. Potter, M.D., Ph.D. 1996. "Vegetables, fruit, and cancer prevention: A review." J Am Dietetic Assoc 96:1027–1039.

Storsrud, S., et al. 1997. "The Oat-Coeliac Study in Gothenburg." 16th International Congress of Nutrition. July 27–August 1, 1997. Montreal, Canada.

Suzuki, I., K. Hashimoto, S. Oikawa, K. Sato, M. Osawa, and T. Yadomae. 1989. "Antitumor and immunomodulating activities of a beta-glucan obtained from liquid-cultured Grifola frondosa." Chem Pharm Bull (Tokyo) 37:410–413.

Tanaka, S., Y. H. Yoon, H. Fukui, M. Tabata, T. Akira, K. Okano, M. Iwai, Y. Iga, and K. Yokoyama. 1989. "Antiulcerogenic compounds isolated from Chinese cinnamon." Planta Med 55:245–248.

Tantaoui-Elaraki, A., and L. Beraoud. 1994. "Inhibition of growth and aflatoxin production in Aspergillus parasiticus by essential oils of selected plant materials." J Environ Pathol Toxicol Oncol 1994; 13(1):67–72.

The Capsaicin Study Group. 1991. "Treatment of painful diabetic neuropathy with topical capsaicin. A multicenter, double-blind, vehicle-controlled study." Arch Intern Med 151:2225–2229.

Truswell, A. S., and Choudhury N. 1998. "Monounsaturated oils do not all have the same effect on plasma cholesterol." Eur J Clin Nutr 52(5):312–315.

Ueland, P. M., et al. 1997. "Homocysteine and cardiovascular disease." 16th International Congress of Nutrition. July 27–August 1, 1997. Montreal, Canada.

Viola, H., C. Wasowski, M. Levi de Stein, C. Wolfman, R. Silveira, F. Dajas, J. H. Medina, and A. C. Paladini. 1995. "Apigenin, a component of Matricaria recutita flowers, is a central benzodiazepine receptors-ligand with anxiolytic effects." Planta Med 61:213–216.

Walsh, G. P. 1997. "Tea and heart disease." Lancet 349:735.

Wei, H., L. Tye, E. Bresnick, and D. F. Birt. 1990. "Inhibitory effect of apigenin, a plant flavonoid, on epidermal ornithine decarboxylase and skin tumor promotion in mice." Cancer Res 50:499–502.

Willett, W. 1997. "Diet and coronary heart disease." 16th International Congress of Nutrition. July 27–August 1, 1997. Montreal, Canada.

Xianli, W. 2004. "Lipophilic and hydrophilic antioxidant capacities of common foods in the United States." J Agric Food Chem Jun 16;52(12):4026–37.

Yagoob, P., et al. 1998. "Effect of olive oil on immune function in middle-aged men." Am J of Clin Nutr 67(1):129–35.

Yamahara, J., Q. R. Huang., Y. H. Li, L. Xu, and H. Fujimura. 1990. "Gastrointestinal motility enhancing effect of ginger and its active constituents." Chem Pharm Bull (Tokyo) 38:430–431.

Yamahara, J., M. Mochizuki, H. Q. Rong, H. Matsuda, and H. Fujimura. 1988. "The anti-ulcer effect in rats of ginger constituents." J Ethnopharmacol 23:299–304.

Yang, Y. C. 2004. "The protective effect of habitual tea consumption on hypertension." Arch Intern Med Jul 26;164(14):1534–40.

Yoshikawa, M., S. Hatakeyama, K. Taniguchi, H. Matuda, and J. Yamahara. 1992. "6-Gingesulfonic acid, a new anti-ulcer principle, and gingerglycolipids A, B, and C, three new monoacyldigalactosylglycerols, from zingiberis rhizoma originating in Taiwan." Chem Pharm Bull (Tokyo) 40:2239–2241.

Yoshikawa, M., S. Yamaguchi, K. Kunimi, H. Matsuda, Y. Okuno, J. Yamahara, and N. Murakami. 1994. "Stomachic principles in ginger. III. An anti-ulcer principle, 6-gingesulfonic acid, and three monoacyldigalactosylglycerols, gingerglycolipids A, B, and C, from Zingiberis Rhizoma originating in Taiwan." Chem Pharm Bull (Tokyo) 42:1226–1230.

Yu, R., J. J. Jiao, J. L. Duh, K. Gudehithlu, T. H. Tan, and A. N. Kong. 1997. "Activation of mitogen-activated protein kinases by green tea polyphenols: potential signaling pathways in the regulation of antioxidant-responsive element-mediated phase II enzyme gene expression." Carcinogenesis 18:451–456.

Zampelas, A., et al. 1998. "Difference in postpriandial lipaemic response between northern and southern Europeans." Atherosclerosis 139(1):83–93.

Zeina, B., M.D., O. Othman, M.D., Ph.D., and S. Al-Assad, M.D. 1996. "Effect of honey versus thyme on Rubella Virus survival in vitro." J Alternative and Complementary Med 2:345–348.

Zheng, G. Q., P. M. Kenney, J. Zhang, and L. K. Lam. 1993. "Chemoprevention of benzo[a]pyrene-induced forestomach cancer in mice by natural phthalides from celery seed oil." Nutr Cancer 19:77–86.

The Recipe Finder

≈✗≈

No one recipe is going to prevent or eliminate any one disease or condition all by itself. But consistently using recipes that have been specifically designed by a nutritionist to include a wide variety of protective nutrients and naturally occurring phytochemicals will help, especially when eaten in conjunction with a balanced diet of fresh fruits, whole grains, and a wide variety of fresh vegetables.

That's why the recipes in this book have been developed by consulting nutritionist Anita Hirsch, M.S., R.D., whose twenty years of developing recipes for *Prevention* Magazine and Prevention Magazine Health Books makes her the grandmother of healthy cooking in the United States. To use Anita's recipes, either flip through the book until one catches your fancy or look down the following table until you see a disease or condition that concerns you. Listed underneath its bold-faced heading, you'll find recipes that Anita has specifically developed to help you prevent or fight that particular problem.

If you're concerned about high cholesterol levels, for example, look down the column until you find the heading "High Cholesterol" in bold-faced type. Then look at the recipes listed under it. Does a batch of Carrot-Oatmeal Drop Cookies sound good? They should. And they're listed there because they contain one or more ingredients that will help keep your cholesterol levels down.

Get the idea? Great. Now get cooking!

Alzheimer's Disease

Broiled Atlantic Mackerel with Ginger and Garlic, 165
Oven-Poached Salmon, 162
Super Sardine Sub, 163

Anxiety

Chamomile Cubes, 15
Refreshing Chamomile and Tonic with Lime, 15

Arthritis

Baked Apples and Sweet Potatoes, 142
Bow Ties with Asparagus, 105
Broiled Atlantic Mackerel with Ginger and Garlic, 165
Cajun Pork Roast Sandwiches, 196
Chile Bean Dip, 213
Grilled Turkey with Ginger Couscous, 207
Honey-Chile Garlic Sauce, 125
Hot and Spicy Ginger Carrot Soup, 207

Celiac Disease

Rice Cakes, 247

Chronic Constipation

Apple-Cranberry Date Crisp, 106
Blueberry-Barley Crisp, 249
Bull's Avocado Chicken Soup, 107
Carrot and Barley Salad, 146
Carrot-Oatmeal Drop Cookies, 35
Charleston Gumbo, 120
Cranberry-Oatmeal Bread, 66
Date and Honey Muffins, 226
Flaxseed Hamburger Rolls, 65
Fruit Compote with Anise, 194
Hearty Kale Soup with Vegetables and
    Soybeans, 131
Oatmeal and Flax Breakfast Cereal, 245
Red Lentils and Bulgur, 247
Refried Beans, 246
Smooth and Creamy Vegetable and
    Lentil Soup, 117
Spicy Vegetarian Minestrone, 205
Three-Bean Salad, 245

Digestive Upset

Apricots Preserved with Honey and
    Cloves, 202
Black Tea with Cloves, 203
Broiled Atlantic Mackerel with Ginger
    and Garlic, 165
Bull's Avocado Chicken Soup, 107
Chilled Artichoke and Rice Salad, 200
Iced Ginger Tea (Homemade Ginger
    Ale), 16
Oven-Poached Salmon, 162
Tummy Soother Tea, 195

Diverticulitis

Barley Bread, 66
Carrot-Oatmeal Drop Cookies, 35
Charleston Gumbo, 120
Chile Bean Dip, 213

Refried Beans, 246
Southern-Style Clam Chowder, 126

Fatigue

Anise-Spiced Biscotti, 194
Caramelized Sweet Peppers and Onions
    with Chicken over Rice, 166
Chicken Stir-Fry with Broccoli and
    Cashews, 167
Curried Vegetables with Turkey, 160
Fruit Compote with Anise, 194
Open-Face Turkey Reuben, 160

Gallstones

Broiled Atlantic Mackerel with Ginger
    and Garlic, 165
Oven-Poached Salmon, 162
Radish and Greens Salad with Orange
    Vinaigrette, 128
Red Cabbage and Beets, 145
Refreshing Fruit Salad, 111
Stir-Fried Artichoke and Scallops with
    Angel Hair Pasta, 104
Super Sardine Sub, 163

Gum (Periodontal) Disease

Apricots Preserved with Honey and
    Cloves, 202
Black Tea with Cloves, 203
Easy Chicken Cacciatore, 208
Flounder with Lemon Thyme Rice, 213
Golden Apple Soup with Wine and
    Thyme, 212
Oregano, Ziti, and Fresh Tomato Salad,
    208

Heart Disease

Acorn Squash Stuffed with Mushrooms
    and Wild Rice, 144
Apple-Cranberry Date Crisp, 106
Apple Raisin Breakfast Squares, 223

Sweet Squash and Onion Stew, 256
Toasted Almond Granola, 254
Toasted Cheese and Veggie Sandwich, 105
Tomato and Chile Cornbread, 110
Tortilla Roll-Ups, 121
Walnut-Coated Baked Apples with
    Blackberry Sauce, 123
Whole Wheat Cinnamon Buns, 201

High Blood Pressure

Baked Apples and Sweet Potatoes, 142
Bow Ties with Asparagus, 105
Broiled Atlantic Mackerel with Ginger
    and Garlic, 165
Cantaloupe and Strawberry Salsa, 108
Cantaloupe with Blueberry-Mint Sauce,
    107
Caponata, 197
Celery Seed Salad Dressing, 197
Celery Slaw, 109
Chilled Watermelon Soup with Ginger, 256
Clam Cakes, 131
Cranberry-Oatmeal Bread, 66
Creamy Vegetable Soup, 198
Crispy Haddock on a Bed of Sautéed
    Julienne Vegetables, 108
Curried Chicken with Apricots, Onions,
    and Rice, 124
Easy Morning Breakfast, 123
Fig Granola Bars, 227
Garlic and Zucchini Fettuccini, 115
Garlic Mashed Potatoes, 142
Oven-Poached Salmon, 162
Pork Loin Chops with Spicy Fruit and
    Rice, 193
Soybean, Corn, and Macaroni Salad, 198
Super Sardine Sub, 163
Toasted Cheese and Veggie Sandwich, 105

High Cholesterol

Apricot-Honey Oat Bar Cookies, 34
Apricots Preserved with Honey and
    Cloves, 202

Barley Bread, 66
Barley-Corn Pancakes, 112
Black Tea with Cloves, 203
Blueberry and Yogurt Breakfast, 200
Blueberry-Barley Crisp, 249
Bow Ties with Asparagus, 105
Broiled Atlantic Mackerel with Ginger
    and Garlic, 165
Broiled Flounder with Honey-Mustard
    Garlic Sauce, 161
Brussels Sprouts in Garlic Butter, 113
Buckwheat, Ground Turkey, and Bow
    Ties, 252
Bull's Avocado Chicken Soup, 107
Cajun Pork Roast Sandwiches, 196
Caponata, 197
Carrot-Oatmeal Drop Cookies, 35
Cauliflower with Ham, Onion, Garlic,
    and Turmeric, 114
Celery Seed Salad Dressing, 197
Charleston Gumbo, 120
Chile Bean Dip, 213
Chilled Watermelon Soup with Ginger,
    256
Cinnamon Applesauce-Raisin Cookies,
    34
Cranberry-Chocolate Chip Cookies, 36
Cranberry-Oatmeal Bread, 66
Creamy Vegetable Soup, 198
Easy Bean-and-Turkey Enchiladas, 225
Fig Granola Bars, 227
French Onion Soup, 127
Fresh Tomato and Onion Pizza, 128
Garlic and Zucchini Fettuccini, 115
Green-and-White Party Dip, 125
Grilled Chicken and Watermelon with
    Sweet-and-Sour Ginger Dressing, 132
Ground Turkey and Rice-Stuffed
    Peppers, 251
Herbed Turkey Burgers with Rosemary,
    210
Honey-Chile Garlic Sauce, 125
Honey-Roasted Onions with Garlic, 126
Indian Spiced Rice with Peas and
    Onions, 248

Jamaican Chicken Thighs with Red
Lentils and Rice, 192
Kale with Spicy Yogurt, 206
Key Lime Pie, 116
Oatmeal and Flax Breakfast Cereal, 245
Oatmeal-Pumpkin Muffins, 255
Orange-Poached Sole, 164
Oriental-Style Chicken Soup with
Cabbage, 114
Oven-Poached Salmon, 162
Peach and Blackberry Crunch, 202
Potato and Lentil Curry, 206
Quick and Easy Mushroom-Spinach
Lasagna, 118
Red Lentils and Bulgur, 247
Refried Beans, 246
Rice Cakes, 247
Shiitake Mushrooms and Rice, 119
Shrimp and Broccoli with Sesame Seeds,
112
South of the Border Pizza, 106
Southern-Style Clam Chowder, 126
Soybean, Corn, and Macaroni Salad, 198
Spicy Spaghetti with Tomatoes and
Cayenne, 195
Stewed Carrots and Tomatoes, 146
Super Sardine Sub, 163
Sweet Potatoes and Cauliflower with
Turmeric, 214
Toasted Almond Granola, 254
Toasted Cheese and Veggie Sandwich,
105
Tomato and Chile Cornbread, 110
Wheat and Barley Pastry, 246
Whole Wheat Cinnamon Buns, 201

Hot Flashes

Cranberry-Chocolate Chip Cookies, 36
Hearty Kale Soup with Vegetables and
Soybeans, 131
Hearty Soy-Corn Soup, 111
Kale with Spicy Yogurt, 206
Popcorn and Roasted Soybeans, 223
Potato and Lentil Curry, 206

Red Lentils and Bulgur, 247
Refried Beans, 246
Three-Bean Salad, 245

Liver Disease

Chile Bean Dip, 213
Chilled Artichoke and Rice Salad, 200
Mediterranean Pita Pizza, 104
Quick and Easy Mushroom-Spinach
Lasagna, 118
Shiitake Mushrooms and Rice, 119
Stir-Fried Artichoke and Scallops with
Angel Hair Pasta, 104
Sweet Potatoes and Cauliflower with
Turmeric, 214

Macular Degeneration

Acorn Squash Stuffed with Mushrooms
and Wild Rice, 144
Apricot-Honey Oat Bar Cookies, 34
Baked Apples and Sweet Potatoes, 142
Barley Borscht, 143
Chicken Marinated in Black Tea, 15
Cinnamon-Pumpkin Pancakes, 255
Curried Chicken with Apricots, Onions,
and Rice, 124
Easy Morning Breakfast, 123
Green-and-White Party Dip, 125
Grilled Chicken with Watermelon and
Sweet-and-Sour Ginger Dressing, 132
Hearty Kale Soup with Vegetables and
Soybeans, 131
Oven-Roasted Pumpkin Chips, 145
Pickled Beets with Vidalia Onions, 204
Quick and Easy Mushroom-Spinach
Lasagna, 118
Red Cabbage and Beets, 145
Spinach and Grapefruit Salad with
Broccoli Sprouts, 109
Sweet Squash and Onion Stew, 256

Migraines

Grilled Turkey with Ginger Couscous, 207
Hot and Spicy Ginger Carrot Soup, 207
Iced Ginger Tea (Homemade Ginger Ale), 16

Nausea

Fruit Snow Cone, 229
Iced Ginger Tea (Homemade Ginger Ale), 16
Refrigerator Iced Tea, 17
Tummy Soother Tea, 195

Osteoporosis

Creamy Chilled Mango Soup, 129
Hearty Soy-Corn Soup, 111
Hot and Spicy Ginger Carrot Soup, 207
Men's Power Shake, 224
Pineapple-Cranberry Dessert, 122
Popcorn and Roasted Soybeans, 223
Radish and Cucumber Yogurt, 120
Smooth and Creamy Vegetable and Lentil Soup, 117

Psoriasis

Broiled Atlantic Mackerel with Ginger and Garlic, 165
Oven-Poached Salmon, 162
Super Sardine Sub, 163

Sinus Headaches

Cajun Pork Roast Sandwiches, 196
Honey-Chile Garlic Sauce, 125
Parsnip Carrot Soup with Tarragon and Dill, 211
Spicy Spaghetti with Tomatoes and Cayenne, 195
Tomato and Chile Cornbread, 110

Sluggish Digestion[1]

Barley Bread, 66
Barley Flour and Dried Cranberry Scones, 250
Barley-Corn Pancakes, 112
Blueberry-Barley Crisp, 249
Bull's Avocado Chicken Soup, 107
Carrot and Barley Salad, 146
Cranberry-Oatmeal Bread, 66
Creamy Chilled Mango Soup, 129
Grilled Turkey with Ginger Couscous, 207
Hot and Spicy Ginger Carrot Soup, 207
Pineapple-Cranberry Dessert, 122
South of the Border Pizza, 106
Wheat and Barley Pastry, 246

Stroke

Acorn Squash Stuffed with Mushrooms and Wild Rice, 144
Apricot-Honey Oat Bar Cookies, 34
Apricots Preserved with Honey and Cloves, 202
Baked Apples and Sweet Potatoes, 142
Black Tea with Cloves, 203
Blueberry and Yogurt Breakfast, 200
Carrot-Oatmeal Drop Cookies, 35
Chai Tea Afternoon Soother, 227
Chile Bean Dip, 213
Cinnamon Applesauce-Raisin Cookies, 34
Cranberry-Oatmeal Bread, 66
Dill and Onion Biscuits, 203
Flax Prairie Bread, 63
Flaxseed Hamburger Rolls, 65
Garlic and Zucchini Fettuccini, 115
Garlic Mashed Potatoes, 142
Grilled Turkey with Ginger Couscous, 207

---

[1] Sluggish digestion refers to a condition in which the gastrointestinal system takes an unusually long time to process food. Particularly common among older folks or those who have regularly relied on harsh laxatives, the problem can result in chronic nausea.

Ulcers

Viral Infections